Lecture Notes in Computer Science   8679

Commenced Publication in 1973
Founding and Former Series Editors:
Gerhard Goos, Juris Hartmanis, and Jan van Leeuwen

Editorial Board

T0212931

Guorong Wu   Daoqiang Zhang
Luping Zhou (Eds.)

Machine Learning in Medical Imaging

5th International Workshop, MLMI 2014
Held in Conjunction with MICCAI 2014
Boston, MA, USA, September 14, 2014
Proceedings

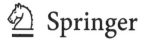 Springer

Volume Editors

Guorong Wu
University of North Carolina at Chapel Hill
Chapel Hill, NC, USA
E-mail: grwu@med.unc.edu

Daoqiang Zhang
Nanjing University of Aeronautics and Astronautics
Nanjing, JiangSu, China
E-mail: dqzhang@nuaa.edu.cn

Luping Zhou
University of Wollongong
Wollongong, NSW, Australia
E-mail: lupingz@uow.edu.au

ISSN 0302-9743   e-ISSN 1611-3349
ISBN 978-3-319-10580-2   e-ISBN 978-3-319-10581-9
DOI 10.1007/978-3-319-10581-9
Springer Cham Heidelberg New York Dordrecht London

Library of Congress Control Number: 2014946444

LNCS Sublibrary: SL 6 – Image Processing, Computer Vision,
Pattern Recognition, and Graphics

Typesetting: Camera-ready by author, data conversion by Scientific Publishing Services, Chennai, India

Printed on acid-free paper

Springer is part of Springer Science+Business Media (www.springer.com)

Preface

The 5th International Workshop on Machine Learning in Medical Imaging (MLMI 2014) was held in the Kresge Auditorium and the Student Center at the Massachusetts Institute of Technology, Cambridge, MA, USA on September 14, 2014, in conjunction with the 17th International Conference on Medical Image Computing and Computer Assisted Intervention (MICCAI).

Machine learning plays an essential role in the medical imaging field, including computer-assisted diagnosis, image segmentation, image registration, image fusion, image-guided therapy, image annotation, and image database retrieval. With advances in medical imaging, new imaging modalities and methodologies, such as cone-beam CT, tomosynthesis, electrical impedance tomography, and new machine learning algorithms/applications, come to the stage for medical imaging. Due to large inter-subject variations and complexities, it is generally difficult to derive analytic formulations or simple equations to represent objects such as lesions and anatomy in medical images. Therefore, tasks in medical imaging require learning from patient data for heuristics and prior knowledge, in order to facilitate the detection/diagnosis of abnormalities in medical images.

The main aim of this MLMI 2014 workshop is to help advance scientific research within the broad field of machine learning in medical imaging. This workshop focuses on major trends and challenges in this area, and presents works aimed to identify new cutting-edge techniques and their use in medical imaging. We hope that the MLMI workshop becomes an important platform for translating research from the bench to the bedside.

The range and level of submissions for this year's meeting were of very high quality. Authors were asked to submit full-length papers for review. A total of 70 papers were submitted to the workshop in response to the call for papers. Each of the 70 papers underwent a rigorous double-blinded peer-review process, with each paper being reviewed by at least two (typically three) reviewers from the Program Committee, composed of 56 well-known experts in the field. Based on the reviewing scores and critiques, the 40 best papers (57%) were accepted for presentation at the workshop and chosen to be included in this Springer LNCS volume. The large variety of machine-learning techniques applied to medical imaging were well represented at the workshop.

We are grateful to the Program Committee for reviewing the submitted papers and giving constructive comments and critique, to the authors for submitting high-quality papers, to the presenters for excellent presentations, and to all the MLMI 2013 attendees who came to Cambridge from all around the world.

July 2014

Guorong Wu
Daoqiang Zhang
Luping Zhou

Organization

Steering Committee

Dinggang Shen	University of North Carolina at Chapel Hill, USA
Pingkun Yan	Philips Research North America, USA
Kenji Suzuki	The University of Chicago, USA
Fei Wang	AliveCorInc, USA

Program Committee

Siamak Ardekani	John Hopkins University, USA
Hidetaka Arimura	Kyusyu University, Japan
Pierrick Bourgeat	CSIRO, Australia
Marleen de Bruijne	University of Copenhagen, Denmark
Weidong (Tom) Cai	The University of Sydney, Australia
Heang-Ping Chan	University of Michigan Medical Center, USA
Rong Chen	The University of Maryland at Baltimore County, USA
Ting Chen	Ventana, USA
Yong Fan	Chinese Academy of Sciences, China
Jurgen Fripp	CSIRO, Australia
Bram van Ginneken	Radboud University Nijmegen Medical Centre, The Netherlands
Ghassan Hamarneh	Simon Fraser University, Canada
Yong He	Beijing Normal University, China
Heng Huang	University of Texas at Arlington, USA
Junzhou Huang	University of Texas, USA
Yaozong Gao	University of North Carolina at Chapel Hill, USA
Xiaoyi Jiang	University of Muenster, Germany
Minjeong Kim	University of North Carolina at Chapel Hill, USA
Byung-Uk Lee	Ewha W. University, Korea
Gang Li	University of North Carolina at Chapel Hill, USA
Yang Li	Allen Institute for Brain Science, USA
Jianming Liang	Arizona State University, USA
Jing Liu	University of California at San Francisco, USA
Xiongbiao Luo	University of Western Ontario, Canada

Table of Contents

Sparsity-Learning-Based Longitudinal MR Image Registration for Early Brain Development

Qian Wang[1], Guorong Wu[2], Li Wang[2],
Pengfei Shi[3], and Weili Lin[2], and Dinggang Shen[2]

[1] Med-X Research Institute, Shanghai Jiao Tong University
[2] Department of Radiology and BRIC, University of North Carolina at Chapel Hill
[3] Department of Automation, Shanghai Jiao Tong University

Abstract. Longitudinal sequences of infant brain MR images are increasingly applied in early brain development studies, while their registration are highly challenging as rapid brain development causes drastic image appearance changes. To this end, we propose a novel sparsity-learning-based strategy to tackle the longitudinal registration of infant subject. *First*, we prepare a set of intermediate sequences, whose longitudinal (voxel-to-voxel) correspondences are established in advance. For each time point of the subject, we *then* utilize sparsity learning to identify its correspondences in the intermediate images at the same age and thus of similar appearances. *Next*, the intermediate sequences are used to bridge the temporal "gaps" between different subject time points, while the sparsity-learning-based correspondence detection is jointly conducted for all subject images to impose the temporal consistency. *Finally*, the deformation field of each subject time point is reconstructed from the spatio-temporal correspondences. Experimental results show that our method is able to achieve the longitudinal registration of the infant subject despite its varying appearances along time.

1 Introduction

Magnetic resonance (MR) imaging provides a non-invasive way to render internal structures of human brains. It has thus been widely applied to numerous applications, including studies upon early brain development. To better monitor the continuous and complicated development patterns in infant brains, many researchers follow the longitudinal experimental design to acquire image data. For example, infant subjects are recruited and scanned via MR imaging every three months apart, e.g., at the gestational ages of 2 weeks, 3 months, 6 months, 9 months, 12 months, etc. All images compose the longitudinal sequences, which are helpful to reveal the common pattern of mankind's early brain development and the uniqueness of each specific subject [1].

Deformable image registration, a major topic in medical image analysis, is fundamentally important to the studies of longitudinal MR images. Once all images in a longitudinal sequence (corresponding to a certain subject) are normalized to a same space (e.g., indicated by a *reference*), we are then able to quantitatively evaluate the temporal changes among brains of different time points.

G. Wu et al. (Eds.): MLMI 2014, LNCS 8679, pp. 1–8, 2014.

To this end, longitudinal (or 4D) registration is more preferred over traditional volumetric (or 3D) image registration. Typically, longitudinal registration considers the alignment of all images in the sequence altogether, and imposes the temporal (smoothness) constraint (TC) upon the deformation fields to reflect the continuous brain development.

The rapid growth of infant brains causes drastic appearance changes in MR images (c.f. Fig. 1), making it hard to establish anatomical correspondences across different time points even for the same subject. Although several longitudinal registration methods are reported [2,3,4,5,6,7], not all of them are capable of handling the appearance "gaps" in longitudinal infant images. Alternatively, logistic regression models are introduced to capture the dynamic appearance changes within the image sequence, while all images are registered together in the longitudinal style [8]. It is also applicable to segment each brain into different tissues [9] first. Then, spatio-temporal correspondences can be detected from features related with the segmentation result, instead of the original intensity, to complete longitudinal registration [10]. However, these methods might be challenged by the large temporal interval (e.g., due to time point missing) in the sequence, which is common for infant image data.

In this paper, we propose a sparsity-learning-based strategy to tackle the dynamic appearance changes and attain longitudinal registration of infant brain MR images. Our solution is to identify spatio-temporal correspondences within the to-be-registered *subject* with helps from a set of *intermediate* sequences, where longitudinal correspondences are pre-established already. Therefore, given a new subject, we only need to utilize sparsity learning to detect correspondences between each subject image and the intermediate images of the same age. After we incorporate temporal information contributed by the intermediate sequences, the spatial-temporal correspondences of the subject would become available. Moreover, for subject voxels that come from different ages but are correspondences to each other, we impose TC and jointly solve for their correspondence detection with respect to the intermediate sequences in sparsity learning. After reconstructing the deformation fields from the detected correspondences, we are able to complete the longitudinal registration of the entire subject sequence.

A major novelty of our method is that we fully bypass the temporal appearance changes in the subject, which prevent us from directly establishing spatio-temporal correspondences. We only need to identify correspondences between each subject image and the intermediate images of the same age, which are similar in appearances. Meanwhile, TC is enforced as we detect correspondences for all subject images jointly and simultaneously. Based on the longitudinal correspondences in the intermediate sequences, the spatial-temporal correspondences can essentially be established for the subject to complete its registration.

2   Method

We attain longitudinal infant image registration based on spatio-temporal correspondences within the subject, which are established by combining (1)

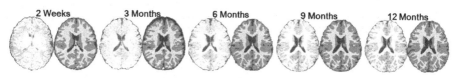

Fig. 1. A sample intermediate sequence of T1 images and the segmented tissues. All images are pre-processed via affine registration to eliminate the scaling effect. Drastic appearance changes are clearly observable throughout the first year of life.

longitudinal correspondences in the intermediate sequences and (2) sparsity-learning-based correspondence detection. To this end, we divide our method into two stages, i.e., the *training* stage and the *application* stage.

- In the *training* stage, we pre-register all intermediate sequences to reveal their longitudinal correspondences, which essentially contribute to bridge the temporal appearance "gaps" across different time points in the subject.
- In the *application* stage, we identify spatio-temporal correspondences for a set of key voxels in the image space, and then reconstruct the dense deformation fields to complete the registration of all subject images. The subject correspondences consist of two parts, i.e., (1) between each subject image and the intermediate images of the same age (blue/cyan lines in Fig. 2), and (2) across the intermediate sequences (dashed pink curve).

The two stages will be detailed in the next. For clarity, we denote the i-th $(i = 1, \cdots , m)$ intermediate sequence as $\mathbf{R}_i = \{R_{it}|t \in n_R\}$ (with t indexing the time point in the set n_R); similarly, the to-be-registered subject is $\mathbf{S} = \{S_t|t \in n_S \subseteq n_R\}$. Since we focus on deformable registration only in this paper, affine registration (via FLIRT [11]) is applied to all images in pre-processing to avoid the scaling effect caused by brain volume enlargement (c.f. Fig. 1).

2.1 Pre-registration of Intermediate Sequences

In the training stage, we pre-register all intermediate images to reveal the spatio-temporal correspondences within each longitudinal sequence. We require that a qualified intermediate sequence should consist of all time points and multiple modalities (i.e., T1, T2, etc.), in contrast to possible time point missing within the subject. The complete (temporal) information in the intermediate sequence enables us to apply the 4D segmentation method [9] and accurately segment each intermediate image into WM, GM, as well as cerebrospinal fluid (CSF) (c.f. Fig. 1). GLIRT [12], a groupwise and longitudinal registration method, is then used to normalize all images to their common space, while TC is enforced to the deformation fields of each sequence simultaneously.

The pre-registration of the intermediate images are based on their tissues, which comes from the 4D segmentation and has passed our visual inspection for quality control. Therefore, though the intensity appearances change drastically in each longitudinal sequence, the spatio-temporal correspondences can still be

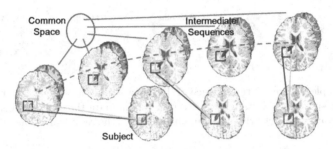

Fig. 2. Each subject image identifies its correspondences (blue/cyan lines) with respect to the intermediate images of the same age. The spatio-temporal correspondences within the subject can be established after combining contributions from the intermediate sequences (dashed pink curve).

matched after all images are deformed to the common space. We denote the deformation field for R_{it} as $\psi_{it}(\cdot)$ and the common space as Ω. Then, given $x \in \Omega$, the two voxels, $\psi_{it}(x)$ in R_{it} and $\psi_{j\tau}(x)$ in $R_{j\tau}$, are regarded as correspondences to each other.

2.2   Initialization of Subject Registration

In the application stage, we also use the common space Ω as the reference to register the subject **S**. We derive an initial deformation field $\phi_t(\cdot)$ for each S_t from the pre-registered intermediate images. Given the time point t, we *first* designate the collection $\{R_{it}\}$ for the intermediate images of the same age. *Then*, we select the most similar intermediate image $\dot{R}_t$ from $\{R_{it}\}$ and register S_t with $\dot{R}_t$. *Finally*, $\phi_t(\cdot)$ (with respect to Ω) can be roughly estimated by composing the deformation fields (1) from $\dot{R}_t$ to Ω and (2) from S_t to $\dot{R}_t$. Note that $\dot{R}_t$ is selected in accordance to the inverse of the intensity difference against S_t. Also, $\dot{R}_t$ is registered to Ω already, while S_t can be registered to $\dot{R}_t$ via most state-of-the-art methods (e.g., diffeomorphic Demons [13]).

2.3   Correspondence Detection via Sparsity Learning

Only a single intermediate image (i.e., $\dot{R}_t$) is utilized by the subject image S_t to initialize its deformation field $\phi_t(\cdot)$ in Section 2.2. However, the simple choice of $\dot{R}_t$ might not be optimal for all voxels in S_t to identify their correspondences with respect to the common space and other subject images under consideration. To this end, we apply the sparsity learning strategy to patch-based image appearances for accurate correspondence detection.

Given the location $x \in \Omega$, its tentative correspondence in S_t is determined as $\phi_t(x)$. We signify $\phi_t(x)$ with its surrounding intensity patch in the vectorized form $\vec{a}_{t,x}^S$. Similarly, we define the signature for any specific intermediate voxel $\psi_{it}(y)$, which is located in R_{it} and associated with $y \in \Omega$ through $\psi_{it}(\cdot)$, as $\vec{a}_{it,y}^R$. A dictionary matrix $\mathbf{A}_t$ is further established for $\phi_t(x)$, as each column vector in $\mathbf{A}_t$ comes from a certain intermediate voxel $\psi_{it}(y)$, or $\vec{a}_{it,y}^R$. Here, we use a search neighborhood $\mathcal{N}(x)$ centered at x, and enumerate all intermediate voxels subject to $y \in \mathcal{N}(x)$ in $\mathbf{A}_t$. Then, we aim to solve

$$\vec{c}_t = \underset{\vec{c}_t}{\arg\min} \frac{1}{2}\|\vec{a}_{t,x}^S - \mathbf{A}_t\vec{c}_t\|_2^2 + \alpha\|\vec{c}_t\|_1,$$

$$\text{s.t.} \quad \vec{c}_t \geq 0. \tag{1}$$

The coefficient vector $\vec{c}_t$ records the linear combination of column vectors in $\mathbf{A}_t$ to approximate the patch-based appearance centered at $\phi_t(x)$ in S_t. The l_1 norm (controlled by the scalar α) encourages that only a limited number of column vectors in $\mathbf{A}_t$ are involved into the sparse representation of $\vec{a}_{t,x}^S$. The intermediate voxels selected in solving (1) are correspondences to $\phi_t(x)$, while the confidences of the correspondences are described by the coefficients in $\vec{c}_t$ [14].

We can utilize the correspondences between S_t and $\{R_{it}\}$ to refresh the correspondences between S_t and Ω, which are conveyed by $\phi_t(\cdot)$. To this end, by denoting the coefficient for $\vec{a}_{it,y}^R$ as $c_t^{(y)}$ in $\vec{c}_t$, we follow

$$\phi_t^{\text{new}}(x) \leftarrow \phi_t^{\text{old}}(x) + \Delta\phi_t(x), \quad \Delta\phi_t(x) = \sum_{y \in \mathcal{N}(x)} c_t^{(y)}\left(\psi_{it}(x) - \psi_{it}(y)\right) \tag{2}$$

to update the deformation field $\phi(\cdot)$ at the location x [15].

2.4 Joint Spatio-Temporal Correspondence Detection

The correspondence detection in Section 2.3 is independent for different subject images. For example, each subject voxel marked by a red patch in Fig. 2 locates two correspondence candidates (in blue and cyan), respectively, from an intermediate image of the same age. If all three marked subject voxels are correspondences (e.g., with respect to the same location $x \in \Omega$), their detected correspondences in the intermediate images (represented by the blue/cyan patches) should also be matched in the common space. Therefore, we are able to impose TC and jointly identify the spatio-temporal correspondences for the subject.

Our purpose is to identify the set $\{\phi_t(x)|x \in \Omega, t \in n_S\}$ such that all its members are spatio-temporal correspondences to each other. To this end, we define the concatenated coefficient vector $\vec{c} = [\cdots, \vec{c}_t^T, \cdots]^T$ and the indexing matrix $\mathbf{I}_t$ such that $\vec{c}_t = \mathbf{I}_t\vec{c}$. Then, we reformulate the problem in (1) as

$$\vec{c} = \underset{\vec{c}}{\arg\min} \sum_{t \in n_S} \left(\frac{1}{2}\|\vec{a}_{t,x}^S - \mathbf{A}_t\mathbf{I}_t\vec{c}\|_2^2 + \alpha\|\mathbf{I}_t\vec{c}\|_1\right) + \sum_{t,t' \in n_S} \frac{\beta}{2}\|\mathbf{I}_t\vec{c} - \mathbf{I}_{t'}\vec{c}\|_2^2,$$

$$\text{s.t.} \quad \vec{c} \geq 0. \tag{3}$$

By increasing β, we encourage $\phi_t(x)$ and $\phi_{t'}(x)$ to have similar representation coefficients based on the dictionaries $\mathbf{A}_t$ and $\mathbf{A}_{t'}$. Then, the spatio-temporal correspondences can be established across subject voxels from different time points (e.g., all three red patches in Fig. 2), due to the existing longitudinal correspondences within the intermediate sequences (e.g., blue/cyan patches). Note that (1) and (3) are both solvable through quadratic programming (QP).

2.5   Implementation Issues

We design a multi-level multi-resolution framework to iteratively optimize the deformation fields in the application stage, based on the detected spatio-temporal correspondences. In each level, voxels that are likely to be on tissue edges are randomly selected as key voxels. We identify the correspondences for each key voxel in all subject images by solving (3). With all key voxels and their incremental displacements in (2), we reconstruct the dense incremental deformation fields via interpolation. The deformation field for each subject image can then be iteratively updated by composing the tentative incremental field [15].

We adopt a low-middle-high level setting and resample images by 2 for two consecutive levels. Each voxel is signified by a $5 \times 5 \times 5$ surrounding patch. The radius of the search neighbourhood $\mathcal{N}(x)$ is 5 voxels in the beginning of each level, and gradually drops to 2 voxels in the end. We set $\alpha = 0.1$ throughout registration. In every level, β starts from 0 in that TC might hinder each subject image correctly identifying its correspondences with respect to the common space. However, β finally reaches 0.12 in the end of each level, as subject images need to refine their spatio-temporal correspondences jointly.

3   Experimental Results

We acquired 9 longitudinal sequences on a Siemens head-only 3T scanner for evaluation. Each sequence consists of images at 2 weeks, 3 months, 6 months, 9 months, and 12 months, respectively. The parameters for T1 images were: 144 sagittal slices, resolution $1 \times 1 \times 1\text{mm}^3$, TR/TE=1900/4.38ms, flip angle=7; T2 images: 64 axial slices, resolution $1.25 \times 1.25 \times 1.95\text{mm}^3$, flip angle=150, TR/TE=7380/119ms; diffusion weighted images: 60 axial slices (thickness 2mm), matrix size=12896, TR/TE=7680/82ms, 42 non-collinear gradients, b=1000s/mm.

We adopted the leave-one-out strategy by using 8 training sequences to register the left subject. All time points and modalities are used for training (particularly for accurate 4D segmentation [9]). In the application stage, we only register the T1 images of three time points (i.e., 2 weeks, 6 months, 12 months), as the other time points are assumed missing to mimic real cases in image acquisition. After completing the longitudinal registration of the subject, we calculated the Dice ratios of segmented tissues, which reflect anatomy overlapping and thus registration quality, between the deformed images of neighbouring time points (i.e., 2-week/6-month and 6-month/12-month) in the subject.

Table 1 provides a detailed report of the Dice ratios. Our method achieved 72.15% (2-week/6-month) and 76.47% (6-month/12-month) in average upon 9 leave-one-out cases. We note that FLIRT is for (input) images after affine yet prior to deformable registration. In our method, we can disable TC, i.e., by letting $\beta = 0$ in (3). However, our results show that TC is helpful to more consistent alignment among different time points and thus higher Dice ratios. Since images of different time points can be regarded as multi-modal data, we also compared with state-of-the-art mutual-information-based registration, where the

Table 1. The Dice ratios (%) of tissues yielded by individual registration schemes

		WM		GM		CSF		Overall	
		Mean	STD.	Mean	STD.	Mean	STD.	Mean	STD.
FLIRT [11]	2-wk/6-mo	69.03	4.74	70.30	2.98	47.78	8.42	62.37	5.38
	6-mo/12-mo	76.17	3.66	79.00	2.94	58.63	4.50	71.27	3.70
Mutual Information	2-wk/6-mo	69.47	4.83	71.91	3.17	50.85	8.62	64.08	5.54
	6-mo/12-mo	77.25	3.59	80.31	3.04	59.66	5.29	72.41	3.97
After Initialization	2-wk/6-mo	77.53	3.98	75.39	2.82	52.30	8.38	68.41	5.06
	6-mo/12-mo	78.97	3.42	77.33	2.66	63.71	5.52	73.34	3.87
Our Method (without TC)	2-wk/6-mo	80.02	3.70	78.56	2.59	54.79	7.95	71.12	4.75
	6-mo/12-mo	82.17	3.16	79.61	2.58	63.85	5.70	75.21	3.81
Our Method (with TC)	2-wk/6-mo	80.93	3.58	79.81	2.41	55.72	7.53	**72.15**	4.51
	6-mo/12-mo	83.81	2.99	81.52	2.32	64.08	5.35	**76.47**	3.55

2-week/12-month image was independently aligned with the 6-month image. In general, our method outperformed all other schemes in the table, demonstrating its capability of longitudinal registration.

In the training stage, all image sequences were registered by GLIRT [12]. The overall 2-week/6-month, 6-month/12-month Dice ratios were $75.16 \pm 4.22\%$, $78.59 \pm 3.47\%$, respectively. It is worth noting that all five time points and multi-modal image data were utilized by GLIRT (as well as its preceding 4D segmentation). The combination of comprehensive data thus leads to more accurate registration and higher Dice ratios. Our method, however, utilizes the intermediate sequences to establish spatio-temporal correspondences within the subject, even though missing time point could exaggerate the temporal appearance "gaps". That is, we regard the longitudinal correspondences in the intermediate sequences as "groundtruth", towards which our method can well approach. We conclude that our method yields high-quality registration results, even though the subject only provides much limited temporal information.

4 Conclusion

We propose a novel longitudinal registration method for infant brain MR images in this paper. To avoid the challenging appearance changes caused by rapid brain development, we use sparsity learning to jointly identify correspondences between all subject images and their respective intermediate images of the same ages. The temporal "gaps" within the subject are filled in by the longitudinal correspondences in the intermediate sequences. In this way, we successfully convert the longitudinal registration of the subject into indirect spatio-temporal correspondence detection powered by the intermediate data. Our experimental results show that the proposed method is capable of registering all subject images in the longitudinal style, even though drastic temporal appearance changes may occur.

References

1. Knickmeyer, R.C., Gouttard, S., Kang, C., Evans, D., Wilber, K., Smith, J.K., Hamer, R.M., Lin, W., Gerig, G., Gilmore, J.H.: A structural mri study of human brain development from birth to 2 years. The Journal of Neuroscience 28(47), 12176–12182 (2008)
2. Aubert-Broche, B., Fonov, V.S., García-Lorenzo, D., Mouiha, A., Guizard, N., Coupé, P., Eskildsen, S.F., Collins, D.L.: A new method for structural volume analysis of longitudinal brain mri data and its application in studying the growth trajectories of anatomical brain structures in childhood. NeuroImage 82, 393–402 (2013)
3. Durrleman, S., Pennec, X., Trouvé, A., Gerig, G., Ayache, N.: Spatiotemporal atlas estimation for developmental delay detection in longitudinal datasets. In: Yang, G.-Z., Hawkes, D., Rueckert, D., Noble, A., Taylor, C. (eds.) MICCAI 2009, Part I. LNCS, vol. 5761, pp. 297–304. Springer, Heidelberg (2009)
4. Holland, D., Dale, A.M.: Nonlinear registration of longitudinal images and measurement of change in regions of interest. Medical Image Analysis 15(4), 489–497 (2011)
5. Qiu, A., Albert, M., Younes, L., Miller, M.I.: Time sequence diffeomorphic metric mapping and parallel transport track time-dependent shape changes. NeuroImage 45(1), S51–S60 (2009)
6. Serag, A., Aljabar, P., Counsell, S., Boardman, J., Hajnal, J.V., Rueckert, D.: Lisa: Longitudinal image registration via spatio-temporal atlases. In: 2012 9th IEEE International Symposium on Biomedical Imaging (ISBI), pp. 334–337. IEEE (2012)
7. Studholme, C., Drapaca, C., Iordanova, B., Cardenas, V.: Deformation-based mapping of volume change from serial brain mri in the presence of local tissue contrast change. IEEE Transactions on Medical Imaging 25(5), 626–639 (2006)
8. Csapo, I., Davis, B., Shi, Y., Sanchez, M., Styner, M., Neithammer, M.: Longitudinal image registration with temporally-dependent image similarity measure. IEEE Transactions on Medical Imaging (2013)
9. Wang, L., Shi, F., Yap, P.T., Gilmore, J.H., Lin, W., Shen, D.: 4D multi-modality tissue segmentation of serial infant images. PloS One 7(9), e44596 (2012)
10. Shen, D., Davatzikos, C.: Measuring temporal morphological changes robustly in brain mr images via 4-dimensional template warping. NeuroImage 21(4), 1508–1517 (2004)
11. Jenkinson, M., Smith, S.: A global optimisation method for robust affine registration of brain images. Medical Image Analysis 5(2), 143–156 (2001)
12. Wu, G., Wang, Q., Shen, D.: Registration of longitudinal brain image sequences with implicit template and spatial–temporal heuristics. Neuroimage 59(1), 404–421 (2012)
13. Vercauteren, T., Pennec, X., Perchant, A., Ayache, N.: Diffeomorphic demons: Efficient non-parametric image registration. NeuroImage 45(1), S61–S72 (2009)
14. Wright, J., Ma, Y., Mairal, J., Sapiro, G., Huang, T.S., Yan, S.: Sparse representation for computer vision and pattern recognition. Proceedings of the IEEE 98(6), 1031–1044 (2010)
15. Wang, Q., Kim, M., Wu, G., Shen, D.: Joint learning of appearance and transformation for predicting brain MR image registration. In: Gee, J.C., Joshi, S., Pohl, K.M., Wells, W.M., Zöllei, L. (eds.) IPMI 2013. LNCS, vol. 7917, pp. 499–510. Springer, Heidelberg (2013)

Graph-Based Label Propagation
in Fetal Brain MR Images

Lisa M. Koch[1], Robert Wright[1], Deniz Vatansever[2], Vanessa Kyriakopoulou[2],
Christina Malamateniou[2], Prachi A. Patkee[2], Mary Rutherford[2],
Joseph V. Hajnal[2], Paul Aljabar[2], and Daniel Rueckert[1]

[1] Biomedical Image Analysis Group, Imperial College London, UK
[2] Division of Imaging Sciences & Biomedical Engineering, King's College London, UK

Abstract. Segmentation of neonatal and fetal brain MR images is a
challenging task due to vast differences in shape and appearance across
age and across subjects. Expert priors for atlas-based segmentation are
often only available for a subset of the population, leading to a reduction
in accuracy for images dissimilar from the atlas set. To alleviate the effects of limited prior information on atlas-based segmentation, we present
a novel semi-supervised learning framework where labels are propagated
among both atlas and test images while modelling the confidence of
propagated information. The method relies on a voxel-wise graph in-
terconnecting similar regions in all images based on a patch similarity
measure. By iteratively allowing information flow from voxels with high
confidence to voxels with lower confidence, segmentations in test images
with low similarity to the atlas set can be improved. The method was
evaluated on 70 fetal brain MR images of subjects at 22–38 weeks gestational age. Particularly for test populations dissimilar from the atlas
population, the proposed method outperformed state-of-the-art patch-
based segmentation.

1 Introduction

Accurate automated segmentation of anatomical structures in MR images of
the neonatal and fetal brain is an important step towards biomarker discovery
for better understanding early brain development. However, segmentation is a
challenging task as the brain undergoes rapid changes in the time before and
after birth, leading to vast differences in its shape and appearance on MR images
across age and across subjects [8].

Atlas-based methods such as multi-atlas label propagation [5] or patch-based
segmentation (PBS) [3] have been successfully applied to the segmentation of
brain MR images, for example on fetal subjects in [4,11]. Both families of methods use expert priors (atlases) to guide the segmentation. However, expert manual segmentations are expensive to obtain and are therefore often available in
small numbers and only for a specific subgroup of the population, for example
for a set of control subjects at a specific age. For a heterogeneous data set, such
as fetal MR images over a wide age range, this means that the atlas set is not

G. Wu et al. (Eds.): MLMI 2014, LNCS 8679, pp. 9–16, 2014.
© Springer International Publishing Switzerland 2014

always representative of the test set to be segmented. As a result, segmentation accuracy declines the more dissimilar the test images are from the priors [1].

To overcome the heterogeneity in terms of shape and appearance across the population, techniques have recently emerged that employ stepwise label propagation, where automatically labelled images or voxels are added to the atlas set and used as priors in subsequent iterations. In [10], a manifold was learned to identify similar images within a data set. Label maps were then propagated through the manifold by applying multi-atlas propagation with segmentation refinement, in each step labelling similar images only. A similar strategy has been applied in computer vision for segmentation propagation in ImageNet [7], a large-scale hierarchichal image database, where labels were propagated to semantically similar object classes. In [2], dense correspondences were established between all images through diffeomorphic registration before propagating labels along locally similar regions. In the above approaches, only similar images or similar regions were labelled during each step, making each individual step less prone to errors. However, it is important to note that no distinction was made between original expert priors and potentially weaker propagated priors. This means that automatically labelled regions contributed to future propagation steps with the same strength and confidence as manually labelled regions, leading to potential accumulation of errors. One step towards accounting for label confidence has been proposed in the computer vision community in [9]. In this approach, annotations were inferred in large, partially annotated image databases through a Markov Random Field formulation enforcing spatial smoothness and consistency among locally similar regions across images. The algorithm distinguishes the strength of manually labelled pixels and propagated information.

The methods presented in the previous paragraph can be viewed as examples of semi-supervised learning, as segmentations are learned from both labelled and unlabelled data. Building on the idea of stepwise label propagation, we propose a novel graph-based label propagation scheme that propagates labels between similar regions in a data set while estimating and accounting for the decreased confidence of propagated information. We formulate the segmentation problem as an information propagation process through a graph that connects similar voxels in the entire population based on patch similarity. Atlas labels are propagated through the graph and the confidence of subsequently labelled voxels decreases with the distance along which the information propagates. By repeatedly allowing information flow from voxels with high confidence to voxels with lower confidence, voxels within the test population are able to contribute to the final segmentation. Thus, test images with poor representation in the atlas set (and therefore low confidence after an initial segmentation step) can be refined in subsequent iterations.

2   Method

The proposed segmentation technique relies on information flow in a graph of interconnected voxels. The set of vertices V consists of all voxels in all images.

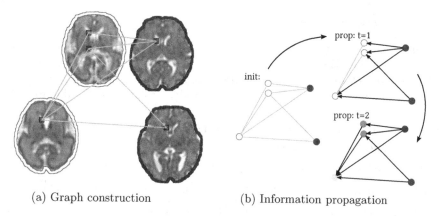

(a) Graph construction   (b) Information propagation

Fig. 1. (a) Similar voxels are interconnected in labelled (green contour) and unlabelled (empty red contour) images. (b) shows vertex initialisation and information propagation. Dark green shades depict high confidence and bold arrows describe active edges. At $t = 1$, labels are available only in the atlas voxels. At $t = 2$, propagated information is available, contributing to the label fusion.

In a data set consisting of R coarsely aligned images with N voxels per image, the graph $G = (V, E)$ is of order $|V| = R \cdot N$. Edges E exist between voxels in corresponding regions of different images. Edge weights w_{ij} are based on the similarity of image patches centred on voxels i and j and aim to express how well label information can be propagated along the edge. Each vertex is assigned a confidence value describing the reliability of its labelling, irrespective of the assigned label probabilities. The confidence is 1 for atlas vertices, 0 for unlabelled vertices, and in the range $(0, 1)$ for vertices labelled in subsequent iterations. Over multiple iterations, information is propagated from vertices with high confidence to vertices with lower confidence. When label probabilities are propagated along an edge, the associated confidence decreases proportionally to the edge weight. Confidence and label probabilities for all voxels in the data at iteration t are described by $\mathbf{c}^{(t)} \in \mathbb{R}^{R \cdot N}$ and $\mathbf{p}_l^{(t)} \in \mathbb{R}^{R \cdot N}$, respectively, where $l \in \{1, \ldots, L, \emptyset\}$ denotes the labels. Unlabelled voxels are described by $l_i = \emptyset$.

2.1 Graph Construction

The graph is constructed such that each voxel (surrounded by a patch) is connected to voxels surrounded by similar patches within a local neighbourhood in the remaining images. To establish the connections w_{ij}, a patch search and pre-selection based on structural similarity, as proposed by [3], is conducted for each voxel i. It is important to note that in the proposed method, similar patches are searched in *all* (labelled and unlabelled) images as shown in Fig. 1a.

A similarity metric is used to describe the weights w_{ij} of edges found during the patch search. Normalised cross correlation (NCC) is invariant to linear intensity changes and fast to compute, making it suitable for patch comparison within a large set of images from subjects of different ages.

2.2   Information Propagation

The following paragraphs describe all aspects of information propagation through the graph: initialisation of the vertex attributes (label probabilities and confidence), the search for propagating neighbours at each iteration, propagation at each iteration, and the final label decision. Key elements are visualised in Fig. 1b.

Initialisation. Before propagating information through the graph, voxel attributes $\mathbf{p}_l$ and $\mathbf{c}$ are initialised. Label probabilities $p_{i,l}^{(0)}$ are set according to the labels at voxel i such that $\sum_{l \in \{1,\dots,L,\emptyset\}} p_{i,l}^{(0)} = 1$. The confidence $c_i^{(0)}$ is set to 1 for voxels in atlas images and 0 for voxels in test images (where $p_{i,\emptyset}^{(0)} = 1$). Neighbourhood sets $V_i^{(t)}$ describe for each vertex which neighbours in the graph propagate information during an iteration. They are initialised as $V_i^{(0)} = \{\}$.

Active Neighbourhood Search. In each iteration, the graph neighbourhood of each vertex is searched for vertices with higher confidence. These vertices are combined with the existing active (propagating) neighbourhood to form $V_i^{(t)}$:

$$V_i^{(t)} = \left\{ j \mid i \sim j, w_{ij} c_j^{(t-1)} > c_i^{(t-1)} \right\} \cup V_i^{(t-1)} \tag{1}$$

$V_i^{(t)}$ is used to propagate information to vertex i and update its existing label probabilities and confidence. Initially, when nodes are either unlabelled ($c_j^{(0)} = 0$) or manually labelled ($c_j^{(0)} = 1$), only atlas voxels propagate information, and only vertices connected to atlas voxels have a non-empty neighbour set $V_i^{(1)}$.

Propagation. For propagation of label probabilities and confidence, the edge weights w_{ij} are transformed with an exponential kernel and a locally and temporally adaptive decay parameter $h_i^{(t)}$. This is done to control the influence of individual neighbours depending on neighbourhood content as proposed in [3]:

$$u_{ij}^{(t)} = \begin{cases} \exp \dfrac{-(1-w_{ij})}{h_i^{(t)}} & \forall i, \forall j \in V_i^{(t)} , \\ 0 & \text{otherwise} \end{cases} \tag{2a}$$

$$h_i^{(t)} = \min_{j \in V_i^{(t)}} (1 - w_{ij}) + \epsilon \tag{2b}$$

The label probabilities $p_{i,l}^{(t)}$ are obtained by averaging the active neighbourhood's labels $p_{j,l}^{(t-1)}$ as in Eq. 3a. Averaging weights are based on the neighbours' confidence $c_j^{(t-1)}$ and the adaptive weights $u_{ij}^{(t)}$ obtained in Eq. 2. The updated confidence $c_i^{(t)}$ is determined by the confidence of the propagating neighbours $c_j^{(t-1)}$ as shown in Eq. 3b. It is calculated as an average of the propagated (and therefore *reduced*) confidence values $w_{ij} c_j^{(t-1)}$, weighted by $u_{ij}^{(t)}$.

$$p_{i,l}^{(t)} = \frac{\sum_{j \in V_i^{(t)}} u_{ij}^{(t)} c_j^{(t-1)} p_{j,l}^{(t-1)}}{\sum_{j \in V_i^{(t)}} u_{ij}^{(t)} c_j^{(t-1)}} \tag{3a}$$

$$c_i^{(t)} = \frac{\sum_{j \in V_i^{(t)}} u_{ij}^{(t)} w_{ij} c_j^{(t-1)}}{\sum_{j \in V_i^{(t)}} u_{ij}^{(t)}} \tag{3b}$$

Convergence and Final Labelling. The active neighbourhood search and propagation step can be interleaved until there are no more changes for any vertex in the graph. This is achieved when for every vertex i, the set of propagating graph neighbours $V_i^{(t)}$ remains constant, i.e. there are no more higher confidence nodes to include in the label fusion. In practice, improvements achieved beyond a few iterations are marginal, as shown in the experiments. At any iteration t, hard labels can be generated from the probabilistic labels $p_{i,l}^{(t)}$ with $l_i^{(t)} = \arg\max_l p_{i,l}^{(t)}$.

2.3 Relationship to Patch-Based Segmentation

In the initial propagation step of the proposed method, the active neighbourhood for each voxel as determined by Eq. 1 consists only of atlas voxels. Since the same patch search strategy as in [3] was used to establish edges in the graph, the set of patches contributing to the label fusion is the same as in PBS. For $t = 1$, the label fusion described in Eq. 3a simplifies to a weighted average of atlas labels based on $u_{ij}^{(1)}$ only. PBS is therefore equivalent to the first iteration of the proposed method except for the choice of similarity measure. While traditional PBS uses an exponential kernel on the sum of squared differences (SSD) to measure patch similarity, the proposed method relies on NCC as described in Eq. 2.

3 Experiments and Results

Experiments were conducted using data from 70 healthy fetal subjects with gestational age (GA) between 22.4–38.7 weeks. All images were acquired on a 1.5T Philips Achieva scanner without sedation. Overlapping T2-weighted slices were acquired in three orthogonal planes. Sequence parameters were repetition time 15,000ms, echo time 160ms, slice thickness 2.5mm, slice gap -1.25mm, excitation flip angle 90° and refocusing flip angle 130°. The images were reconstructed [6] and preprocessed as described in [11]. They were then affinely aligned, resampled to $0.85 \times 0.85 \times 0.85$mm^3 and normalised to the intensity range $[0, 100]$. Manual segmentations of the lateral ventricle were available for all subjects.

For each experiment, the data were split into a small atlas set and a test set consisting of the remaining images. To investigate the problem of unrepresentative atlas sets, the subjects were split so that the atlas set consisted of the n oldest subjects in the dataset. We refrained from performing cross-validation as its usefulness is limited in the setting at hand, where the atlas and test population are expected to show systematic differences. To build the propagation graph, for each voxel connections were searched in a local neighbourhood of $5 \times 5 \times 5$ voxels,

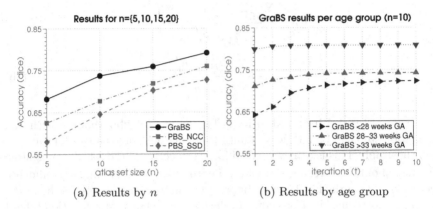

(a) Results by n (b) Results by age group

Fig. 2. Results for GraBS, PBS_NCC and PBS_SSD. (a) Influence of atlas set size on segmentation accuracy across methods. (b) Influence of iterative refinement on GraBS accuracy, evaluated for young, medium, and old subjects.

and a patch size of $5 \times 5 \times 5$ voxels was used to calculate the edge weights. The parameters were manually selected to achieve optimal results for PBS on the fetal data. The graph was constructed for voxels within a region of interest around the lateral ventricle, determined by a union and subsequent dilation of all manual segmentations. This lead to a dimensionality of $|V| \approx 2.7 \cdot 10^6, |E| \approx 2.9 \cdot 10^9$. The proposed graph-based segmentation method (subsequently referred to as 'GraBS') was compared to PBS using NCC (PBS_NCC, equivalent to the first iteration of GraBS) and PBS using SSD (PBS_SSD, as in [3]). All experiments were run with the same parameter set for fair comparison. Segmentation accuracy in the labelled regions is measured by the Dice coefficient. All quantitative results are reported with the median and interquartile range. As the results are not normally distributed, statistical significance is measured using the two-sided Wilcoxon signed-rank test and is reported for $p < 10^{-6}$.

Results. The experiment was run for atlas set sizes $n = \{5, 10, 15, 20\}$. Figure 2a shows the segmentation results of GraBS after 10 iterations and the baseline (PBS_NCC and PBS_SSD), evaluated on the whole test population. As expected [5], segmentation accuracy improved when using more atlases. GraBS outperformed the baseline for each n and was able to match the performance of PBS using smaller atlas sets. Due to the unbalanced split and heterogeneous data, the achieved performance for all methods in this experiment setup does not match the results observed in [3].

To test the ability of the proposed method to propagate labels from older subjects to younger subjects, a more detailed analysis for different age groups is presented for $n = 10$. Results are examined separately for young (<28 weeks GA), medium (28–33 weeks GA), and old (>33 weeks GA) subjects. Example segmentations in each age group are shown in Fig. 3. Table 1 summarises the achieved Dice coefficients for all methods and Fig. 2b presents the performance of the proposed method for each iteration. All methods achieved consistently better

Table 1. Dice coefficients by age group for atlas size $n = 10$. For GraBS, Dice coefficients after 10 iterations are reported. Statistically significant improvements of GraBS over PBS_NCC and PBS_SSD are marked with $*$ and $\dagger$ respectively.

Method	Young	Medium	Old
GraBS	**0.72 (0.63–0.76)*†**	**0.74 (0.70–0.78)*†**	0.81 (0.74–0.86)
PBS_NCC	0.64 (0.57–0.68)	0.71 (0.66–0.77)	0.80 (0.74–0.85)
PBS_SSD	0.58 (0.53–0.63)	0.68 (0.61–0.73)	0.76 (0.73–0.82)

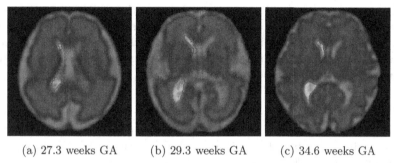

(a) 27.3 weeks GA   (b) 29.3 weeks GA   (c) 34.6 weeks GA

Fig. 3. Example segmentations for randomly chosen subjects from the young (a), medium (b), and old (c) population. The label probability map for the lateral ventricle is indicated in green, manual segmentations are outlined in red.

results for older test subjects, i.e. those more similar to the atlas set. For medium subjects and more prominently for young ones, strong improvements could be achieved with GraBS in the first few refinement steps. As seen in Table 1, the Dice coefficients of the proposed method were significantly higher compared to PBS_NCC and PBS_SSD for the young and medium population.

4   Discussion and Conclusion

We propose a novel stepwise label propagation scheme that incorporates the notion of label confidence. It extends patch-based segmentation [3] to a semi-supervised learning framework where both atlases and test images contribute to the final segmentation results. The proposed method iteratively refines segmentations of images with poor representation in the atlas set. It thus addresses the segmentation problem in heterogeneous data with limited expert priors, often relevant in perinatal MR imaging.

Due to the challenging data and an experiment setup which often reflects reality (a small atlas set consisting of images that do not represent well the entire test population), the resulting Dice coefficients are not comparable to results obtained in [3]. However, experiments show that especially for images least similar to the atlas set, i.e. very young subjects, segmentation accuracy could be increased considerably with the proposed refinement steps. For the older population, iterative refinement did not improve the segmentations significantly. This is expected, as MR images of old subjects are well represented by an atlas set consisting of similarly aged subjects. In these images, test patches are strongly and directly connected to patches in the atlas set, yielding high confidence segmentations after the first iteration, which is equivalent to PBS. By formulating the segmentation problem as an extension of PBS and thus keeping the proposed method closely related to the baseline method, the effectiveness of using label confidence to propagate weakened priors can be measured. However, these restrictions lead to a high dimensional problem with many redundant edges in the connectivity graph. Future work will aim to exploit the graph structure and explore sparsification techniques to reduce the graph dimensionality and computational complexity. This will improve scalability of the method for application to larger datasets and whole brain segmentation. The proposed framework may also be suitable for segmentation tasks in other populations with heterogeneous imaging data and limited manual labels, such as neonates or dementia patients with varying degrees of disease progression.

References

1. Aljabar, P., Heckemann, R.A., Hammers, A., Hajnal, J.V., Rueckert, D.: Multi-atlas based segmentation of brain images: atlas selection and its effect on accuracy. NeuroImage 46(3), 726–738 (2009)
2. Cardoso, M.J., Wolz, R., Modat, M., Fox, N.C., Rueckert, D., Ourselin, S.: Geodesic information flows. In: Ayache, N., Delingette, H., Golland, P., Mori, K. (eds.) MICCAI 2012, Part II. LNCS, vol. 7511, pp. 262–270. Springer, Heidelberg (2012)
3. Coupé, P., Manjón, J.V., Fonov, V., Pruessner, J., Robles, M., Collins, D.L.: Patch-based segmentation using expert priors: application to hippocampus and ventricle segmentation. NeuroImage 54(2), 940–954 (2011)
4. Habas, P.A., Kim, K., Rousseau, F., Glenn, O.A., Barkovich, A.J., Studholme, C.: Atlas-based segmentation of developing tissues in the human brain with quantitative validation in young fetuses. Hum. Brain Mapp. 31(9), 1348–1358 (2010)
5. Heckemann, R.A., Hajnal, J.V., Aljabar, P., Rueckert, D., Hammers, A.: Automatic anatomical brain MRI segmentation combining label propagation and decision fusion. NeuroImage 33(1), 115–126 (2006)
6. Jiang, S., Xue, H., Glover, A., Rutherford, M., Rueckert, D., Hajnal, J.V.: MRI of moving subjects using multislice snapshot images with volume reconstruction. IEEE Trans. Med. Imag. 26(7), 967–980 (2007)
7. Kuettel, D., Guillaumin, M., Ferrari, V.: Segmentation propagation in ImageNet. In: Fitzgibbon, A., Lazebnik, S., Perona, P., Sato, Y., Schmid, C. (eds.) ECCV 2012, Part VII. LNCS, vol. 7578, pp. 459–473. Springer, Heidelberg (2012)
8. Prayer, D., Kasprian, G., Krampl, E., Ulm, B., Witzani, L., Prayer, L., Brugger, P.: MRI of normal fetal brain development. Eur. J. Radiol. 57(2), 199–216 (2006)
9. Rubinstein, M., Liu, C., Freeman, W.T.: Annotation propagation in large image databases via dense image correspondence. In: Fitzgibbon, A., Lazebnik, S., Perona, P., Sato, Y., Schmid, C. (eds.) ECCV 2012, Part III. LNCS, vol. 7574, pp. 85–99. Springer, Heidelberg (2012)
10. Wolz, R., Aljabar, P., Hajnal, J.V., Hammers, A., Rueckert, D.: LEAP: learning embeddings for atlas propagation. NeuroImage 49(2), 1316–1325 (2010)
11. Wright, R., Vatansever, D., Kyriakopoulou, V.: Age dependent fetal MR segmentation using manual and automated approaches. In: MICCAI 2012 PaPI Workshop, pp. 97–104 (2012)

Deep Learning Based Automatic Immune Cell Detection for Immunohistochemistry Images

Ting Chen and Christophe Chefd'hotel

Ventana Medical Systems, Inc. A Member of the Roche Group, USA, 94043

Abstract. Immunohistochemistry (IHC) staining is a widely used technique in the diagnosis of abnormal cells such as cancer. For instance, it can be used to determine the distribution and localization of the differentially expressed biomarkers of immune cells (such as T-cells or B-cells) in cancerous tissue for an immune response study. Typically, the immunological data of interest includes the type, density and location of the immune cells within the tumor samples; this data is of particular interest to pathologists for accurate patient survival prediction. However, to manually count each subset of immune cells under a bright-field microscope for each piece of IHC stained tissue is usually extremely tedious and time consuming. This makes automatic detection very attractive, but it can be very challenging due to the wide variety of cell appearances resulting from different tissue types, block cuttings, and staining processes. This paper presents a novel method for automatic immune cell counting on digitally scanned images of IHC stained slides. The method first uses a sparse color unmixing technique to separate the IHC image into multiple color channels that correspond to different cell structures. Since the immune cell biomarkers that we are interested in are membrane markers, the detection problem is formulated into a deep learning framework using the membrane image channel. The algorithm is evaluated on a clinical data set containing a large number of IHC slides and demonstrates more effective detection than the existing technique and the result is also in accordance with the human observer's output.

1 Introduction

Immunohistochemistry (IHC) slide staining has the advantage of identifying proteins in cells of a tissue section, and hence is widely used to study of the distribution and localization of different cell types in a biological tissue such as cancerous cells and immune cells. For example, tumors often contain infiltrates of immune cells, which may prevent the development of tumors or favor the outgrowth of tumors [1]. In this scenario, multiple biomarkers are used to target different types of immune cells and the population distribution of each type are compared with the clinical outcomes of the patients. As an emerging research topic of tremendous interest in pathology and immunology, an "immune profile" studies the correlation between the immune response and the growth and recurrences of human tumors. However, a prerequisite of an immune profile

G. Wu et al. (Eds.): MLMI 2014, LNCS 8679, pp. 17–24, 2014.

study requires the human observer to manually locate and count the number of different immune cells within selected lymph node regions, which may contain hundreds to thousands of cells. This is an extremely tedious and time consuming process and the results are also subject to intra- and inter-individual variability. In order to avoid the tedium involved in manual counting, a technique that is able to automatically and reliably detect different types of immune cells is of great research and clinical interest.

Typically, a tissue slide is stained by an IHC diagnostic assay with a cluster of differentiation (CD) protein markers identifying the immune cells and the nucleus marker Hematoxylin (HTX) marking the nuclei. The stained slide is then imaged using a CCD color camera mounted on a microscope or a scanner. The acquired RGB color image is a mixture of the immune cell membrane and the universal cell nuclear biomarker expressions. Several techniques have been proposed in the literature to detect such cells. Most of the techniques are based on image processing methods that capture the symmetric information of the cell appearance features. For instance, in [2] Pavin *et al.* proposed an iterative voting method to cluster and group non-convex perceptual circular symmetries along the radial line of an object, and demonstrated its efficacy in the detection of nucleus which presents a round blob shape. Xin *et al.* in [3] extended Pavin's method by adding a shifted Gaussian kernel at the center of the voting area and showed improved detection for overlapping cells. Machine learning techniques have also been explored in literature for cell detection. A statistical model matching method learned from structured SVM was proposed in [4] to identify the cell-like regions. However, all of the three aforementioned techniques are limited to nucleus rather than cell membrane detection. Since the most popular immune cell markers, such as CD3 and CD8 for universal T-cells and cytotoxic T-cells respectively, are membrane markers, the stain appears as a ring instead of a blob. Another machine learning based system using SIFT, Random Forests, and Hierarchical Clustering was developed by Mualla *et al.* in [5] for *unstained* cell imaging which has the properties of maintaining sufficient contrast of cell boundaries. In this work, the SIFT key-points are classified into cells and backgrounds, and all the key-points within each cell are linked together using hierarchical clustering. The system was validated on a large data set, and has shown robustness and stability. However, it is non-trivial to extend it to detect immune cells in IHC stained images.

Recently, an automatic CD8 cytotoxic T-cell counting algorithm was proposed by Niazi *et al.* in [6], wherein normalized multi-scale difference of Gaussian is used to detect the candidate regions, and the color and intensity information is applied to fuse the results. This image processing and rule-based technique has a potential robustness concern due to the great diversity exhibited in terms of cell shape and size. Meanwhile, deep learning techniques, such as Convolutional Neural Networks (CNN) [7], have evidenced great success in mitosis cell detection from histology images stained with Hematoxylin and Eosin [8].This serves as a valuable source of inspiration for developing a new learning-based immune cell detection algorithm as the hard mitosis cell detection problem also suffers from large appearance variation and high complexity. As a powerful pixel classifier, CNN takes the image patch centered at each pixel as input and provides the classification label for each patch. The advantage of CNN is that the feature descriptors are automatically learned as the kernel matrices in the convolution layers, therefore, less effort is needed in designing sophisticated features for immune cells.

In this paper, we propose an automatic immune cell detection framework for IHC images. The algorithm first unmixes the RGB image into different color channels corresponding to the different cell structures. CNN is then trained using the immune cell marker image channel and produces a probability response map of the immune cell locations. Finally, we apply non-max suppression to obtain the centroids of the cells. There is very little published literature for IHC image analysis due to the limited data availability. As the major contribution of this paper, we are the first to propose an immune cell counting algorithm based on sparse color unmixing and deep learning, and demonstrate a RGB image unmixing algorithm potentially working for more than three stains as well as a new, important application of the CNN algorithm.

2   Methodology

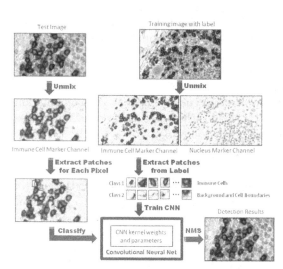

Fig. 1. The framework of the algorithm

In this section, we present the methodology of our algorithm. We begin with illustrating the basic framework in Fig.1. In the analysis of the cancerous tissues, different biomarkers are specified to one or more types of immune cells. For instance, CD3 is a known universal marker for all T-cells and CD8 only stains the membranes of cytotoxic T-cells. To detect the T-cells, the IHC image is first unmixed into HTX and T-cell marker channels. The pixels in the T-cell channel are then classified into foreground and background using CNN, the output of which is a probability map. Finally, we apply non-max suppression to the probability map and obtain the T-cell centroids.

2.1   Color Unmixing

There are several techniques available in the literature to unmix each pixel of the RGB image into multiple biologically meaningful channels corresponding to different stain colors. As the most widely used method in the digital pathology domain, Ruifrok *et al.* developed an unmixing algorithm [9] to unmix the RGB image with up to three stains in the converted optical density space. Given the reference color vectors $x_i \in R^3$ of the pure stains, the method assumes that each pixel of the color mixture $a \in R^3$ is a linear combination of the pure stain colors and solves a linear system to obtain the combination weights $b \in R^M$. The linear system is denoted as $a = Xb$, where $X = [x_1, \ldots, x_M], M \leq 3$ is the matrix of reference colors. Most of the effort in reported literature is for multi-spectral image unmixing [10] which is not applicable for RGB images. *To the best of our knowledge, a technique that is able to reliably unmix more than three colors from a RGB image has never been reported in literature.* In this paper, we extended Ruifrok's method by providing the L_1 norm constraint for b due to the fact that only a small number of stains exist at each pixel. With the sparse constraint, we obtain the following advantages: (1) the linear system is no longer deficient and thus can potentially unmix more than three colors, (2) background noise is greatly suppressed in the unmixed channels due to the sparsity regularization which leads to a larger signal noise ratio.

In a pre-processing step, the RGB image I is converted into the optical density (OD) space using the formula $O_c = -\log(\frac{I_c}{I_{0,c}})$ derived from Beer's law; this is based on the fact that the optical density is proportional to the stain concentration. Here c is the index of the RGB color channels, I_0 is the RGB value of the white points and O is the optical density image obtained. As in [9], O will be the image to work with in the rest of the paper.

Let $\mathbf{a}$ be a pixel of O and it is a 3-dimensional column vector corresponding to the OD values converted from RGB. There are M biomarkers available in a multiplex IHC slide corresponding to M stain colors. Let $\mathbf{b}$ be the combination weight vector of the stains; $b_m, m = 1, \ldots, M$ is the m_{th} element of $\mathbf{b}$. The sparse unmixing problem is then formulated as the following:

$$\min_{\mathbf{b}} ||\mathbf{a} - X\mathbf{b}||_2^2 + \lambda ||\mathbf{b}||_1. \tag{1}$$

Each column of X corresponds to a reference stain color sampled from the control slide of pure stain. Existing techniques such as LASSO can be used to solve Eqn. 1, and can achieve better unmixing results than in [9] in terms of robustness and accuracy.

Note that instead of working in the unmixed immune cell marker channel, the detection algorithm proposed in this paper is also applicable to the absorbance image of I. However, the noisy HTX channel (Fig.5) may lead to a false positive detection of immune cells. As accurate unmixing provides an accurate separation of the two stains with less cross-talk among different channels, we therefore work in the unmixed T-cell marker channel which has sufficient information about cell membranes.

2.2   Cell Detection

The accurate detection of immune cells is a challenging task due to the large variation of data caused by a variety of issues, such as different tissue types, tissue section cuttings, chemical staining artifacts, and scanner focus problems, etc. Fig.2 shows some example fields of view (FOVs) from the whole slide images and the tissue cutting problem.

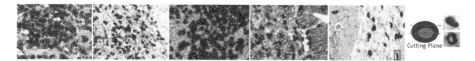

Fig. 2. Example FOVs demonstrate the data variations. The boxes show the staining artifacts and the cell shape variations due to cutting. The figure on the right shows the blob and ring shape cells from different cuttings.

Given an input RGB image I, sparse color unmixing is used to unmix the image into immune cell markers and nucleus marker channels, denoted as I_{dab} and I_{htx}, respectively. I_{dab} is then

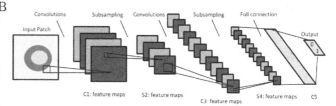

Fig. 3. The architecture of CNN for membrane detection

used as the input image for learning the detector. The immune cell detection problem is formulated as classifying each pixel of I_{dab} into two classes, positive for the centroids of the immune cells and negative for the rest. More specifically, let P be the training data and Y be the set of labels, where (p_n, y_n) are drawn randomly from $P \times Y$ based on some unknown distribution. In this application, P is the set of patch images centered at each pixel of I_{dab} and Y is a binary set containing two labels $\{+1, -1\}$. We have ground truth immune cell locations manually labeled by the pathologist, wherein the coordinates of the cell centroids are recorded. The positive class of training data consists of k by k-pixel image patches centered at the pixels within a d-pixel neighborhood of the recorded coordinates. The non-immune cell class contains all the image patches centered at pixels sampled from the boundaries of the cells and the background.

A convolutional neural network (CNN) is trained given the training data (patches and their corresponding labels). CNN is basically a neural network with the sequence of alternating convolutional layers and sub-sampling layers, followed by the fully connected layers, which can be trained by a

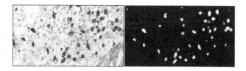

Fig. 4. The test image and its probability map from CNN

back-propagation algorithm (Fig.3). CNN has the advantages of automatically learning the feature descriptors which are invariant to small translation and distortion from the training image patches. The convolution layer convolves the input patch with a kernel matrix; the output is passed to a continuous and differentiable activation function. The kernel matrix is part of the parameter set to be learned in CNN. The sub-sampling layer reduces the size of the image by a coarse sampling or max-pooling. The fully connected layer is similar to a typical neural network designed to generate probabilistic labels for each class.

In the testing stage, we first unmix the test RGB image $\bar{I}$ to obtain $\bar{I}_{dab}$, then apply the trained CNN classifier to the patches centered at each pixel of the test image $\bar{I}_{dab}$. Let $y = \mathcal{C}(p)$ denote the CNN classifier that takes the patch p as input and produces the probabilistic label y for the patch, here $y \in [0,1]$. Hence, a probability map M as shown in Fig.4 is created for each test image, in which higher probability means that the pixel is more likely to be the centroid of the immune cell. Non-maximum suppression (NMS) [11] is typically used for the local maximum search, i.e. finding the pixel with the value that is greater than all its neighbors. Therefore, we apply NMS to the probability map to yield the final detection.

3   Experiments

In this section, we empirically validate our immune cell detection algorithm, and compare it to the existing technique and human observer's output.

3.1   Data Set and Experiment Setting

A clinical data set containing several different cancer tissue samples was used to test the proposed approach. The data set contains 42 fields of view (FOVs) which

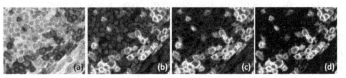

Fig. 5. Unmixing of the RGB image. (a) input image I. (b) input image in absorbance space. (c) I_{dab} from Ruifrok's method [9]. (d) I_{dab} from sparse unmixing.

were scanned under 20X magnification. The tissues were stained with the following assay: DAB for the immune cell markers and HTX for the nucleus marker. We have two types of T-cell markers in our data set, the universal T-cell marker CD3 and the cytotoxic T-cell marker CD8. As both are membrane markers with DAB staining, they have a similar appearance. Hence, the same detection algorithm can be used for both cases. Among the 42 FOVs, 10 were randomly selected by the pathologist for manual counting for quality control purposes, and these images were reserved for testing only. We first selected 3 images out of the remaining 32 FOVs, and manually annotated the positive and negative pixels. This yielded 491 positive samples and 539 negative annotated samples. To generate more training data, we sampled the patches around the 2-pixel neighborhood of the annotation, also flipped and rotated the patches, and finally created 17355 training patches in all. For all the experiments, the sparse regularization parameter λ was set to be 0.5.

3.2   Comparisons of Detection Algorithms

We first compared the sparse unmixing with Ruifrok's unmixing algorithm and showed that the sparse unmixing leads to better results with less backgound noise. Fig.5 shows the input RGB image, its absorbance transformed image and the unmixed immune cell channel from both methods.

To train a CNN classifier, we used the following network configuration. The size of the image patch was set to be 27 by 27. We used I_{dab} as the input layer and set 2 convolution layers with both kernel sizes being 6 by 6. 10 epochs were used for training and we finally obtained the training error 0.008. Example detection results are shown in Fig.6. We compared with iterative voting based method [2] for immune cell detection. The algorithm tends to accumulate votes around the centroid of the ring, hence it has the potential to fail if the immune cell shows a solid elliptical shape due to the angle at which the tissue sample was cut (Fig.2). It also has the disadvantage of being sensitive to local gradient changes, since local votes will be accumulated near the boundary of the blob. See Fig. 6 for the examples. The iterative voting based method obtained two local maximums near the boundary of the elliptical blob. Note that we also improved the iterative voting algorithm by filtering out false positive detections near the ring boundaries caused by the local votes using the binary mask of the immune cell marker image channel. As both blob and ring shape immune cells can be included in the training of CNN, the proposed algorithm is more robust in detecting both types of cells.

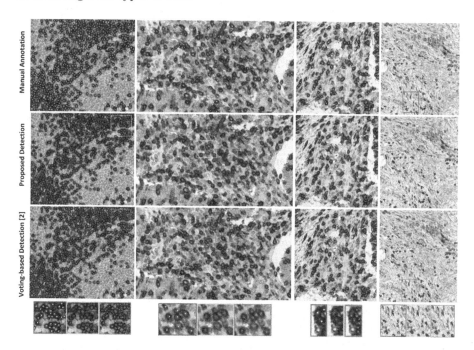

Fig. 6. First row: manual annotation. Second row: detection using the proposed method. Third row: detection using iterative voting based method [2].

3.3   Comparison to Human Observer's Counts

We have 10 FOVs manually annotated by a human observer. To measure the accuracy of the proposed detection algorithm, we compared the algorithm counts with the manual counts and obtained correlation coefficients as high as 0.9949. The average count difference is 17.19 cells per FOV; the number of cells in each FOV is between 200 to 300. This demonstrates that the automatic immune cell detection algorithm proposed in this paper is in concordance with the human's output. As more annotations become available, we believe that it is possible to train the algorithm to follow the human observer's behavior even more reliably.

4   Conclusion

In this paper, we introduced an automatic immune cell detection algorithm for IHC images to assist the clinical immune profile studies. Sparse color unmixing algorithm was proposed to unmix the RGB image into different biologically meaningful color channels. The cell detector was trained using a convolutional neural network in the immune cell marker image channel. The experiments using clinical data demonstrate the efficacy of the proposed algorithm in terms of accuracy, stability, and robustness when compared to the existing techniques and human observer.

References

1. Galon, J., et al.: Type, Density, and Location of Immune Cells Within Human Colorectal Tumors Predict Clinical Outcome. Science 313(5795), 1960–1964 (2006)
2. Parvin, B., et al.: Iterative Voting for Inference of Structural Saliency and Characterization of Subcellular Events. IEEE Trans. Image Processing 16(3), 615–623 (2007)
3. Xin, Q., et al.: Iterative Voting for Inference of Structural Saliency and Characterization of Subcellular Events. IEEE Trans. Biomedical Engineering 59(3), 754–765 (2011)
4. Arteta, C., Lempitsky, V., Noble, J.A., Zisserman, A.: Learning to Detect Cells Using Non-overlapping Extremal Regions. In: Ayache, N., Delingette, H., Golland, P., Mori, K. (eds.) MICCAI 2012, Part I. LNCS, vol. 7510, pp. 348–356. Springer, Heidelberg (2012)
5. Mualla, F., et al.: Automatic Cell Detection in Bright-Field Microscope Images Using SIFT, Random Forests, and Hierarchical Clustering. IEEE Trans. Medical Imaging 32(12), 2274–2286 (2013)
6. Niazi, M.K.K., et al.: An Automated Method for Counting Cytotoxic T-cells from CD8 Stained Images of Renal Biopsies. In: SPIE, vol. 8676 (2013)
7. LeCun, Y., et al.: Gradient-based Learning Applied to Document Recognition. Proceedings of the IEEE 86(11), 2278–2324 (1998)
8. Cireşan, D.C., Giusti, A., Gambardella, L.M., Schmidhuber, J.: Mitosis Detection in Breast Cancer Histology Images with Deep Neural Networks. In: Mori, K., Sakuma, I., Sato, Y., Barillot, C., Navab, N. (eds.) MICCAI 2013, Part II. LNCS, vol. 8150, pp. 411–418. Springer, Heidelberg (2013)
9. Ruifrok, A.C., et al.: Quantification of Histochemical Staining by Color Deconvolution. Anal. Quant. Cytol. Histol. 23, 291–299 (2001)
10. Kesheva, N.: A Survey of Spectral Unmixing Algorithms. Lincoln Laboratory Journal 14(1), 55–78 (2003)
11. Lindeberg, T.: Edge Detection and Ridge Detection with Automatic Scale Selection. In: CVPR, pp. 465–470 (1996)

Stacked Multiscale Feature Learning for Domain Independent Medical Image Segmentation

Ryan Kiros, Karteek Popuri, Dana Cobzas, and Martin Jagersand

University of Alberta, Canada

Abstract. In this work we propose a feature-based segmentation approach that is domain independent. While most existing approaches are based on application-specific hand-crafted features, we propose a framework for learning features from data itself at multiple scales and depth. Our features can be easily integrated into classifiers or energy-based segmentation algorithms. We test the performance of our proposed method on two MICCAI grand challenges, obtaining the top score on VESSEL12 and competitive performance on BRATS2012.

1 Introduction

The choice of image representation plays a crucial role in the success of medical image segmentation algorithms. Most existing methods utilize hand-crafted features incorporated into an energy-based segmentation method or into a machine learning classifier. Commonly, energy-based methods utilize engineered features such as Gabor filters for texture-based segmentation [1], while machine learning approaches use many more simple features like Haar or steerable filters leaving the classification method to disambiguate the ones that are significant for the segmentation task. Popular examples of machine learning methods are ones based on decision trees [2] or random forests [3]. Some methods use very specialized filters designed for a particular task, such as extracting linear structures based on eigenvalues of the image Hessian matrix [4].

Recently there has been much interest within the machine learning and computer vision communities to automatically learn feature representations from scratch. Feature learning methods are general, while hand-crafted features require a certain insight and understanding of the given image data to be analyzed, thus they are often not optimal when applied to a new dataset. Moreover, feature learning algorithms can benefit from many unlabeled examples, even those that may come from a different distribution than the target data [5]. Features can be learned either in an unsupervised setting or in a joint end-to-end system trained with supervision. Successful applications have included object recognition [6] [7], scene parsing and segmentation [8], annotation and retrieval [9], multimodal applications [10] and large-scale learning [11]. What these methods have in common is the emphasis on learning hierarchical representations as opposed to single-layer algorithms such as sparse coding.

Unfortunately, most of the above methods are not directly applicable to medical imaging tasks as they often assume the use of natural images and require a

G. Wu et al. (Eds.): MLMI 2014, LNCS 8679, pp. 25–32, 2014.

Table 1. A comparison of different feature learning architectures for application to medical image segmentation: Y is yes, N is no and S is sometimes. Multi-scale and multi-depth methods can often improve performance while patch-based and stagewise learning improve speed. Here sparse coding eefers to any method that aims to learn a filter bank with a sparsity cost.

Method	Patch-based	Multi-scale	Multi-depth	Stagewise
Sparse coding	Y	N	N	Y
Convolutional sparse coding	N	N	N	Y
Convolutional networks	N	S	Y	N
Proposed approach	Y	Y	Y	Y

large number of labeled examples to be effective. There exist few feature learning methods applied to medical data like the segmentation of linear [12] and curvilinear [13] structures; segmentation of electron microscopy (EM) images [14] and a recent work on MS lesions segmentation [15]. In this paper we propose a framework that is domain independent and utilizes features learned from multiple scales and depth. The key features that make our method fast and thus suitable for medical data are detailed below and can be summarized as: (1) patch-based, (2) stage-based system and a (3) fast dictionary learning method.

Table 1 summarizes and distinguishes four types of feature learning architectures. Simpler single layer sparse coding methods like [15] also use patches but with no scales or depth. Convolutional sparse coding algorithms, such as those used by [12],[16] and [13], differ from standard sparse coding methods as convolution is incorporated into the optimization procedure. The third architecture describes convolutional networks, used by [14] for EM segmentation, which are learned jointly with supervision. While convolutional networks are often very effective, jointly training the whole model can be time consuming. Furthermore, convolutional networks require many labeled examples in order to avoid overfitting. The last architectures illustrates our proposed framework. Features are learned one stage at a time using patch-based learning at multiple scales. Since the model does not require joint learning, features can be learned efficiently and quickly. Our framework is the first to utilize the "encoding versus training" principle of [17] in the context of image segmentation. The emphasis of this work is the importance of the feature encoding as opposed to the filter learning algorithm itself. Due to this, we suggest that more expensive convolutional filter learning is unnecessary, so long as a proper encoding is performed after learning.

Experimentally we demonstrate that the same algorithm can be used to obtain strong performance on two completely different medical segmentation tasks. We report superior results on the vessel segmentation of the lung (VESSEL12) challenge data and competitive performance on multimodal brain tumor segmentation (BRATS2012) data. Furthermore, our system is able to learn features in under ten minutes on both challenges. Code for our approach will be released upon publication.

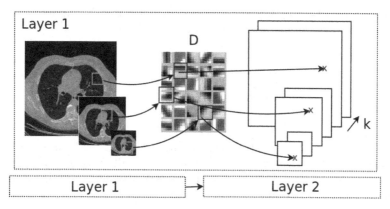

Fig. 1. Visualization of our feature learning approach. Each volume slice is scaled using a Gaussian pyramid. Patches are extracted at each scale to learn a dictionary D using OMP. Convolution is performed over all scales with the dictionary filters, resulting in Γk feature maps. After training the first layer, the feature maps can then be used as input to a second layer.

2   Method

We assume we are given m volumes with s modalities $\{\{V^{(j)}\}_{j=1}^s\}_{i=1}^m$, where each $V_i^{(j)} \in \mathbb{R}^{n_V \times n_H \times n}$. $n_V \times n_H$ is the spatial dimension of a slice and n is the number of slices. For simplicity, we assume that each volume $V_i^{(j)}$ has dimensionality $n_V \times n_H \times n$ although this is not needed. As a specific example, brain tumor segmentation tasks can use $s = 4$ modalites consisting of FLAIR, T1, T2 and post-Gadolinium T1. The general outline of our feature learning framework is as follows:

- Extract multimodal patches at multiple scales using a Gaussian pyramid.
- Learn a filter bank using orthogonal matching pursuit.
- Convolutionally extract feature maps using the learned filters as kernels.
- Repeat the above steps, using the computed features maps as input to another layer. The number of feature maps (next layer modalities) corresponds to the number of filters.

In each of the following subsections, we describe the above operations in detail.

2.1   Pre-Processing and Dictionary Learning

Given a volume V, a Gaussian pyramid with Γ scales is applied to each modality of each slice. Let $\{p^{(1)}, \ldots, p^{(m_P)}\}$ denote a set of m_P patches randomly extracted from the scaled volumes. Each patch $p^{(l)}$ is of spatial dimension $r \times c \times s$ where $r \times c$ is the receptive field size. These patches are then flattened into column vectors. Per patch contrast normalization and patch-wise mean subtraction is performed. For dictionary learning we use orthogonal matching pursuit (OMP). OMP aims to solve the following optimization problem:

$$\underset{D,x^{(i)}}{\text{minimize}} \quad \sum_{i=1}^{m_P} ||Dx^{(i)} - p^{(i)}||_2^2$$
$$\text{subject to} \quad ||D^{(l)}||_2^2 = 1, \forall l \tag{1}$$
$$||x^{(i)}||_0 \le q, \forall i$$

where $D \in \mathbb{R}^{n_P \times k}$ and $D^{(l)}$ is the l-th column of D. Optimization is done using alternation over the dictionary D and codes x. For all our experiments we set $q = 1$, which reduces to a form of gain-shape vector quantization. In particular, given a dictionary D, an index κ is chosen as

$$\kappa = \underset{l}{\text{argmax}} |D^{(l)^T} p^{(i)}| \tag{2}$$

for which the κ-th index of $x^{(i)}$ is set as $x_\kappa^{(i)} = D^{(\kappa)^T} p^{(i)}$ with all other indices left as zero in order to satisfy the constraint $||x^{(i)}||_0 \le 1$ for all i. Given the one-hot codes X, the dictionary is easily updated by first solving the unconstrained problem, followed by re-normalization to satisfy the constraint $||D^{(l)}||_2^2 = 1$ for all l.

2.2 Convolutional Feature Extraction

Let T_j^γ denote a volume slice of modality j and scale γ. Each $r \times c \times s$ patch in T_j^γ is pre-processed by contrast normalization and mean subtraction. Let $D_j^{(l)} \in \mathbb{R}^{r \times c}$ denote the l-th basis for modality j of D. We will define the feature encoding for basis l as:

$$f_l^\gamma = \sum_{j=1}^{s} T_j^\gamma * D_j^{(l)} \tag{3}$$

where $*$ denotes convolution. The resulting feature maps $\{f_l^\gamma\}_{l=1}^k$ are of the same spatial dimensions as T_j^γ. The feature maps are finally upsampled to the original $n_V \times n_H$ spatial dimension. Figure 1 illustrates our approach.

2.3 Stacking Multiple Layers

Our described setup for feature learning has involved scaling, dictionary learning and convolutional extraction. Just as the volumes slices were inputs to a first layer with s modalities, the upsampled output feature maps $\{\{f_l^\gamma\}_{\gamma=1}^{\Gamma}\}_{l=1}^{k}$ may be seen as inputs to a second layer but with Γk modalities. The same described operations are applied a second time resulting in additional second layer output feature maps. These groups of feature maps can be concatenated together resulting in a total number of $\Gamma_1 k_1 + \Gamma_2 k_2$ feature maps, where Γ_1, k_1 are the number of first layer scales and filters while Γ_2, k_2 are the number of second layer scales and filters. Thus each pixel in a volume slice can be represented as a $\Gamma_1 k_1 + \Gamma_2 k_2$ dimensional feature vector.

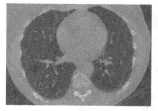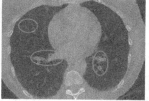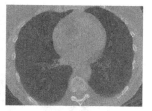

Fig. 2. Visualizing the importance of scale and depth for vessel segmentation

3   Experiments

We perform experimental evaluation using data from two MICCAI grad challenges: vessel segmentation of the lung[1] and multimodal brain tumor segmentation[2].

3.1   Vessel Segmentation

The vessel segmentation challenge consists of 20 volumes of CT scans to segment with 3 additional volumes that include 882 labeled pixels based on the agreement of at least 3 experts. Each slice is of size 512×512 with each volume containing a few hundred slices. We performed feature learning with 2 depths, 6 scales, a receptive field size of 5×5, 32 first layer filters and 64 second layer filters. The final feature vector is thus of size $6 \times (32+64) = 576$. In order to perform segmentation, we extracted features for the existing labeled pixels and trained a L2-regularized logistic regression classifier, using 10-fold cross validation in order to tune the L2 hyperparameter. Each pixel of a new slice is then classified, resulting in a probability of whether or not the pixel is a vessel. For our submission to the challenge, the probabilities are scaled and rounded to unsigned 8-bit integers as requested.

Table 2. The top 5 results from the VESSEL12 challenge leaderboard

Team	Method type	score
our method	feature learning + classification	**0.986**
LKEBChina	Krissian-inspired vesselness	0.984
FME_LungVessels	Frangi vesselness + region growing	0.984
LKEBChina	Krissian-inspired vesselness with bi-Gaussian kernel	0.981
FME_LungVessels	Frangi vesselness + region growing (raw)	0.981

Figure 2 illustrates the importance of adding depth and scale to segmentation. The first image is the original CT scan. The second image shows segmentation

---

[1] http://vessel12.grand-challenge.org/
[2] http://www2.imm.dtu.dk/projects/BRATS2012/

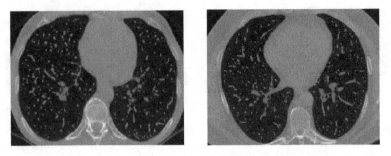

Fig. 3. Sample vessel segmentation results

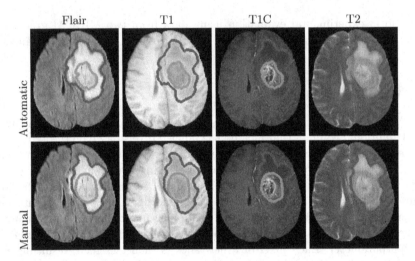

Fig. 4. Sample brain tumor segmentation results

when neither depth nor scale is added while the third image shows segmentation with added depth and scale. Without scale, larger vessels are less likely to be segmented while without depth, segmentation is much more scattered and less contiguous. For visualization purposes, a pixel is labeled as being a vessel if the probability of a vessel given the pixel features is greater than 0.5.

Table 2 shows the top 5 performing methods on the VESSEL12 challenge. Our proposed method tops all existing approaches. The top performing methods in the competition are largely based on the use of Frangi [4] and Krissian vesselness [18] all of which derive structural properties from the eigenvalues of the Hessian.

3.2   Brain Tumor Segmentation

To emphasize that the proposed method is domain independent, we evaluated it on the BRATS2012 multimodal brain tumor segmentation challenge, a dataset that has totally different properties and segmentation task than the vessel data. Due to BRATS2012 site maintenance, the test volume labels were unavailable at the time we did our experiments. Instead we perform evaluation using leave-one-out cross validation on the training set. Two types of tumour data are evaluated: high-grade and low-grade. Each volume voxel is labeled as being one of three classes: tumor, edema and other. We utilized our approach with one scale and two depths, with 16 bases in each depth for a total of 32 features. A 2 hidden layer network with dropout [19] is used to make predictions. Within each training fold, 10-fold cross validation is used to select the dropout parameters.

Table 3. Comparison against the top two performers in the BRATS2012 competition. HG and LG stand for high-grade and low-grade, respectively.

Team	region	mean dice coeff.	region	mean dice coeff.
our method	HG edema	0.485	LG edema	0.250
Bauer et al.	HG edema	0.536	LG edema	0.179
Zikic et al.	HG edema	**0.598**	LG edema	**0.324**
our method	HG tumor	0.470	LG tumor	**0.406**
Bauer et al.	HG tumor	**0.512**	LG tumor	0.332
Zikic et al.	HG tumor	0.476	LG tumor	0.339
our method	HG GTV	0.720	LG GTV	0.494

Table 3 shows our results in comparison to the top 2 methods in the competition. We note again that out comparison is not on the same held-out data. None the less, our results are competitive with the top performing methods.

4   Conclusion

In this paper we proposed a domain independent approach for segmenting medical images. Our approaches involves learning feature representations at multiple scales and depths which are compatible with existing classification and energy-based segmentation methods. We obtain the best performing result on the VESSEL12 challenge and competitive results on the BRATS2012 multimodal brain tumor segmentation challenge. For future work we intend to further evaluate our approach on additional grand challenge problems. We also intend to study various transfer learning scenarios between domains and modalities.

References

1. Paragios, N., Deriche, R.: Geodesic active regions and level set methods for supervised texture segmentation. IJCV 50(3), 223–247 (2002)
2. Zheng, Y., Barbu, A., Georgescu, B., Scheuering, M., Comaniciu, D.: Four-chamber heart modeling and automatic segmentation for 3D cardiac ct volumes using marginal space learning and steerable features. IEEE Trans. Medical Imaging 27(11), 1668–1681 (2008)
3. Criminisi, A., Robertson, D., Konukoglu, E., Shotton, J., Pathak, S., White, S., Siddiqui, K.: Regression forests for efficient anatomy detection and localization in computed tomography scans. Medical Image Analysis (2013)

4. Frangi, A.F., Niessen, W.J., Vincken, K.L., Viergever, M.A.: Multiscale vessel enhancement filtering. In: Wells, W.M., Colchester, A.C.F., Delp, S.L. (eds.) MICCAI 1998. LNCS, vol. 1496, pp. 130–137. Springer, Heidelberg (1998)
5. Raina, R., Battle, A., Lee, H., Packer, B., Ng, A.Y.: Self-taught learning: transfer learning from unlabeled data. In: ICML, pp. 759–766 (2007)
6. Bo, L., Ren, X., Fox, D.: Unsupervised Feature Learning for RGB-D Based Object Recognition. In: ISER (June 2012)
7. Krizhevsky, A., Sutskever, I., Hinton, G.: Imagenet classification with deep convolutional neural networks. In: NIPS, pp. 1106–1114 (2012)
8. Farabet, C., Couprie, C., Najman, L., LeCun, Y.: Scene parsing with multiscale feature learning, purity trees, and optimal covers. In: ICML (2012)
9. Kiros, R., Szepesvari, C.: Deep representations and codes for image auto-annotation. In: NIPS, pp. 917–925 (2012)
10. Srivastava, N., Salakhutdinov, R.: Multimodal learning with deep boltzmann machines. In: NIPS, pp. 2231–2239 (2012)
11. Dean, J., Corrado, G., Monga, R., Chen, K., Devin, M., Le, Q., Mao, M., Ranzato, M., Senior, A., Tucker, P., Yang, K., Ng, A.: Large scale distributed deep networks. In: NIPS, pp. 1232–1240 (2012)
12. Rigamonti, R., Lepetit, V.: Accurate and efficient linear structure segmentation by leveraging ad hoc features with learned filters. In: Ayache, N., Delingette, H., Golland, P., Mori, K. (eds.) MICCAI 2012, Part I. LNCS, vol. 7510, pp. 189–197. Springer, Heidelberg (2012)
13. Becker, C., Rigamonti, R., Lepetit, V., Fua, P.: Supervised feature learning for curvilinear structure segmentation. In: Mori, K., Sakuma, I., Sato, Y., Barillot, C., Navab, N. (eds.) MICCAI 2013, Part I. LNCS, vol. 8149, pp. 526–533. Springer, Heidelberg (2013)
14. Ciresan, D., Giusti, A., Schmidhuber, J., et al.: Deep neural networks segment neuronal membranes in electron microscopy images. In: NIPS, pp. 2852–2860 (2012)
15. Weiss, N., Rueckert, D., Rao, A.: Multiple sclerosis lesion segmentation using dictionary learning and sparse coding. In: Mori, K., Sakuma, I., Sato, Y., Barillot, C., Navab, N. (eds.) MICCAI 2013, Part I. LNCS, vol. 8149, pp. 735–742. Springer, Heidelberg (2013)
16. Rigamonti, R., Türetken, E., González, G., Fua, P., Lepetit, V.: Filter learning for linear structure segmentation. Technical report, EPFL (2011)
17. Coates, A., Ng, A.Y.: The importance of encoding versus training with sparse coding and vector quantization. In: ICML, vol. 8, p. 10 (2011)
18. Krissian, K., Malandain, G., Ayache, N., Vaillant, R., Trousset, Y.: Model-based detection of tubular structures in 3D images. Computer Vision and Image Understanding 80(2), 130–171 (2000)
19. Hinton, G.E., Srivastava, N., Krizhevsky, A., Sutskever, I., Salakhutdinov, R.R.: Improving neural networks by preventing co-adaptation of feature detectors. arXiv preprint arXiv:1207.0580 (2012)

Detection of Mammographic Masses
by Content-Based Image Retrieval

Menglin Jiang[1], Shaoting Zhang[2], and Dimitris N. Metaxas[1]

[1] Department of Computer Science, Rutgers University, Piscataway, NJ, USA
[2] Department of Computer Science, UNC Charlotte, Charlotte, NC, USA

Abstract. Computer-aided diagnosis (CAD) of mammographic masses is important yet challenging, since masses have large variation in shape and size and are often indistinguishable from surrounding tissue. As an alternative solution, content-based image retrieval (CBIR) techniques can facilitate the diagnosis by finding visually similar cases. However, they still need radiologists to identify suspicious regions in the query case. To overcome the drawbacks of both kinds of methods, we propose a CAD approach that integrates image retrieval with learning-based mass detection. Specifically, a query mammogram is first matched with a database of exemplar masses, getting a series of similarity maps. Then these maps are subtracted by discriminatively learned thresholds to eliminate noise. At last, individual similarity maps are aggregated, and local maxima in the final map are selected as masses. By utilizing a large database, our approach can effectively detect masses despite their variation. Moreover, it bypasses the identification of suspicious regions by radiologists. Experiments are conducted on 500 mammograms randomly selected from the digital database for screening mammography (DDSM) using receiver operating characteristic (ROC) analysis. The proposed approach achieves a promising ROC area index $A_z = 0.91$, and outperforms two traditional classifier-based CAD methods.

1 Introduction

For years, mammography has played a key role in diagnosis of breast cancer, the second leading cause of cancer-related death among women. The major indicators of breast cancer are masses and microcalcifications. Generally speaking, the detection of mammographic masses is even more challenging than that of microcalcifications, since masses vary substantially in shape, margin, size and usually have obscure boundaries. Consequently, a considerable portion of retrospectively visible masses is missed by radiologists, and biopsies are frequently conducted on normal tissues or benign lesions [1].

Due to the clinical significance and great challenge of mammographic mass detection, numerous computer-aided diagnosis (CAD) methods have been proposed to facilitate this procedure. A majority of these approaches first segment a query mammogram into several regions, then extract certain features from each region, and finally classify these regions as mass or normal tissue using the extracted features and pre-trained classifiers [4,13,18]. However, it is very difficult for classifiers to model all the training masses, and they are likely to miss

G. Wu et al. (Eds.): MLMI 2014, LNCS 8679, pp. 33–41, 2014.

masses of "uncommon" appearance or sizes [13]. Besides, their performance may be affected by the obscure boundaries of masses [18], since most of them need to perform image segmentation before mass detection.

As an intuitive alternative, content-based image retrieval (CBIR) techniques have gradually gained their popularity. Specifically, these methods first prompt radiologists to label a region of interest (ROI) in the query case, then compare it with ROIs extracted from previously diagnosed cases, and finally return the most relevant cases along with the likelihood of a lesion in the query [7,11]. Compared with classifier-based approaches, CBIR-based CAD methods could provide more clinical evidence to assist the diagnosis. Especially, the recent progress of scalable CBIR techniques has been a catalyst for the increase of such CAD systems [6, 20]. Nevertheless, they are semi-automatic and rely heavily on radiologist-specified ROI. A nonrepresentative region, e.g. a normal region in a malignant mammogram, will lead to wrong diagnosis.

To overcome the above drawbacks, inspired by [16], we propose a CAD method that combines image retrieval with discriminative learning, which is illustrated in Fig. 1. In particular, a large database of exemplar mammographic masses is constructed, and a query mammogram is matched with each exemplar to compute a series of similarity maps. A similarity map describes the probabilities of a mass centered at each pixel in the query mammogram. Second, each similarity map is subtracted by a discriminatively learned threshold to remove non-mass regions. Finally, individual similarity maps are summed up, and masses are detected by simply choosing local maxima in the aggregated map. Our approach has several advantages over traditional classifier-based methods. First, it could detect unusual masses as long as there are several similar exemplars in the database. Second, the obscure mass boundary problem is eliminated, since no segmentation is required. Third, our method returns not only a detection result but also the most similar diagnosed cases, which are valuable to the interpretation of current case. The presented approach is also superior to CBIR-based methods regarding that it does not need artificial labeling of suspicious regions. Therefore it provides radiologists with "double reading" aid automatically.

2   Methodology

In this section, we first introduce the similarity matching between query mammogram and exemplar masses, then present the refinement of similarity maps based on discriminative learning, and finally describe how to detect masses using these similarity maps. The overview of our approach is shown in Fig. 1.

2.1   Local Feature Voting-Based Image Retrieval

Our approach builds upon the "bag of words" (BoW) framework [2, 6, 15–17], which describes an image with a series of quantized local features. The local feature we choose here is scale-invariant feature transform (SIFT) [8]. SIFT has been successfully applied to medical image retrieval and analysis [2,6], owing to its excellent robustness and discriminability.

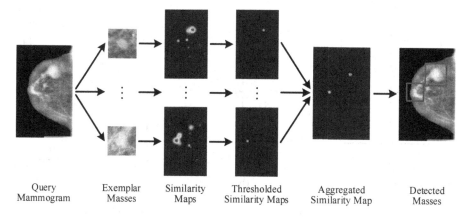

| Query
Mammogram | Exemplar
Masses | Similarity
Maps | Thresholded
Similarity Maps | Aggregated
Similarity Map | Detected
Masses |

Fig. 1. Overview of the proposed approach

During offline stage, a large set of SIFT features extracted from a separate database are used to train a visual vocabulary (VOC) through k-means clustering. After that, SIFT features are extracted from exemplar database D, then quantized using this VOC. Each SIFT feature is represented by the ID of its nearest visual word (cluster center), and an exemplar mass is characterized by all the quantized SIFT features along with their locations. During online stage, given a mammogram q in the query set Q, SIFT features are extracted and quantized using the same VOC. Following [15,16], each exemplar d is matched with q to calculate a similarity score $sim(q,d)$ and a similarity map $\boldsymbol{S}(q,d)$, where $\boldsymbol{S}(q,d)[x,y]$ indicates the similarity between a region of q centered at (x,y) and d.

Formally speaking, q is represented as a BoW, $q = \{v_i^q\}_{i=1}^m$, where v_i^q denotes its i-th quantized feature. Similarly, d is represented as $d = \{v_j^d\}_{j=1}^n$. Supposing d is transformed to $d_{\alpha,s}$ after rotation α and scale s, and $d_{\alpha,s}$ matches a region in q denoted as $q_{\alpha,s}$, then their features should match with each other and have similar locations relative to their centers. For a given pair of matched features $v_i^q = v_j^d = v$, the center of $q_{\alpha,s}$, denoted as c_i^q, can be localized based on the locations of v_i^q and v_j^d:

$$l_{ci}^q = l_{vi}^q - s \cdot \boldsymbol{R} \cdot l_{vj}^d, \quad \boldsymbol{R} = \begin{bmatrix} \cos\alpha & -\sin\alpha \\ \sin\alpha & \cos\alpha \end{bmatrix}, \tag{1}$$

where l_{vj}^d is the location of v_j^d relative to the center of d, α and s are transformation parameters, l_{vi}^q and l_{ci}^q are the absolute locations of v_i^q and c_i^q respectively.

After localizing c_i^q, v_i^q can cast its vote. To resist gentle nonrigid deformation, v_i^q votes in favor of not only c_i^q but also c_i^q's neighbors. c_i^q earns a full vote, and each neighbor gains a vote shrinked by a Gaussian weight:

$$\boldsymbol{S}(q,d_{\alpha,s})[x_{ci}^q + \delta x, y_{ci}^q + \delta y] + = \frac{idf^2(v)}{tf(v,q) \cdot tf(v,d)} \cdot \exp\left(-\frac{\delta x^2 + \delta y^2}{\sigma^2}\right), \tag{2}$$

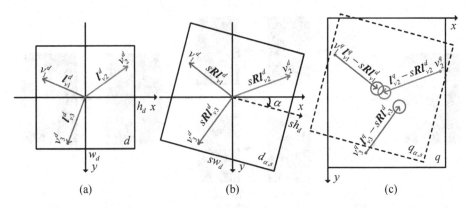

Fig. 2. Illustration of local feature voting-based similarity measure. Note that only one pair of (α, s) is used here, whereas 64 pairs are used in practice. (a) An exemplar mass d. (b) d is virtually transformed to $d_{\alpha,s}$. (c) A query mammogram q with three features v_1^q, v_2^q and v_3^q matched with v_1^d, v_2^d and v_3^d respectively. v_1^q and v_2^q vote for nearby centers, whereas v_3^q is a noise and votes for a wrong center. $q_{\alpha,s}$ is localized by finding the maximum value in $\boldsymbol{S}(q, d_{\alpha,s})$.

where $(x_{ci}^q, y_{ci}^q) = \boldsymbol{l}_{ci}^q$ is the location of c_i^q, $(\delta x, \delta y)$ is the deviation from c_i^q to its neighbor and satisfies $\delta x^2 + \delta y^2 \leqslant r^2$, $tf(v, q)$ and $tf(v, d)$ are the term frequencies (TFs) of v in q and d respectively, and $idf(v)$ is the inverse document frequency (IDF) of v. TF-IDF [14] is widely adopted in BoW-based CBIR methods. It reflects the importance of a visual word to an image in a collection of images. The vote score in Eq. (2) is defined based on the observation that visual words occurring rarely in the whole database (with high IDF) are more informative, and visual words occurring frequently in a single mammogram (with high TF) are less informative.

The cumulative votes of all matched pairs generate a similarity map $\boldsymbol{S}(q, d_{\alpha,s})$. The center of $q_{\alpha,s}$ is localized by finding the maximum value in $\boldsymbol{S}(q, d_{\alpha,s})$. This value represents the similarity between q and $d_{\alpha,s}$, and is denoted as $sim(q, d_{\alpha,s})$. For the robustness to rotation and scale transformations, d is virtually transformed using every combination of 8 α (from 0 to $7\pi/4$) and 8 s (from $1/2$ to 2). Among all the 64 similarity maps, the one with highest similarity score is selected. The chosen similarity map and score serve as the similarity map and score between q and d, which are referred to as $\boldsymbol{S}(q, d)$ and $sim(q, d)$ respectively:

$$sim(q, d) = \max_{\alpha,s} \max_{x,y} \boldsymbol{S}(q, d_{\alpha,s})[x, y] . \tag{3}$$

Let (x^*, y^*) and (α^*, s^*) be the parameters that maximize Eq. (3), then the query mass is localized at (x^*, y^*). Calculation of $\boldsymbol{S}(q, d_{\alpha,s})$ and $sim(q, d_{\alpha,s})$ is illustrated in Fig. 2.

The above image retrieval approach has several advantages. First, it performs mass retrieval and localization simultaneously. Second, it is robust to translation, rotation and scale transformations of masses. Last, without resort to sliding window-based scanning, our approach is computationally efficient.

2.2   Learning Similarity Thresholds

With the quantization of local features for fast retrieval, their discriminative power is weakened. Therefore some non-mass regions may receive high similarity scores, as shown in the third column of Fig. 1. To solve this problem, following [16], we subtract a similarity score $sim(q,d)$ by a pre-trained threshold θ_d:

$$\overline{sim}(q,d) = \begin{cases} sim(q,d) - \theta_d, & if \ sim(q,d) > \theta_d \\ 0 & , otherwise \end{cases} \qquad (4)$$

where $\overline{sim}(q,d)$ denotes the gated similarity score between q and d.

After applying the thresholds, only those exemplars with positive similarity scores are kept. For each remaining exemplar d, its similarity map $\boldsymbol{S}(q,d)$ is also gated, resulting in $\bar{\boldsymbol{S}}(q,d)$:

$$\bar{\boldsymbol{S}}(q,d)[x,y] = \begin{cases} \boldsymbol{S}(q,d)[x,y] - \theta_d, & if \ \boldsymbol{S}(q,d)[x,y] > \theta_d \\ 0 & , otherwise \end{cases} \qquad (5)$$

As demonstrated in the fourth column of Fig. 1, most noise in the similarity maps could be successfully eliminated.

In order to learn all the thresholds, a group of mammograms depicting healthy breasts are collected to form a negative query set $\tilde{Q}$. For each exemplar d, its threshold is chosen as the maximum similarity score between d and any negative query $\tilde{q} \in \tilde{Q}$:

$$\theta_d = \max_{\tilde{q} \in \tilde{Q}} sim(\tilde{q}, d) . \qquad (6)$$

It is worth pointing out that the above threshold scheme can be interpreted as Naive Bayes classification [16]. Each gated similarity score $\overline{sim}(q,d)$ is regarded as the output of a simple classifier, where a positive score indicates a mass. The threshold θ_d learned in Eq. (6) satisfies the constraint that no negative query $\tilde{q} \in \tilde{Q}$ is mistaken for a positive one by d. In the meantime, it maximizes the likelihood that a positive query is correctly detected.

2.3   Detection of Masses

After obtaining all the exemplars with positive similarity scores $\overline{sim}(q,d)$, we sum up their similarity maps $\bar{\boldsymbol{S}}(q,d)$ to calculate the final similarity map of q, denoted as $\hat{\boldsymbol{S}}(q)$:

$$\hat{\boldsymbol{S}}(q) = \sum_{d:\overline{sim}(q,d)>0} \bar{\boldsymbol{S}}(q,d). \qquad (7)$$

Then, non-maximum suppression is exploited to find the local maxima in $\hat{\boldsymbol{S}}(q)$, and masses are asserted around these maxima points. Finally, each mass is localized based on its supporting exemplars. Let (x^*, y^*) be the center of an asserted mass, the individual similarity maps $\bar{\boldsymbol{S}}(q,d)$ contributing to $\hat{\boldsymbol{S}}(q)[x^*, y^*]$ can be identified. Remember that in Subsection 2.1, the mass region is localized when calculating $\boldsymbol{S}(q,d)$. The final mass region is determined as the per-component median of the regions corresponding to all supporting exemplars. An example is provided in the fifth and sixth columns of Fig. 1.

It is noteworthy that during the above detection and localization process, the supporting exemplars for each detected mass are also found. These exemplars, along with their diagnosed pathologies, can be displayed to the radiologists. Such clinical evidence is a by-product of our method.

3   Experiments

Our experiment dataset is constructed from the digital database for screening mammography (DDSM) [5], which is currently the largest public mammogram database. DDSM is comprised of 2,604 cases, and every case consists of four views, i.e. LEFT-CC, LEFT-MLO, RIGHT-CC and RIGHT-MLO. The masses have diverse shapes, sizes, margins, breast densities as well as patients' races and ages, and are associated with annotations labeled by experienced radiologists. To build our dataset, mammograms are first mapped from grey level to optical density to eliminate visual difference caused by different scanners. Second, normalized mammograms are processed for better visual quality using inver-

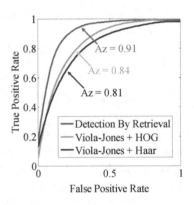

Fig. 3. ROC performance of the three evaluated methods

sion, breast segmentation, and contrast enhancement. Third, 2,021 ROIs centered at masses are extracted to form an exemplar database D. Finally, 500 mammograms containing masses are randomly selected as query set Q. Besides, 500 mammograms depicting healthy breasts compose a negative query set $\tilde{Q}$, which is utilized to train the similarity threshold θ_d for each exemplar mass $d \in D$. D, Q and $\tilde{Q}$ are randomly selected from different cases.

As a point of reference, we also implement two classifier-based CAD methods. Both methods adopt a cascade of boosted classifiers [19]. This framework, usually referred to as "Viola-Jones", is widely used in general object detection and also achieves promising results in mammographic lesion detection [12]. The first method employs the same Haar feature as [19], and the second one utilizes histogram of oriented gradient (HOG) [3] to better describe mass appearance and shape. HOG and its variations demonstrate excellent performance in the latest works on mammographic mass detection and segmentation [9,10].

All the methods are evaluated using receiver operating characteristic (ROC) curve and ROC area index A_z, which are shown in Fig. 3. The proposed approach significantly outperforms the Viola-Jones methods. It achieves an A_z value as high as 0.91, whereas the A_z values of the other two methods are 0.84 and 0.81. Detailed results show that the Viola-Jones methods miss most of the "uncommon" masses, which is expected since classifiers can hardly recognize minority features extracted from the exemplar database. On the contrary, our approach could precisely detect and localize these masses as long as there are a few similar exemplar masses. Remember that in addition to better detection performance, our method also provides users with visually similar cases and associated pathologies. Such information can further improve the accuracy of radiologists' diagnosis. An example can be found in Fig. 4. The query mammogram contains a malignant mass of great size, lobulated shape and obscure boundary. There are only several similar masses in the exemplar database, which cannot be modeled by classifiers. Consequently, the Viola-Jones methods fail to detect this mass. Nevertheless, these exemplars are sufficient to vote the mass using our approach.

It is worth mentioning that a considerable portion of false positives is caused by the visual similarity between malignant masses and normal regions with bright cores and spiculated boundaries. A possible solution is to filter out these regions through an additional mass validation step. In particular, a series of annotated mammograms depicting either healthy or abnormal breasts should be collected to make up a validation database V. Then, an asserted mass q is matched with each validation mammogram using the same similarity measure explained in Subsection 2.1. A true positive is expected to discover some masses in V, while a false positive is likely to find normal tissues or localize masses inaccurately. Therefore a validation score can be calculated for q based on how much its retrieved regions overlap with the annotated mass regions in V. And q is reported only if its score is higher than a validation threshold θ_V.

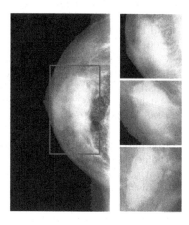

Fig. 4. A query mammogram with a malignant mass (left) and its top 3 supporting exemplar masses retrieved by our approach (right)

4   Conclusion

During the past decades, various CAD approaches have been presented to assist mammographic mass detection, which are based on classifiers or CBIR techniques. Nevertheless, either category has its limitations. In this paper, image retrieval and discriminative classifiers are unified to complement each other. In particular, a query mammogram is matched with each exemplar mass using a local feature voting scheme, achieving mass retrieval and localization simultaneously. Then, discriminatively learned thresholds are employed to prune non-mass regions, which can be regarded as Naive Bayes classification. Finally, thresholded similarity maps are accumulated, and masses are detected by finding local maxima in the aggregated map. Compared with classifier-based CAD methods, the proposed approach could handle unusual masses by using a large exemplar database. In addition, it solves the obscure mass boundary problem, and provides radiologists with relevant diagnosed cases. Compared with CBIR-based methods, it doesn't rely on radiologist-labeled suspicious regions and serves as a fully automated double reading aid. A large dataset is built from DDSM, and experiments show the effectiveness of our method. Further endeavors will be devoted to remove false positives through mass validation.

References

1. Birdwell, R.L., Ikeda, D.M., O'Shaughnessy, K.F., Sickles, E.A.: Mammographic characteristics of 115 missed cancers later detected with screening mammography and the potential utility of computer-aided detection. Radiology 219(1), 192–202 (2001)
2. Caicedo, J.C., Cruz, A., Gonzalez, F.A.: Histopathology image classification using bag of features and kernel functions. In: Combi, C., Shahar, Y., Abu-Hanna, A. (eds.) AIME 2009. LNCS, vol. 5651, pp. 126–135. Springer, Heidelberg (2009)
3. Dalal, N., Triggs, B.: Histograms of oriented gradients for human detection. In: Proc. IEEE CVPR, pp. 886–893 (2005)
4. Ganesan, K., Acharya, U.R., Chua, C.K., Min, L.C., Abraham, K.T., Ng, K.H.: Computer-aided breast cancer detection using mammograms: A review. IEEE Rev. Biomed. Eng. 6, 77–98 (2013)
5. Heath, M., Bowyer, K., Kopans, D., Kegelmeyer Jr., W.P., Moore, R., Chang, K., Munishkumaran, S.: Current status of the digital database for screening mammography. In: Digital Mammography, pp. 457–460. Springer, Netherlands (1998)
6. Jiang, M., Zhang, S., Liu, J., Shen, T., Metaxas, D.N.: Computer-aided diagnosis of mammographic masses using vocabulary tree-based image retrieval. In: Proc. IEEE ISBI (2014)
7. Kumar, A., Kim, J., Cai, W., Fulham, M., Feng, D.: Content-based medical image retrieval: A survey of applications to multidimensional and multimodality data. J. Digit. Imaging 26(6), 1025–1039 (2013)
8. Lowe, D.G.: Distinctive image features from scale-invariant keypoints. Int. J. Comput. Vis. 60(2), 91–110 (2004)
9. Molinara, M., Marrocco, C., Tortorella, F.: A boosting-based approach to refine the segmentation of masses in mammography. In: Petrosino, A. (ed.) ICIAP 2013, Part II. LNCS, vol. 8157, pp. 572–580. Springer, Heidelberg (2013)
10. Moura, D.C., Guevara-López, M.Á.: An evaluation of image descriptors combined with clinical data for breast cancer diagnosis. Int. J. Comput. Assist. Radiol. Surg. 8(4), 561–574 (2013)
11. Müller, H., Michoux, N., Bandon, D., Geissbühler, A.: A review of content-based image retrieval systems in medical applications - clinical benefits and future directions. Int. J. Med. Inform. 73(1), 1–23 (2004)
12. Nemoto, M., Shimizu, A., Kobatake, H., Takeo, H., Nawano, S.: Study on cascade classification in abnormal shadow detection for mammograms. In: Astley, S.M., Brady, M., Rose, C., Zwiggelaar, R. (eds.) IWDM 2006. LNCS, vol. 4046, pp. 324–331. Springer, Heidelberg (2006)
13. Oliver, A., Freixenet, J., Martí, J., Pérez, E., Pont, J., Denton, E.R.E., Zwiggelaar, R.: A review of automatic mass detection and segmentation in mammographic images. Med. Image Anal. 14(2), 87–110 (2010)
14. Salton, G., Buckley, C.: Term-weighting approaches in automatic text retrieval. Inf. Process. Manag. 24(5), 513–523 (1988)

15. Shen, X., Lin, Z., Brandt, J., Avidan, S., Wu, Y.: Object retrieval and localization with spatially-constrained similarity measure and k-nn re-ranking. In: Proc. IEEE CVPR, pp. 3013–3020 (2012)
16. Shen, X., Lin, Z., Brandt, J., Wu, Y.: Detecting and aligning faces by image retrieval. In: Proc. IEEE CVPR, pp. 3460–3467 (2013)
17. Sivic, J., Zisserman, A.: Video google: A text retrieval approach to object matching in videos. In: Proc. IEEE ICCV, pp. 1470–1477 (2003)
18. Tang, J., Rangayyan, R.M., Xu, J., El Naqa, I., Yang, Y.: Computer-aided detection and diagnosis of breast cancer with mammography: Recent advances. IEEE Trans. Inf. Technol. Biomed. 13(2), 236–251 (2009)
19. Viola, P.A., Jones, M.J.: Rapid object detection using a boosted cascade of simple features. In: Proc. IEEE CVPR, pp. I–511–I–518 (2001)
20. Zhang, X., Liu, W., Zhang, S.: Mining histopathological images via hashing-based scalable image retrieval. In: Proc. IEEE ISBI (2014)

Inferring Sources of Dementia Progression with Network Diffusion Model

Chenhui Hu[1,2], Xue Hua[3], Paul M. Thompson[4],
Georges El Fakhri[1], and Quanzheng Li[1]

[1] Center for Advanced Medical Imaging Science, Massachusetts General Hospital
[2] School of Engineering and Applied Sciences, Harvard University
[3] Keck School of Medicine, USC
[4] Dept. of Neurology, UCLA

Abstract. Pinpointing the sources of dementia is crucial to the effective treatment of neurodegenerative diseases. In this paper, we model the dementia progression by a diffusive model over the brain network with sparse impulsive stimulations. By solving inverse problems, we localize the possible origins of Alzheimer's disease based on a large set of repeated magnetic resonance imaging (MRI) scans in ADNI. The distribution of the sources averaged over the sample population is evaluated. We find that the dementia sources have different concentrations in the brain lobes for Alzheimer's disease (AD) patients and mild cognitive impairment (MCI) subjects, indicating possible switch of the dementia driving mechanism. Our model provides a quantitative way to perform explanatory analysis of the dynamics of dementia.

Keywords: Sources of dementia, network diffusion, brain morphology, longitudinal study, MRI, Alzheimer's disease.

1 Introduction

As a collective term describing symptoms of severe cognitive decline, *dementia* affects 35.6 million people worldwide. About 50% to 80% of dementia is due to Alzheimer's disease (AD), a progressive neurodegenerative disease without cure since the cause and progression of AD are not well understood. To reveal the pathology of AD, the *amyloid* and *tau* hypotheses have been proposed. They postulate that the disease begins in the gray matter with accumulation of misfolded beta-amyloid and/or tau protein and progresses along extant fiber pathways [1]. The progression results in gross atrophy of the affected brain regions, containing degeneration in the temporal lobe and parietal lobe, and parts of the frontal cortex and cingulate gyrus [2].

Recently, a network diffusion model was used to characterize the propagation of dementia [3]. The transmission of disease agents like misfolded beta-amyloid and tau protein was modeled as a diffusive mechanism mediated by the *brain connectivity network* [4]. The authors effectively predicted spatially distinct "persistent modes" capturing the patterns of dementia by this model. Moreover,

G. Wu et al. (Eds.): MLMI 2014, LNCS 8679, pp. 42–49, 2014.

prevalence rates forecasted by the model strongly agree with published data. Later, it was demonstrated that network diffusion could accurately model the relationship between structural and functional brain connectivity networks [5].

In this work, we infer sources of dementia progression using a network diffusion model with *sparse impulsive stimulations*. The study of brain disease agents attributed the cause of dementia to a few seed regions in the brain [6]. We introduce sparse impulsive stimulations arriving at different time to the seed regions that drive the atrophy. Based on this, we propose a network diffusion model that simultaneously describes the propagation of dementia and the dynamics of the seed effect. In practice, we fit the amplitudes of the input impulses and the diffusion speed to the observed data. Numerical simulations demonstrated that we were able to recover the input impulses at the source nodes. Next, we evaluated the longitudinal MRI dataset in ADNI with this model. We extracted the average atrophy level at each brain region and inferred the dementia source distributions of both AD patients and MCI subjects.

Two primary differences between summarized source distributions of the AD and MCI groups were the lower contrast of the distribution and the denser sources in the temporal lobe for MCI. We found that the dementia progression was more evidently driven by a set of leading brain regions in AD than MCI. Moreover, there was a shift of dominant dementia sources from the temporal lobe and cerebellum for MCI to the central brain regions, frontal lobe and the border between parietal lobe and occipital lobe for AD, consistent with former findings in [7,8]. Since MCI subjects have high chances to develop AD, the different patterns in the source distributions of MCI and AD may indicate the evolution of the dementia progression mechanism. The results may help better understand the dynamics of the brain and design targeted treatments to dementia.

2   Inferring Dementia Sources with Diffusion Model

As in [3], we model dementia progression as a diffusion process on a brain network $\mathcal{G} = (\mathcal{V}, \mathcal{E}, W)$, where $\mathcal{V}$ and $\mathcal{E}$ are the node set and the edge set, accordingly. Node $v_i \in \mathcal{V}$ represents the i-th brain region (cortical or subcortical gray matter structure) and edge $(i, j) \in \mathcal{E}$ represents a connected region pair (v_i, v_j) by white-mater fiber pathways. W is a symmetric weight matrix with W_{ij} quantifying the connection strength between regions v_i and v_j. The amount of disease agent transmitting from an *affected* region v_i to an *unaffected* region v_j is proportional to the product of the disease factor concentration x_i and the inter-region connection strength W_{ij}. Adversely, a reverse diffusion from v_j to v_i proportional to $W_{ji}x_j$ exists. Assuming undirected pathways, the diffusion process could be captured by the first-order differential equation

$$\frac{dx_i}{dt} = -\beta \sum_j W_{ij}(x_i - x_j). \tag{1}$$

Here $\beta \geq 0$ is a constant controlling the speed of diffusion. In [5], a refined version of Eq. (1) is raised by performing the normalization $\mathcal{W} = D^{-1/2}WD^{-1/2}$, where D is the diagonal matrix with the i-th diagonal element $D_{ii} = \sum_j W_{ij}$.

Suppose the disease factors at time t in the network are represented by the vector $\mathbf{x}(t) = \{x(v,t), v \in \mathcal{V}\}$ for all the nodes, then the diffusion process can be rewritten as the following "*network heat equation*"

$$\frac{d\mathbf{x}(t)}{dt} = -\beta \mathcal{L} \mathbf{x}(t), \tag{2}$$

where $\mathcal{L} \triangleq I - \mathcal{W}$ is the (normalized) graph Laplacian matrix. Eq. (2) has an explicit solution $\mathbf{x}(t) = \exp(-\beta \mathcal{L} t) \mathbf{x}(0)$. Throughout this paper, we consider continuous systems while t could also be restricted to discrete values.

We model the sources of dementia by a series of impulsive stimulations expressed by $\mathbf{s}(t) = \sum_{t_{ij} \leq t} c_{ij} \delta(t - t_{ij}) \mathbf{e}_i$, where c_{ij} is the amplitude of the impulse at node i at the j-th time step t_{ij}. Note that $\delta(\cdot)$ is the dirac delta function; $\mathbf{e}_i$ is a standard basis in $\mathbb{R}^{|\mathcal{V}|}$ with the i-th element being nonzero. By adding the input, we update Eq. (2) to $\frac{d\mathbf{x}(t)}{dt} = -\beta \mathcal{L} \mathbf{x}(t) + \mathbf{s}(t)$, with the solution

$$\mathbf{x}(t) = e^{-\beta \mathcal{L} t} \mathbf{x}(0) + \sum_{t_{ij} \leq t} c_{ij} e^{-\beta \mathcal{L}(t - t_{ij})} \mathbf{e}_i. \tag{3}$$

In reality, the dynamics in Eq. (3) might not be followed exactly due to the unavoidable modeling error. Hence, usually $\boldsymbol{\theta}$ could not be directly solved from Eq. (3). It motivates us to fit the observed data $\mathbf{y}(t)$ to the diffusive model by

$$\min_{\boldsymbol{\theta}} \left\| \mathbf{y}(t) - e^{-\beta \mathcal{L} t} \mathbf{y}(0) - \sum_{t_{ij} \leq t} c_{ij} e^{-\beta \mathcal{L}(t - t_{ij})} \mathbf{e}_i \right\|_2^2, \tag{4}$$

where the indicators of the unknown parameters take values $i = 1, \cdots, N$ and $j = 1, \cdots, K$. There are $2NK + 1$ parameters to be fitted in above formula compared with the dimension N of the observed data, which may make the gradient descent methods to search the optimal solution unstable.

To solve the inverse problem more robustly, we simplify the model of the input disease factor by restricting the arrival time on integer time steps $1, 2, \cdots, K = \lfloor t \rfloor$, meaning that $t_{ik} = k$ for any node i and integer $k \in \{1, \cdots, K\}$. This is reasonable, since in practice often we only want to determine the sources up to a certain time resolution. Let $\widetilde{\mathbf{y}}_\beta(t) = \mathbf{y}(t) - e^{-\beta \mathcal{L} t} \mathbf{y}(0)$ and $\mathbf{h}_{ij}(\beta) = e^{-\beta \mathcal{L}(t - t_{ij})} \mathbf{e}_i$, then the minimization in Eq. (4) could be replaced by

$$\min_{\beta, c_{ij}} \left\| \widetilde{\mathbf{y}}_\beta(t) - \sum_{i=1}^{N} \sum_{j=1}^{K} c_{ij} \mathbf{h}_{ij}(\beta) \right\|_2^2. \tag{5}$$

The above procedure can be treated as a linear regression parameterized by β. To obtain a unique solution, we enforce the l_1-sparsity constraint:

$$\min_{\beta, c_{ij}} \left\| \widetilde{\mathbf{y}}_\beta(t) - H(\beta) \mathbf{c} \right\|_2^2 + \alpha |\mathbf{c}|_1, \tag{6}$$

where $H = (\boldsymbol{h}_{1,1}, \boldsymbol{h}_{1,2}, \cdots, \boldsymbol{h}_{N,K})$ is a $N \times NK$ matrix and $\mathbf{c} = (c_{1,1}, c_{1,2}, \cdots, c_{N,K})^T$ is a column vector storing all the amplitudes of the impulses; α is a spareness control parameter. If β is known, then the optimization can be effectively solved by the coordinate descent learning or the active-set algorithm [9]. When β is unknown, the overall estimation task becomes hard. We propose a two-stage algorithm with an initial stage and a refined stage. For the inference problem in Eq. (6), we first adopt the following iterative algorithm:

Algorithm 1. Solving the Parameterized Lasso Problem

---

1. Given $0 < \varepsilon_1, \varepsilon_2, < 1$. Initialize any feasible $\beta^{(1)}, \{c_{ij}^{(1)}\}$.
2. For $k = 1, 2, \cdots$
   2.1 Find a descent direction d in Eq. (6) given $\beta = \beta^{(k)}$ using algorithms in [9].
   2.2 Update $\{c_{ij}^{(k+1)}\} = \{c_{ij}^{(k)}\} - \varepsilon_1 d$.
   2.2 Update $\beta^{(k+1)} = \beta^{(k)} - \varepsilon_2 f^T g$, with
   $$f = \widetilde{y}_{\beta^{(k)}}(t) - H(\beta^{(k)}) c^{(k+1)},$$
   $$g = e^{-\beta^{(k)} \mathcal{L}t} \mathcal{L}t x(0) + \sum_{i,j} c_{ij}^{(k+1)} (t - t_{ij}) \mathcal{L} h_{ij}(\beta^k).$$

Each time when applying the above algorithm, we obtain an estimate of the impulsive inputs since the last observation and β. In the end, there will be several estimates of β, namely $\widehat{\beta}_1, \cdots, \widehat{\beta}_K$. We average them to get a refined version $\widehat{\beta} = \frac{1}{K} \sum_{i=1}^{K} \widehat{\beta}_i$. Next, we treat $\beta = \widehat{\beta}$ in Eq. (6) and solve the problem. 5-fold cross-validation is performed for tuning the regularization parameter α at both the initial stage and refined stage.

3   Numerical Simulations

We evaluated the inference algorithm by simulations on a random geometric network. We arbitrarily spread 100 nodes in a unit square area and drew edges between node pairs when their Euclidean distances were less than 0.2 (see Fig. 1). Unit weight was assigned to each edge. Then, we imported 4 impulsive stimulations $c_{10,0} = 1, c_{40,0} = 0.6, c_{51,9} = 0.2, c_{40,19} = 0.1$ with c_{ij} signifying the input at node i at the j-th time step. Observations with Gaussian noise were made at three time steps $t = 6, 12, 24$, where the standard deviation of the noise was 10^{-3}. In Fig. 1, we visualized the observations on the network with heat maps.

In the first row of Fig. 2, the input impulses were displayed during time periods: $t = [0, 6], [6, 12], [12, 24]$, respectively. In each period, we plotted out c_{ij} in the order of $c_{1,1}, \cdots, c_{1,K}, \cdots, c_{N,K}$. We first ran Algorithm 1 and obtained the estimation results in the second row of Fig. 2. It appeared that the locations of the sources were correctly detected. However, the amplitudes and arrival times of the impulses were not well estimated. For instance, during $t = 6 \sim 12$, the recovered impulse had an index 651, meaning that the estimated arrival time was $t = 12$ at node 51. Meanwhile, we knew that the true arrival time was $t = 9$ at node 51. The impulse locations during other two time periods were correctly detected too. Then, we applied the refinement step to get a better estimate of β. The improved results were shown in the third row of the plot, from which we observed that although a true impulse seemed to be split into bunches of multiple recovered impulses, the cumulative value and arrival time were better preserved. For example, in Fig. 2(b), the summation of the amplitudes at node 51 was 0.2103, close to the true amplitude 0.2; in Fig. 2(c), the aggregated amplitudes at node 40 was 0.1079, which was near the truth 0.1 as well.

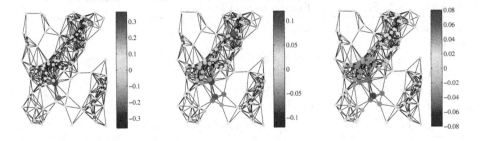

Fig. 1. From left to right are the observations of a diffusion process on a 100-node random geometric network at time $t = 6, 12, 24$. Edges built across nearby nodes have unit weights. The sizes and colors both indicate the scales of the noisy measurements.

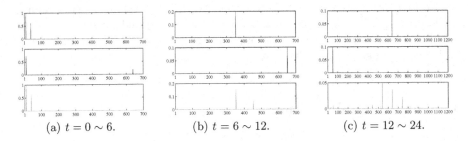

(a) $t = 0 \sim 6$.   **(b)** $t = 6 \sim 12$.   **(c)** $t = 12 \sim 24$.

Fig. 2. Inference results on the simulated data. From above to bottom, the rows correspond to the truth, direct estimate, refined estimate of the impulsive amplitudes c_{ij}; from left to right, the columns illustrate the results based on the observations at $t = 6, 12, 24$, respectively. The x-axes and y-axes denote t_{ij} and the amplitude.

4   Evaluation on ADNI Data

We employed our diffusion source inference method and the tensor-based morphometry (TBM) [10] to analyze the Alzheimer's Disease Neuroimaging Initiative (ADNI-1) dataset. The full ADNI-1 dataset contained sequential brain MRI scans from 188 AD patients, 400 individuals with MCI, and 229 healthy elderly controls. Subjects were scanned at screening and followed up at 6, 12, 18 (MCI only), 24, and 36 months (MCI and normal only). To adjust for linear shifts in head position, the follow-up scan was linearly registered to its matching screening scan via 9-parameter (9P) registration. By warping the 9P-registered follow-up scans to match the corresponding screening scan, individual Jacobian maps were produced to estimate 3D patterns of structural brain change over time. The Jacobian determinants illustrate regions of ventricular/CSF expansion (*i.e.*, with $\det J(r) > 1$), or brain tissue loss/atrophy (*i.e.*, with $\det J(r) < 1$) over time.

We first constructed the brain connectivity network and extracted the brain atrophy measurements from the Jacobian deformation maps. The Jacobian maps in the 6, 12, 24 month were registered to the 116 region automated anatomic labeling (AAL) atlas. In parallel, we built a 116-node weighted brain network by

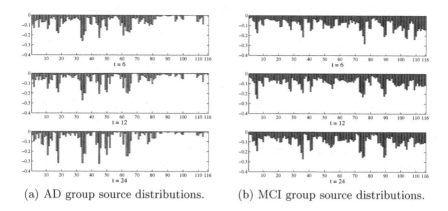

(a) AD group source distributions.   (b) MCI group source distributions.

Fig. 3. Average source distributions recovered at three time steps (t = 6, 12, 24 months). Horizontal axes of the subplots denote the ROI index of the AAL template; vertical axes of the charts signify the normalized cumulative atrophy imported to a certain brain region since last observation averaged over population.

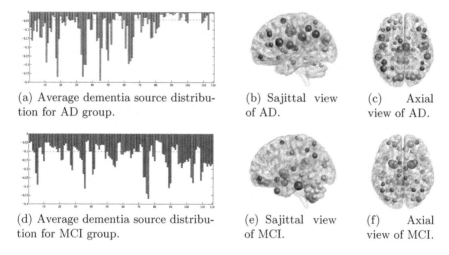

(a) Average dementia source distribution for AD group.

(b) Sajittal view of AD.

(c)   Axial view of AD.

(d) Average dementia source distribution for MCI group.

(e) Sajittal view of MCI.

(f)   Axial view of MCI.

Fig. 4. Estimated total dementia source distributions averaged over the two groups. Dotted lines in (a) and (d) delineate the thresholds above which there are 60 brain regions. (b-c) and (e-f) show the sagittal and axial views of these ROIs with significant atrophy, where sizes of the color-balls are proportional to the atrophy levels.

treating each region of interest (ROI) as a node and assigning weight between brain region i and j according to $W_{ij} = \frac{1}{d(i,j)}$, if $d(i,j) < 40$; $W_{ij} = 0$ otherwise, where d_{ij} is the Euclidean distance between the i-th and j-th ROI centers. From [11], we knew that this simple construction approximates the functional and anatomical brain network topologies very well. Next, averaged brain deformation level within every ROI was calculated. The original deformation maps were downsampled to 116 dimensional vectors with postive/negative numbers signify expansion/shrinkage of the regions. We set positive average deformation values to zero, since we only wanted to consider the brain atrophy. The truncated data were regarded as the observations of the dementia progression over the brain connectivity network, namely $y(t)$ in Eq. (4).

We ran our diffusion source inference algorithm for the AD and MCI groups by keeping the regularization factor α in Eq. (6) the same. From cross-validations, we found that $\alpha \in [10^{-4}, 10^{-5}]$ was favorable. Here we choose $\alpha = 10^{-4}$. At $t = 6$ month, we replaced $y(0) = 0$ and $t = 6$ in Eq. (4). Arrival times and locations of the impulsive stimulations of dementia were estimated via solving this optimization for every individual. The resulted amplitude sequence c_{ij} for $i = 1, \cdots, N$ and $j = 1, \cdots, K$, were folded up and summed over each ROI to give the cumulative atrophy input $\widetilde{c}_i$ at the i-th region: $\widetilde{c}_i = \sum_{j=1}^{K} c_{ij}$. Thus, $\widetilde{c} = (\widetilde{c}_1, \cdots, \widetilde{c}_N)$ describes the dementia source distribution of the subject. To obtain a meaningful summary of the atrophy sources across the group, we normalized $\widetilde{c}$ such that the maximum absolute value of its elements was one. The normalized source distributions for both groups were displayed in the first row of Fig. 3. Next, we inferred the sources coming into play during the time intervals $t \in [6, 12]$ and $t \in [12, 24]$ by treating $y(6)$ and $y(12)$ as initial conditions. Those results were in the second and third rows of Fig. 3. We observed that the envelopes of the source distributions obtained at different time for a certain group were close to each other, which might signify that the dementia was due to stimulations at a constant set of regions.

To obtain an atrophy source map for every group, we further added up the source distributions $\widetilde{c}$ estimated at the three time steps. The total dementia source distributions were presented on the left panels of Fig. 4. Two main differences between the AD and MCI groups were the lower contrast of the distribution as well as the denser sources in the temporal lobe for MCI. To quantify the contrast of the source distributions, we calculated the ratio ρ between the sum of top 60 leading source regions and that of the rest regions. It turned out that $\rho_{AD} = 8.97$ compared with $\rho_{MCI} = 2.70$, meaning that the dementia progression was more evidently driven by a set of leading brain regions in AD than MCI. We also examined the difference of the distributions over brain lobes. Using BrainNet Viewer [12], we displayed the center locations of the 60 major dementia sources inside the 3D brain mesh in Fig. 4. We observed that the dominant dementia sources overlap with the hubs of the functional brain network [12], namely the bilateral Rolandic operculum, bilateral superior temporal gyrus, right supplementary motor area, right temporal pole, and right supramarginal gyrus, which were primarily located at the association and subcortical regions. On the whole, there was a shift of dominant dementia sources from the temporal lobe and cerebellum for MCI to the central brain regions, frontal lobe and the border between parietal lobe and occipital lobe for AD. This phenomenon is consistent with former findings in [7,8]. Since MCI subjects have high chances to develop AD, the different patterns in the source distributions of MCI and AD may indicate the evolution of the dementia progression mechanism.

5   Conclusion

We presented a diffusive model on network to trace back the sources of a diffusion process. Numerical simulations demonstrated that it was possible to estimate the locations of the sources and arrival times of the input impulses. Possible origins of Alzheimer's disease were found by using the longitudinal MRI dataset provided by ADNI. The average distributions of the dementia sources had different concentrations in the brain lobes for AD patients and MCI subjects, indicating possible transformation of the dementia driving mechanism. Our method enables the quantitative assessment of the dementia causes, which may help discover better targeted treatments of the disease.

References

1. Goedert, M., Clavaguera, F., Tolnay, M.: The propagation of prion-like protein inclusions in neurodegenerative diseases. Trends in Neurosciences 33(7), 317–325 (2010)
2. Wenk, G.L.: Neuropathologic changes in Alzheimers disease. J. Clin. Psychiatry 64(suppl. 9), 7–10 (2003)
3. Raj, A., Kuceyeski, A., Weiner, M.: A network diffusion model of disease progression in dementia. Neuron 73(6), 1204–1215 (2012)
4. Bassett, D.S., Bullmore, E.T.: Human brain networks in health and disease. Current Opinion in Neurology 22(4), 340 (2009)
5. Abdelnour, F., Voss, H.U., Raj, A.: Network diffusion accurately models the relationship between structural and functional brain connectivity networks. Neuroimage (in press)
6. Jucker, M., Walker, L.C.: Self-propagation of pathogenic protein aggregates in neurodegenerative diseases. Nature 501(7465), 45–51 (2013)
7. Thompson, P.M., Hayashi, K.M., Zubicaray, G.D., Janke, A.L., Rose, S.E., Semple, J.: Dynamics of gray matter loss in Alzheimer's disease. The Journal of Neuroscience 23(3), 994–1005 (2003)
8. Sabuncu, M.R., Desikan, R.S., Sepulcre, J., Yeo, B.T.T., Liu, H., Schmansky, N.J.: The dynamics of cortical and hippocampal atrophy in Alzheimer disease. Archives of Neurology 68(8), 1040–1048 (2011)
9. Schmidt, M., Fung, G., Rosales, R.: Fast optimization methods for L1 regularization: A comparative study and two new approaches. In: Kok, J.N., Koronacki, J., Lopez de Mantaras, R., Matwin, S., Mladenič, D., Skowron, A. (eds.) ECML 2007. LNCS (LNAI), vol. 4701, pp. 286–297. Springer, Heidelberg (2007)
10. Hua, X., Lee, S., Yanovsky, I., Leow, A., Chou, Y., Ho, A.: Optimizing power to track brain degeneration in Alzheimer's disease and mild cognitive impairment with tensor-based morphometry: an ADNI study of 515 subjects. NeuroImage 48, 668–681 (2009)
11. Alexander-Bloch, A.F., Vértes, P.E., Stidd, R., Lalonde, F., Clasen, L., Rapoport, J.: The anatomical distance of functional connections predicts brain network topology in health and schizophrenia. Cereb. Cortex 23(1), 127–138 (2013)
12. Xia, M., Wang, J., He, Y.: BrainNet Viewer: a network visualization tool for human brain connectomics. PLoS One 8(7), e68910 (2013)

3D Intervertebral Disc Localization and Segmentation from MR Images by Data-Driven Regression and Classification

Cheng Chen[1], D. Belavy[2], and Guoyan Zheng[1]

[1] Institute for Surgical Technology and Biomechanics,
University of Bern, Switzerland
{cheng.chen,guoyan.zheng}@istb.unibe.ch
[2] Department of Radiology, Charite University Medicine Berlin, Germany

Abstract. In this paper we propose a new fully-automatic method for localizing and segmenting 3D intervertebral discs from MR images, where the two problems are solved in a unified data-driven regression and classification framework. We estimate the output (image displacements for localization, or fg/bg labels for segmentation) of image points by exploiting both training data and geometric constraints simultaneously. The problem is formulated in a unified objective function which is then solved globally and efficiently. We validate our method on MR images of 25 patients. Taking manually labeled data as the ground truth, our method achieves a mean localization error of 1.3 mm, a mean Dice metric of 87%, and a mean surface distance of 1.3 mm. Our method can be applied to other localization and segmentation tasks.

1 Introduction

In clinical practice, accurate identifying of intervertebral discs (IVD) is very important for diagnosis and operation planning of spine pathologies. In this paper we propose a fully automatic method to localize and segment 3D IVDs from MR image with a unified regression and classification framework.

In literature, different methods have been proposed for IVD localization [1,2] and segmentation [5,6,7,8,9]. In [1], the IVDs were localized and labeled by a probabilistic model considering image intensity and geometric constraints. Corso et al. [2] enforced the inter-disc distance constraint to improve the label accuracy. Glocker et al. applied the Random Forest regression [3] and classification [4] methods, although their localization target is the vertebrae instead of IVD.

For IVD segmentation, existing methods are based on watershed algorithm [5], atlas registration [6], graph cuts with geometric priors from neighboring discs [7], template matching and statistic shape model [8], or anisotropic oriented flux detection [9]. All of these methods except [8] work only on 2D sagittal images.

Recently, a new data-driven optimization method [10] was proposed for landmark localization. Inspired by this, in this paper we make four contributions. (1): We extend the method into segmentation domain, where we estimate the

G. Wu et al. (Eds.): MLMI 2014, LNCS 8679, pp. 50–58, 2014.
© Springer International Publishing Switzerland 2014

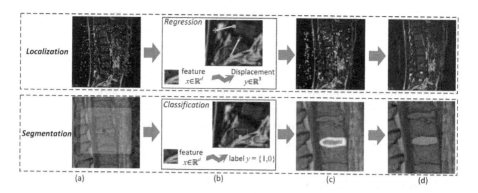

Fig. 1. Pipeline overview our method. Top: localization. Bottom: segmentation.

foreground/background label of image points instead of displacements. (2): We introduce a new constraint for segmentation which ensures the neighborhood smoothness. (3): We unify our localization and segmentation solutions into one unified framework, where we estimate output values (displacements or labels) on image locations. (4): We verified our method on MR images.

2 Data-Driven Regression/Classification Method

2.1 Overview

The localization and segmentation problems are formulated as in Fig. 1. Given an image, we consider a set of points (Fig. 1(a)): for localization task these are some randomly sampled points (green dots), and for segmentation these are all voxels inside a region of interest (yellow box). Each of these points can be represented by its visual feature calculated in a small image neighborhood (the green dash box in Fig. 1(b)). Then, we want to estimate the output values for each point. In the case of localization, the output is the displacement vector from the point to the target position (e.g. disc center), which makes it a *regression* problem. Each point makes a vote relative to itself (Fig. 1(c)) and a score map can be estimated by aggregating these votes (Fig. 1(d)). For segmentation, we estimate the fg/bg label of each voxel (Fig. 1(c)), which is a soft *classification* problem. The binary segmentation is then derived from the soft labels (Fig. 1(d)).

Notations. Suppose that N points are sampled on the training images, and let $\{x_i\}_{i=1...N}$ denote the features calcuated at these points, where $x_i \in \mathbb{R}^d$. We denote $X = [x_1...x_N] \in \mathbb{R}^{N \times d}$. We use $\{y\}_{i=1...N}$ to denote the output value of the training points, i.e. $y_i \in \mathbb{R}^3$ for localization, and $y_i \in \{0,1\}$ for segmentation. The training images are annotated, so that the ground-truth output values of training points are known as $\{y_i^{GT}\}_{i=1...N}$, and we denote $Y^{GT} = [y_1^{GT}...y_N^{GT}]$.

Given a new image, we randomly sample N' points at locations $\{c'\}_{i=1...N'}$, whose features are $\{x'\}_{i=1...N'}$. We denote $X' = [x'_1...x'_{N'}]$. The task is to compute the output values for these points $\{y'\}_{i=1...N'}$. We write $Y' = [y'_1...y'_{N'}]$.

We solve for Y' by optimizing an objective function as below. Please refer to the supplementary material for a complete mathematical treatment.

2.2   Objective Function

First, we construct a matrix $\tilde{Y} = [Y, Y']$ which is the composition of training and test outputs. Although we want to compute Y', our objective function is defined on $\tilde{Y}$. In this way we can encode the relations between training and test data in a uniform way. After solving for the optimal $\tilde{Y}$, we simply take its right part as $Y' = \tilde{Y}Q$, where Q is a $\begin{pmatrix} \mathbf{0} & \mathbf{1} \end{pmatrix}^T$ matrix selecting the right part.

1. Ground-truth Consistence E_g. The output of the training points, which is the left part of $\tilde{Y}$, should be consistent with the ground-truth. With a (0,1) matrix P selecting the left part of $\tilde{Y}$, we define the penalty of violation as:

$$E_g(\tilde{Y}) = \frac{1}{N}\|Y - Y^{GT}\|_F^2 = \frac{1}{N}\|\tilde{Y}P - Y^{GT}\|_F^2 \tag{1}$$

2. Feature Proximity Consistence E_f. The ith column of $\tilde{Y}$, $\mathrm{col}_i(\tilde{Y})$, encodes the output of the ith point (either a training or a test point). We construct a binary similarity matrix $S \in \{0,1\}^{(N+N')\times(N+N')}$, where $S_{ij} = 1$ iff the ith and jth points are mutually k nearest neighbors *in the feature space*. A natural assumption is that points with similar features should have similar outputs:

$$E_f(\tilde{Y}) = \frac{1}{\sum_{i \neq j} S_{ij}} \sum_{i \neq j} S_{ij}\|\mathrm{col}_i(\tilde{Y}) - \mathrm{col}_j(\tilde{Y})\|_F^2 \tag{2}$$

For each pair of points (i, j), E_f introduces a high penalty if they are similar in the feature space (i.e. $S_{ij} = 1$) but the output are very different (i.e. $\|\mathrm{col}_i(\tilde{Y}) - \mathrm{col}_j(\tilde{Y})\|$ is big). Denoting L_S as the Laplacian matrix of S, we can write:

$$E_f(\tilde{Y}) = \mathrm{Tr}\left(\tilde{Y}L_S\tilde{Y}^\top\right) \tag{3}$$

3. Point Subtractive Constraint E_s. In the case of localization, y_i' and y_j' are displacements from two test points c_i' and c_j' to the (unknown) target location. From triangle geometry we have $y_i' - y_j' = c_j' - c_i'$. Therefore, we want to minimize:

$$E_s^{i,j}(Y') = \|(y_i' - y_j') - (c_j' - c_i')\|_2^2 = \|Y'u_{i,j} - \Delta c_{j,i}\|_F^2 \tag{4}$$

where $u_{i,j}$ is a N' dimensional vector whose ith element is 1, jth element is -1, and all others are 0s, and $\Delta c_{j,i} = c_j' - c_i'$. Adding these constraints together:

$$E_s(\tilde{Y}) = \frac{1}{N'(N'-1)} \sum_{i \neq j} E_s^{i,j}(Y') = \frac{1}{N'(N'-1)}\|\tilde{Y}QU - \Delta C\|_F^2 \tag{5}$$

where $U = [..., u_{i,j}, ...]$ and $\Delta C = [..., \Delta c_{j,i}, ...]$ are matrices of column vectors.

4. Point Neighborhood Constraint E_n. In the case of segmentation, y_i' is the label of the ith point. A natural assumption is that the segmentation should be smooth, i.e. neighboring points should have similar labels. Therefore, if we define a neighboring system $\mathcal{N}$, we would want to minimize:

$$E_n(\tilde{Y}) = \frac{1}{|\mathcal{N}|} \sum_{(i,j)\in\mathcal{N}} \|y_i' - y_j'\|_F^2 \tag{6}$$

If we define A as the neighbor affinity matrix, where $A_{i,j} = 1$ iff only $(i,j) \in \mathcal{N}$, and we denote L_A as the Laplacian matrix of A, we can write E_n as:

$$E_n(\tilde{Y}) = \mathrm{Tr}\left(Y'L_A(Y')^\top\right) = \mathrm{Tr}\left(\tilde{Y}QL_AQ^\top\tilde{Y}^\top\right) \tag{7}$$

The Objective Function. Our objective function consists of the above terms:

$$E(\tilde{Y}) = E_g(\tilde{Y}) + \alpha E_f(\tilde{Y}) + \beta E_s(\tilde{Y}) + \gamma E_n(\tilde{Y}) \tag{8}$$

where the terms are defined in Eqs. (1), (3), (5) and (7), with their respective importance controlled by parameters α, β and γ. Note that E_s is defined only for localization ($\gamma = 0$), and E_n is only defined for segmentation ($\beta = 0$).

Optimization. Without loss of generality, we relax the binary requirement of labels in the segmentation case, and let labels y to be continuous. It is not difficult to prove that Eq. (8) is convex, with gradient given by:

$$\begin{aligned}
\frac{\partial E(\tilde{Y})}{\partial \tilde{Y}} &= \tilde{Y}\left(\frac{1}{N}PP^\top + \alpha L_S + \beta\frac{1}{N'(N'-1)}QUU^\top Q^\top + \gamma QL_AQ^\top\right) \\
&- \frac{1}{N}Y^{GT}P^\top - \frac{\beta}{N'(N'-1)}\Delta CU^\top Q^\top
\end{aligned} \tag{9}$$

For the globally optimal $\tilde{Y}$, we can either solve the equation $\frac{\partial E(\tilde{Y})}{\partial \tilde{Y}} = 0$ in closed form, or use gradient descent from the initialization given by k-nn search.

Discussion. E_g ensures the consistency with the ground-truth data. E_f propagates outputs from training data to test data based on feature proximity. The key contribution is that in E_s and E_n we exploit different pairwise geometric constraints to regularize the output values being estimated, which are not exploited in other methods, such as [3]. These MRF-like neighboring constraints are encoded compactly in our objective function which can be solved globally.

3 Application to IVD Localization and Segmentation

We applied our method to IVD, where we first localize the disc centers, and then segment the discs. Without loss of generality, we consider 7 discs T11-L5 and number them reversely from 1 (L5) to 7 (T11). Note that for both localization and segmentation, the training and prediction are done separately for each IVD, which means that the presence of other IVDs outside T11-L5 will not affect our method as those IVDs will not generate significant response.

Localization of disc centers

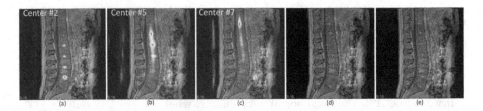

Fig. 2. The first step of localization. (a)-(c): Score images of three disc centers 2, 5 and 7. (d): The mode of each score image. (e): After HMM optimization. For (d) and (e), the red crosses are ground-truth center locations and the greens are detected centers.

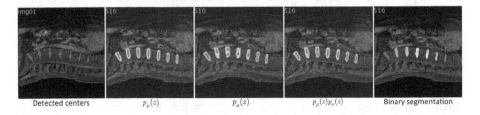

Fig. 3. The segmentation process after the disc centers are detected

For each disc center, the method in Section 2 will sample a set of points over the image and produce a set of votes. We aggregate these discrete votes to produce a continuous soft score map by considering each vote as a small Gaussian distribution [10]. Therefore, for each image, 7 score maps are produced.

We detect the disc centers in a two-step coarse-to-fine way. In the first step, points are sampled over the entire image to search for the disc centers, as in Fig. 2. Due to the repetitive pattern, the produced score maps are multimodal with potential ambiguities. For example, in Fig. 2(d) the center 5 is confused with center 6 if we simply take mode of its score map. To improve the robustness, the score maps are treated as observation probabilities and are fed to an HMM model encoding the prior geometric information of neighboring disc centers as in [3]. In the second step, we fine-tune the center locations by sampling points only in a local region around the centers initialized from the first step.

Segmentation of Discs

The segmentation of a disc is performed after its center is detected at location $z_0 = (u_0, v_0, w_0)$. The process is shown in Fig. 3. To save space, we superimpose the visualization of the 7 discs on a single image, but the segmentation is conducted separately for each disc. For each pixel location $z = (u, v, w)$, we compute two probabilities of it being the foreground of a disc: $p_p(z)$, the prior probability, and $p_o(z)$, the observation probability. $p_p(z)$ is the probability of being the foreground given the offset from the disc center $z - z_0$, which is estimated using the parzen window method from the annotated training data. On the other hand, $p_o(z)$ is calculated by the data-driven estimation method in Section 2. Since $p_p(z)$ is much cheaper to calculate and serve as a good pre-filter

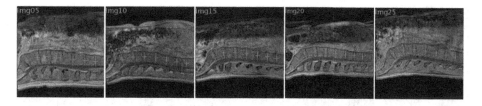

Fig. 4. The qualitative localization result on some images (the 18th sagittal slice)

Table 1. Quantitative evaluation of disc center localization

	Median	Mean	Std.	Min.	Max.
Ours	1.3	1.3	0.6	0.2	3.0
Random Forest [3]	1.6	2.7	6.2	0.3	40.6

of the potential foreground pixels, we first calculate $p_p(z)$ over all pixels around the disc center, and then we only consider voxels where $p_p(z)$ is not zero, on which $p_o(z)$ is then calculated. The final probability of each pixel is then given by $p(z) = p_p(z)p_o(z)$. The final binary segmentation is derived by thresholding the probability map and only keeping the largest connected component.

4   Experiments

Data
We validate our method on MR images of 25 patients. Each patient was scanned with 1.5 Tesla MRI scanner of Siemens. Dixon protocol was used to reconstruct four aligned high-resolution 3D volumes during one data acquisition: in-phase, opposed-phase, fat and water images. We manually annotated the intervertebral discs in water images of all subjects, resulting in 175 discs in total. The ground-truth disc centers are defined as disc centroids. The study is conducted in a leave-one-out manner. In each round data of 1 subject is chosen for testing and data of the remaining 24 subjects are used for training purpose.

Implementation Details
We use the neighborhood intensity vector as the visual feature of sampled image points. Specifically, we draw a cube (of edge size 3cm for localization and 1cm for segmentation) centered on the point. The cube is then evenly divided into $4 \times 4 \times 4$ blocks, and the mean intensities in each block are concatenated to form a 64 dimensional feature. As our data contains 4 channels, we concatenate the vector from all channels to form a 256 dimensional final feature vector. For parameter selection, we fix $\alpha = 0.01, \beta = 0.001, \gamma = 0$ for localization, and $\alpha = 0.01, \beta = 0, \gamma = 0.01$ for segmentation. Our unoptimized Matlab implementation requires on average 3.5 minutes to finish both localization and segmentation of one subject. Please note that all our operations are done in 3D space. However, to ease visualization, the figures in the following sections are presented in 2D sagittal slices.

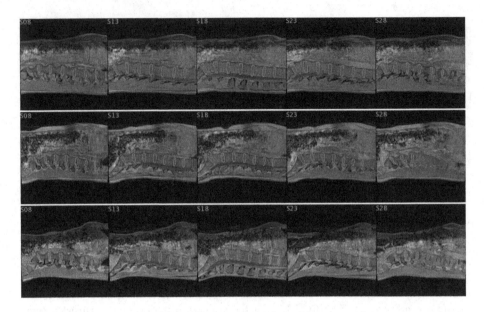

Fig. 5. Segmentation result on three images. We visualize the result on the 8th, 13th, 18th, 23th, 28th sagittal slices. Red: ground-truth contour. Green: our results.

Localization Result

Fig. 4 shows some qualitative results of disc center localization (only the 18th sagittal slice is shown), where the red crosses are ground-truth and the green ones are the detected centers. We also conducted quantitative evaluation as in Table 1, where the evaluation metric is the Euclidean distance from the detected disc centers to the ground-truth. We get a mean localization error of 1.3mm. We also compare our results with the Random Forest based method [3]. To make the comparison fair, we use the same parameters (e.g. the same features...) and the same HMM optimization process for both methods. From the result we can see that we do get better results.

Segmentation Result

We show our qualitative segmentation result on randomly selected three images in Fig. 5. We visualize the results by superimposing the contours of ground-truth discs and those of our results on five sagittal slices (slices 8,13,18,23 and 28). The red contours are ground-truth and the green ones are our results.

For quantitative evaluation, we employ two metrics: the Dice metric which measures the percentage of correctly identified pixels, and the average physical distance from the ground-truth disc surface and the segmented surface. The results are summarized in Table 2. We achieve a mean Dice of 87% and a mean SurfDist of 1.3mm. We note that Neubert et al. [8] reported a mean Dice of 76%-80% in their 3D IVD segmentation paper on a different dataset.

Table 2. Quantitative evaluation of disc segmentation. The unit of SurfDist is mm.

	Median	Mean	Std.	Min.	Max.
Dice (3D)	87%	87%	3%	76%	92%
SurfDist (3D)	1.3	1.3	0.2	1.0	2.4
Dice (sagittal)	91%	90%	4%	72%	96%
SurfDist (sagittal)	0.7	0.7	0.3	0.3	1.6

Since most existing methods work only on 2D sagittal slices, for comparison we also calculate the 2D versions of the metrics by using only the 18th slice (in most cases it is the centered sagittal slice), where we achieve a mean Dice of 90% and SurfDist of 0.7mm. We note that in [7] they reported a mean Dice of 88% in the case of 2D IVD segmentation on a different dataset.

5 Conclusions

We have proposed a unified framework for localization and segmentation tasks of medical images. We estimate outputs (displacements or labels) on image points by considering both training data and geometric constraints. Applied to the intervertebral disc case on MR data, our method achieves good results. Our method can be generally applied to other localization and segmentation tasks, and in the future, we plan to conduct more studies on different types of images.

References

1. Schmidt, S., Kappes, J.H., Bergtholdt, M., Pekar, V., Dries, S.P.M., Bystrov, D., Schnörr, C.: Spine detection and labeling using a parts-based graphical model. In: Karssemeijer, N., Lelieveldt, B. (eds.) IPMI 2007. LNCS, vol. 4584, pp. 122–133. Springer, Heidelberg (2007)
2. Corso, J.J., Alomari, R.S., Chaudhary, V.: Lumbar disc localization and labeling with a probabilistic model on both pixel and object features. In: Metaxas, D., Axel, L., Fichtinger, G., Székely, G. (eds.) MICCAI 2008, Part I. LNCS, vol. 5241, pp. 202–210. Springer, Heidelberg (2008)
3. Glocker, B., Feulner, J., Criminisi, A., Haynor, D.R., Konukoglu, E.: Automatic localization and identification of vertebrae in arbitrary field-of-view CT scans. In: Ayache, N., Delingette, H., Golland, P., Mori, K. (eds.) MICCAI 2012, Part III. LNCS, vol. 7512, pp. 590–598. Springer, Heidelberg (2012)
4. Glocker, B., Zikic, D., Konukoglu, E., Haynor, D.R., Criminisi, A.: Vertebrae localization in pathological spine CT via dense classification from sparse annotations. In: Mori, K., Sakuma, I., Sato, Y., Barillot, C., Navab, N. (eds.) MICCAI 2013, Part II. LNCS, vol. 8150, pp. 262–270. Springer, Heidelberg (2013)
5. Chevrefils, C., Cheriet, F., Aubin, C.E., Grimard, G.: Texture analysis for automatic segmentation of intervertebral disks of scoliotic spines from mr images. IEEE Trans. on Information Technology in Biomedicine 13, 608–620 (2009)

6. Michopoulou, S.K., Costaridou, L., Panagiotopoulos, E., Speller, R., Panayiotakis, G., Todd-Pokropek, A.: Atalas-based segmentation of degenerated lumbar intervertebral discs from mr images of the spine. IEEE Trans. on Biomedical Engineering 56(9), 2225–2231 (2009)
7. Ben Ayed, I., Punithakumar, K., Garvin, G., Romano, W., Li, S.: Graph cuts with invariant object-interaction priors: Application to intervertebral disc segmentation. In: Székely, G., Hahn, H.K. (eds.) IPMI 2011. LNCS, vol. 6801, pp. 221–232. Springer, Heidelberg (2011)
8. Neubert, A., Fripp, J., Shen, K., Salvado, O., Schwarz, R., Lauer, L., Engstrom, C., Crozier, S.: Automatic 3D segmentation of vertebral bodies and intervertebral discs from mri. In: International Conference on Ditial Imaging Computing: Techniques and Applications (2011)
9. Law, M.W.K., Tay, K., Leung, A., Garvin, G.J., Li, S.: Intervertebral disc segmentation in mr images using anisotropic oriented flux. Medical Image Analysis 17, 43–61 (2013)
10. Chen, C., Xie, W., Franke, J., Grutzner, P.A., Nolte, L.-P., Zheng, G.: Automatic x-ray landmark detection and shape segmentation via data-driven joint estimation of image displacements. Medical Image Analysis 18, 487–499 (2014)

Exploring Compact Representation of SICE Matrices for Functional Brain Network Classification

Jianjia Zhang, Luping Zhou, Lei Wang, and Wanqing Li

University of Wollongong, Wollongong, 2522, Australia
jz163@uowmail.edu.au, {lupingz,leiw,wanqing}@uow.edu.au

Abstract. Recently, sparse inverse covariance matrix (SICE matrix) has been used as a representation of brain connectivity to classify Alzheimer's disease and normal controls. However, its high dimensionality can adversely affect the classification performance. Considering the underlying manifold where SICE matrices reside and the common patterns shared by brain connectivity across subjects, we propose to explore the lower dimensional intrinsic components of SICE matrix for compact representation. This leads to significant improvements of brain connectivity classification. Moreover, to cater for the requirement of both discrimination and interpretation in neuroimage analysis, we develop a novel pre-image estimation algorithm to make the obtained connectivity components anatomically interpretable. The advantages of our method have been well demonstrated on both synthetic and real rs-fMRI data sets.

1 Introduction

Early and precise diagnosis of Alzheimer's disease (AD), especially at its early warning stage: Mild Cognitive Impairment (MCI), enables treatments to delay or even avoid cognitive symptoms. Constructing and classifying functional brain networks based on resting-state functional Magnetic Resonance Imaging (rs-fMRI) holds great promise for this purpose. Many methods have been proposed to model brain network based on rs-fMRI time series by identifying network nodes and inferring functional connectivity (FC) between the nodes. The nodes are often defined as anatomically separated brain regions of interest (ROIs) and the FC between two nodes is conventionally defined as the correlation of time series associated with the two nodes. However, it has been argued that partial correlation could be a better choice of FC since it measures the correlation of two nodes by regressing out the effects from all other nodes [1]. This often results in a more accurate estimate of network structure. Sparse inverse covariance estimation (SICE) is a principled method for partial correlation estimation, which often produces a stable estimation due to the L_1-norm regularization. The result of SICE is an inverse covariance matrix, and each of its off-diagonal entries indicates the partial correlation between two nodes. For brevity, we call it "SICE matrix" throughout this paper.

SICE matrix can be used as a representation to classify brain connectivity. A direct approach could be to vectorize each SICE matrix, as in [2]. However, when using it to train a classifier to separate AD from normal controls (NC), the problem of "curse of

G. Wu et al. (Eds.): MLMI 2014, LNCS 8679, pp. 59–67, 2014.

dimensionality" will occur since the dimensionality of the vector ($d \times d^1$ for network with d notes, for example, $d = 90$) is usually much larger than the number of training subjects, which is often tens for each class. An alternative approach is to summarize a $d \times d$ SICE matrix into lower dimensional graphical features such as hubs [3] or local clustering coefficient (LCC) [4]. Nevertheless, these approaches have the risk of losing useful information in the SICE matrices. This paper aims to address the high dimensionality issue of SICE matrix by extracting compact representation for classification.

As an inverse covariance matrix, SICE matrix is symmetric positive definite (SPD). This inherent property restricts SICE matrices to a lower-dimensional Riemannian manifold rather than the full $d \times d$ dimensional Euclidean space. In the community of medical image, the Riemannian manifold has been widely used for DTI analysis [5], shape statistics [6] and functional-connectivity detection [7]. Moreover, considering the fact that the brain connectivity patterns are generally similar across different subjects, the SICE matrices representing brain connectivity should concentrate on an even smaller subset of this manifold. In other words, the intrinsic degree of freedom of these SICE matrices is much lower than the apparent dimensions of $d \times d$. These two factors motivate us to seek a compact representation that better reflects the underlying distribution of the SICE matrices.

Principal component analysis (PCA), the commonly used unsupervised dimensionality reduction method, is our default option. However, a linear PCA is expected not to work well for manifold-constrained SICE matrices. Recently, advances have been made on measuring the similarity of SPD matrices. In particular, two SPD kernels, Stein kernel [8] and Log-Euclidean kernel [9], have been proposed. Both of them implicitly embed the Riemannian manifold of SPD matrices to a kernel-induced feature space $\mathcal{F}$. They offer better measurement than their counterparts in Euclidean space and require less computation than Riemannian metric, as detailed in [8]. In this paper, we take advantage of the two kernels to conduct a kernel PCA. This brings forth two advantages: i). It produces a compact representation that can mitigate the curse of dimensionality and thus improves the generalization. ii). The extracted leading eigenvectors in $\mathcal{F}$ reveal the intrinsic structure of the SICE matrices, and hence, assist brain network analysis.

Although our approach mentioned above could significantly improve the classification accuracy, another problem arises: how to interpret the obtained results anatomically? This is important in neuroimage analysis, as it could possibly help to reveal the disease mechanisms behind. Since SPD-kernel PCA is implicitly carried out in $\mathcal{F}$, estimating the pre-image of the objects, say, leading eigenvectors obtained by kernel PCA in $\mathcal{F}$, is very challenging. Existing pre-image methods [10,11] require explicit distance mapping between the input space and $\mathcal{F}$, which is intractable for SPD kernels. To solve this problem, we further propose a novel pre-image method for the SPD kernel and use it to gain an insight into SICE-based brain network analysis. To verify our approach, we conduct extensive experimental study on synthetic data set and rs-fMRI data from ADNI. The result well demonstrates the effectiveness and advantages of our approach.

---

[1] To be precise, the number of variables is $\frac{d(d-1)}{2}$ because the SICE matrix is symmetric and its diagonal entries are not used.

2 Constructing Brain Network Using SICE

Let $\{\mathbf{x}_1, \mathbf{x}_2, \cdots, \mathbf{x}_M\}$ be a time series of length M, where $\mathbf{x}_i$ is a d-dimensional vector, corresponding to an observation of d brain nodes. Following the literature of SICE, $\mathbf{x}_i$ is assumed to follow a Gaussian distribution $\mathcal{N}(\boldsymbol{\mu}, \boldsymbol{\Sigma})$. Each off-diagonal entry of $\boldsymbol{\Sigma}^{-1}$ indicates the partial correlation between two nodes by eliminating the effect of all other nodes. For example, $\boldsymbol{\Sigma}_{ij}^{-1}$ will be zero if nodes i and j are independent of each other when conditioned on the other nodes. In this sense, $\boldsymbol{\Sigma}_{ij}^{-1}$ can be interpreted as the existence and strength of the connectivity between nodes i and j. The estimation of $\mathbf{S} = \boldsymbol{\Sigma}^{-1}$ can be obtained by maximizing the penalized log-likelihood:

$$\mathbf{S}^* = \arg\max_{\mathbf{S} \succ 0} \quad \log\left(\det(\mathbf{S})\right) - tr(\mathbf{CS}) - \lambda \|\mathbf{S}\|_1 \qquad (1)$$

where $\mathbf{C}$ is the sample-based covariance; $\det(\cdot)$, $tr(\cdot)$ and $\|\cdot\|_1$ denote the determinant, trace and the sum of the absolute values of the entries of a matrix. $\|\mathbf{S}\|_1$ imposes sparsity to achieve more reliable estimation by considering the fact that a brain region often has limited direct connections with other brain regions in neurological activities. The tradeoff between the degree of sparsity and the log-likelihood estimation of $\mathbf{S}$ is controlled by the regularization parameter λ. The maximization problem in Eq. (1) can be efficiently solved by the off-the-shelf package such as SLEP [12].

3 Proposed Method

3.1 SICE Representation Using SPD-Kernel Based PCA

The SICE method is applied to N subjects to obtain $\{\mathbf{S}_1, \mathbf{S}_2, \cdots, \mathbf{S}_N\}$, where $\mathbf{S}_i \in \mathrm{Sym}_d^+$ is the obtained SICE matrix for the i-th subject. Sym_d^+ denotes the set of $d \times d$ SPD matrices. As known, Sym_d^+ forms a Riemannian manifold in the Euclidean space $\mathbb{R}^{d \times d}$ [8]. To effectively measure the similarity of two SICE matrices, Riemannian metrics that respect the specific manifold structure should be used [9]. However, directly using Riemannian metrics usually leads to unaffordable computational cost. SPD kernels implicitly map the Riemannian manifold of SPD matrices to a high-dimensional kernel-induced feature space $\mathcal{F}$. They are computationally more efficient than Riemannian metrics and also well maintain the measurement accuracy. We consider two recently proposed SPD kernels: Stein kernel [8] and Log-Euclidean kernel [9] in our study. Stein kernel measures the similarity between two SPD matrices $\mathbf{S}_i$ and $\mathbf{S}_j$ as:

$$k(\mathbf{S}_i, \mathbf{S}_j) = \exp\left(-\theta \cdot S\left(\mathbf{S}_i, \mathbf{S}_j\right)\right) \qquad (2)$$

where θ is a positive scalar within the range of $\{\frac{1}{2}, \frac{2}{2}, \frac{3}{2}, \cdots, \frac{(d-1)}{2}\} \cup \left(\frac{(d-1)}{2}, +\infty\right)$ to guarantee Stein kernel to be a Mercer kernel. $S(\mathbf{S}_i, \mathbf{S}_j)$ is S-Divergence defined as

$$S(\mathbf{S}_i, \mathbf{S}_j) = \log\left(\det\left(\frac{\mathbf{S}_i + \mathbf{S}_j}{2}\right)\right) - \frac{1}{2}\log\left(\det(\mathbf{S}_i \mathbf{S}_j)\right). \qquad (3)$$

Log-Euclidean kernel is another commonly used SPD kernel defined as: $k(\mathbf{S}_i, \mathbf{S}_j) = \exp\left(-\theta \cdot d^2(\mathbf{S}_i, \mathbf{S}_j)\right)$ with $d(\mathbf{S}_i, \mathbf{S}_j) = \|\log(\mathbf{S}_i) - \log(\mathbf{S}_j)\|_F$. The parameter $\theta \in \mathbb{R}^+$ and $\|\cdot\|_F$ denotes the Frobenius matrix norm.

Although having detailed differences for each individual, human brains do share common connectivity patterns across different subjects. Therefore, SICE matrices, as a representation of brain networks, shall have similar structure across subjects. This makes them only occupy a small subset of the manifold. Taking advantage of this, we aim to extract new representation to compactly represent SICE matrices. Linear PCA is expected not to work well for these SICE matrices because it cannot consider the manifold structure. By integrating SPD kernels into kernel PCA, we can effectively account for the manifold structure of SICE matrices when performing dimension reduction.

Let $\{\mathbf{S}_i\}_{i=1}^{N}$ be a training set, where $\mathbf{S}_i \in \mathrm{Sym}_d^{+}$. We define $\Phi(\cdot) : \mathrm{Sym}_d^{+} \mapsto \mathcal{F}$ and it is induced by a SPD kernel denoted by $k(\cdot, \cdot)$. Without loss of generality, it is assumed that $\Phi(\mathbf{S}_i)$ is centered, i.e. $\sum_{i=1}^{N} \Phi(\mathbf{S}_i) = \mathbf{0}$. Then a $N \times N$ kernel matrix $\mathbf{K}$ can be obtained by applying $k(\cdot, \cdot)$ to $\mathbf{S}_i, \cdots, \mathbf{S}_N$, where $\mathbf{K}_{ij} = \langle \Phi(\mathbf{S}_i), \Phi(\mathbf{S}_j) \rangle = k(\mathbf{S}_i, \mathbf{S}_j)$. In our study, $k(\cdot, \cdot)$ will be Stein kernel or Log-Euclidean kernel. Kernel PCA first performs the eigen-decomposition: $\mathbf{K} = \mathbf{U}\mathbf{\Lambda}\mathbf{U}^{\top}$. The i-th column of $\mathbf{U}$, denoted by $\mathbf{u}_i$, is the i-th eigenvector, and $\mathbf{\Lambda} = \mathrm{diag}(\lambda_1, \lambda_2, \cdots, \lambda_N)$, where λ_i corresponds to the i-th eigenvalue in a descending order. Let $\mathbf{\Sigma}_{\Phi}$ denote the covariance matrix computed by $\{\Phi(\mathbf{S}_i)\}_{i=1}^{N}$ in $\mathcal{F}$. The m-th eigenvector of $\mathbf{\Sigma}_{\Phi}$ can be expressed as $\mathbf{v}_m = \frac{1}{\sqrt{\lambda_m}}\mathbf{\Phi}\mathbf{u}_m$, where $\mathbf{\Phi} = [\Phi(\mathbf{S}_1), \Phi(\mathbf{S}_2), \ldots, \Phi(\mathbf{S}_N)]$. Analogous to linear PCA, $\Phi(\mathbf{S})$ can then be projected onto the top m eigenvectors to obtain a m-dimensional principal component vector $\boldsymbol{\alpha} = \mathbf{V}_m^{\top}\Phi(\mathbf{S})$, where $\mathbf{V}_m = [\mathbf{v}_1, \mathbf{v}_2, \cdots, \mathbf{v}_m]$. Note that the i-th component of $\boldsymbol{\alpha}$ is $\mathbf{v}_i^{\top}\Phi(\mathbf{S})$. With the kernel trick, it can be computed as $\mathbf{v}_i^{\top}\Phi(\mathbf{S}) = \lambda_m \mathbf{u}_m^{\top}\mathbf{k}_{\mathbf{S}}$, where $\mathbf{k}_{\mathbf{S}} = [k(\mathbf{S}, \mathbf{S}_1), k(\mathbf{S}, \mathbf{S}_2), \ldots, k(\mathbf{S}, \mathbf{S}_N)]^{\top}$. Once $\boldsymbol{\alpha}$ is obtained as a new representation for each SICE matrix, a SVM or k-NN classifier can be trained on $\boldsymbol{\alpha}$ with class labels.

3.2   Pre-image Estimation

As will be shown in the experimental study, the principal components $\boldsymbol{\alpha}$ extracted by the above SPD-kernel PCA achieve superior classification performance. Note that $\boldsymbol{\alpha}$ is fundamentally determined by the eigenvectors which capture the underlying structure of SICE matrices in $\mathcal{F}$. Therefore, the analysis of the leading eigenvectors is equally important for the interpretation of classification result and the exploration of knowledge about brain connectivity structure. However, the eigenvectors are extracted in $\mathcal{F}$ via an implicit kernel mapping, and thus cannot be readily used for analysis in the input space Sym_d^{+}. To tackle this issue, we can try to recover the SPD matrix in the input space that corresponds to a feature vector (be it a single eigenvector or their linear combinations) in $\mathcal{F}$, which is known as "pre-image" problem in the literature [10,11]. Unfortunately, existing pre-image methods, such as those in [10,11], cannot be applied to SPD kernels, because they require an explicit mapping between the distance in $\mathcal{F}$ and the distance in the input space, which is unavailable for SPD kernels. In the following, we develop a novel pre-image method for SPD kernels to address this issue.

Let $\Phi_m(\mathbf{S})$ denote the projection of $\Phi(\mathbf{S})$ into the subspace spanned by the leading m eigenvectors in $\mathcal{F}$, that is, $\Phi_m(\mathbf{S}) = \mathbf{V}_m\boldsymbol{\alpha}$. The aim is to find a pre-image $\hat{\mathbf{S}}$ in Sym_d^{+} which best satisfies $\Phi(\hat{\mathbf{S}}) = \Phi_m(\mathbf{S})$. Considering the fact that Riemannian manifold is locally homeomorphic with Euclidean space, we model $\hat{\mathbf{S}}$ by a convex combination of its neighboring SICE matrices. Similar to [10], we assume that if $\Phi(\mathbf{S}_i)$ and $\Phi(\mathbf{S}_j)$ is close in $\mathcal{F}$, $\mathbf{S}_i$ and $\mathbf{S}_j$ shall also be close in Sym_d^+. With this assumption, the neighbors of $\hat{\mathbf{S}}$ can be obtained by finding the neighbors of $\Phi_m(\mathbf{S})$ in $\mathcal{F}$.

Specifically, $\hat{\mathbf{S}}$ is estimated as follows: i) Find a set of nearest neighbors $\Omega = \{\mathbf{S}_j\}_{j=1}^L$ for $\hat{\mathbf{S}}$ from the training set $\{\mathbf{S}_i\}_{i=1}^N$ by sorting the distance in Eq.(4),

$$d^2(\Phi_m(\mathbf{S}), \Phi(\mathbf{S}_i)) = ||\Phi_m(\mathbf{S}) - \Phi(\mathbf{S}_i)||^2$$
$$= (\mathbf{k_S} - 2\mathbf{k_{S_i}})\mathbf{Mk_S} + k(\mathbf{S}_i, \mathbf{S}_i) \qquad (4)$$

where $\mathbf{M} = \sum_{i=1}^m \frac{1}{\lambda_i}\mathbf{u}_i\mathbf{u}_i^\top$; ii) Model $\hat{\mathbf{S}}$ by a convex combination (to guarantee SPD of $\hat{\mathbf{S}}$) of its neighbors $\sum_{j=1}^L w_j\mathbf{S}_j$, where $\mathbf{S}_j \in \Omega$, $w_j \geq 0$, and $\sum_{j=1}^L w_j = 1$. Defining $\mathbf{w} = [w_1, w_2, \cdots, w_L]^\top$, the optimal $\mathbf{w}$ can be obtained as:

$$\mathbf{w}^* = \arg\min_{w_j \geq 0;\ \sum w_j = 1} d^2\left(\Phi_m(\mathbf{S}), \Phi\left(\sum_{\mathbf{S}_j \in \Omega} w_j\mathbf{S}_j\right)\right) \qquad (5)$$

Note that when estimating the pre-image of an eigenvector, we can simply set $\Phi_m(\mathbf{S})$ as $\mathbf{v}_m$. In this case, Eq.(4) reduces to $1 + k(\mathbf{S}_i, \mathbf{S}_i) - \frac{2}{\lambda_m}\mathbf{u}_m^\top\mathbf{k_{S_i}}$. The pre-image of $\mathbf{v}_m$ reveals the underlying structure of the SICE matrices in $\mathcal{F}$ and could enable us to analyze the building blocks of these SICE matrices in Sym_d^+. Algorithm 1 outlines the overall algorithm.

Algorithm 1. Pre-image estimation for $\Phi_m(\mathbf{S})$ in $\mathcal{F}$

Input: A training set $\{\mathbf{S}_i\}_{i=1}^N$, m, $\mathbf{S}$;
Output: Pre-image $\hat{\mathbf{S}}$
1: Find L neighbors $\Omega = \{\mathbf{S}_j\}_{j=1}^L$ for $\hat{\mathbf{S}}$ by sorting $d^2(\Phi_m(\mathbf{S}), \Phi(\mathbf{S}_i)), i = 1, \cdots, N$;
2: Solving $\mathbf{w}^* = \arg\min_{w_j \geq 0; \sum w_j = 1;} d^2(\Phi_m(\mathbf{S}), \Phi(\sum_{\mathbf{S}_j \in \Omega} w_j\mathbf{S}_j))$
3: **return** $\hat{\mathbf{S}} = \sum_{j=1}^L w_j\mathbf{S}_j$;

---

4 Experimental Study

4.1 Data Preprocessing and Experimental Settings

Rs-fMRI data of 44 MCI and 38 NC subjects downloaded from ADNI website are used in our study. The data are acquired on a 3 Tesla (Philips) scanner with TR/TE set as 3000/30 ms and flip angle of $80°$. Each series has 140 volumes, and each volume consists of 48 slices of image matrices with dimensions 64×64 with voxel size of $3.31 \times 3.31 \times 3.31\ mm^3$. The preprocessing is carried out using SPM8 and DPARSFA [13]. The first 10 volumes of each series are discarded for signal equilibrium. Slice timing, head motion correction and MNI space normalization are performed. Participants with too much head motion are excluded. The normalized brain images are warped into AAL atlas to obtain 90 ROIs as nodes. The ROI mean time series are extracted and then band-pass filtered to obtain the most discriminative sub-band by following [4].

The functional connectivity (FC) networks of 82 participants are obtained by SICE using SLEP [12], with sparse level set as $\lambda = [0.1 : 0.1 : 0.9]$. For comparison, constrained sparse linear regression (SLR) [4] is also used to learn FC networks with the same setting. FC networks constructed by SICE and SLR are called "SICE matrices" and "SLR matrices" respectively. To make full use of the limited number of subjects, leave-one-out procedure is used for training and test. All parameters, including λ, number of eigenvectors m, k of k-NN, θ in LogEuclidean kernel (LEK) or Stein kernel (SK) and the regularization parameter of SVMs, are tuned by cross-validation on training set. Since SVMs are sensitive to parameter tuning when training samples are scarce, we mainly use linear SVMs and LCC methods as baseline and focus on k-NN.

4.2 Experimental Result

The experiment has three parts: i) to evaluate classification methods using original SICE or SLR matrices; ii) to evaluate linear PCA and the proposed SPD-kernel PCA methods for classification; iii) to evaluate the effect of our proposed pre-image method. The classification results of the three parts are summarized in Tables 1, 2, 3, respectively.

As shown in Table 1, when applied to original SICE or SLR matrices, SPD kernels (LEK and SK) outperform linear kernel. Specifically, linear kernel produces poor classification performance ($< 60\%$) on both vectorized SICE and SLR matrices. This is largely due to the "curse of dimensionality" caused by their high dimensionality. When LEK and SK are applied to SICE matrices, 61% and 63.4% are obtained, indicating that applying SPD kernels are helpful[2]. The lower-dimensional graphical feature LCC from original SICE or SLR matrices achieves 65.9%. Compared to LCC, we can see that merely applying SPD kernels on SICE matrices for classification is not good enough.

Table 2 shows the result of extracting compact representation of SICE or SLR matrices for classification. When linear PCA is applied to vectorized SICE or SLR matrices to extract the top m principal components (PCs) as features, the classification accuracy reaches 67% for both matrices, which is significantly better than all methods in Table 1. This indicates the power of compact representation and also preliminarily justifies our idea of exploring the lower intrinsic dimensions of the SICE matrices. By further taking the SPD property into account and using SPD-kernel PCA to extract the PCs, the classification accuracy is boosted up to 68.3% for LEK and 72% for SK. This well demonstrates that: i) the obtained compact representation can effectively improve the generalization of the classifier in the case of limited training samples. ii) It is important to consider the manifold property of SICE matrices to obtain more representative PCs than those in linear PCA. Cross-referencing the two tables, SPD-kernel PCA achieves the best classification performance, which is at least 14.7% higher than the linear kernel method and 6% higher than LCC.

We perform the proposed pre-image method to estimate the pre-image of $\Phi_m(\mathbf{S})$ on both synthetic and real rs-fMRI data sets. The synthetic data set allows the comparison of pre-image with the ground truth covariance matrix in Sym_d^+, which is not available for real rs-fMRI data. The synthetic data are generated as follows: i) 82 similar covariance matrices $\{\boldsymbol{\Sigma}_i\}_{i=1}^{82}$, $\boldsymbol{\Sigma}_i \in \mathrm{Sym}_{90}^+$, are generated as ground truth (refer to supplementary material for details); ii) 82 sets of 130 vectors are randomly sampled from the normal distribution $\mathcal{N}(\mathbf{0}, \boldsymbol{\Sigma}_i)$; iii) sample-based covariance matrix $\hat{\boldsymbol{\Sigma}}_i$ is estimated by using these 130 vectors; iv) Apply the SICE method to $\hat{\boldsymbol{\Sigma}}_i$ to obtain $\{\mathbf{S}_i\}_{i=1}^{82}$

---

[2] Noting that SLR matrices are not necessarily SPD, SPD kernels are therefore not applied.

Table 1. Classification accuracy (in %) on directly using SICE/SLR matrices

	Linear kernel		LCC		LEK	SK
	k-NN	SVMs	k-NN	SVMs	k-NN	k-NN
SLR [4]	53.7	52.4	65.9	64.6	-	-
SICE	57.3	57.3	65.9	60	61	63.4

Table 2. k-NN accuracy (in %) of PCA and kernel PCA methods on SICE/SLR matrices

	Linear PCs	LEK PCs (proposed)	SK PCs (proposed)
SLR [4]	67.1	-	-
SICE	67.1	68.3	**72**

Table 3. k-NN accuracy (in %) on original SICE/SLR matrices and pre-images of $\Phi_m(\mathbf{S})$

	SLR [4]	SICE	SK pre-image(proposed)	LEK pre-image(proposed)
Linear kernel	53.7	57.3	**67.1**	**68.3**
LCC	65.9	65.9	**67.1**	**67.1**

and use it as the training set for Algorithm 1; v) Estimate the pre-image $\hat{\mathbf{S}}$ of $\Phi_m(\mathbf{S})$ (with $m = 10$) for a randomly selected SICE matrix $\mathbf{S}$. We then calculate the KL divergence between the ground truth distribution $\mathcal{N}(\mathbf{0}, \mathbf{\Sigma})$ and $\mathcal{N}(\mathbf{0}, \hat{\mathbf{S}}^{-1})$. It is interesting to find that the KL divergence significantly reduces to 5.14, compared with 19.05 between $\mathcal{N}(\mathbf{0}, \mathbf{\Sigma})$ and $\mathcal{N}(\mathbf{0}, \mathbf{S}^{-1})$ (See supplementary material for illustration). Table 3 shows the result on rs-fMRI data. The pre-images of $\Phi_m(\mathbf{S}_i)$, $\mathbf{S}_i \in \{\mathbf{S}_i\}_{i=1}^N$ obtained by either SK or LEK consistently outperform the original SICE or SLR matrices in classifications with either linear kernel or LCC. These result may suggest that the pre-images seem to be more reliable than the original SICE matrix when minor components in $\mathcal{F}$ are removed, bringing some kind of denoising effect.

We also estimate the pre-image of each eigenvector in $\mathcal{F}$ for anatomical analysis. The pre-images of top 4 eigenvectors, which pose the most significant variance of SICE matrices in $\mathcal{F}$, are visualized in Fig.1. We observe that: i) In the first three pre-images, there are strong intra-lobe connections, especially in the occipital lobe; ii) In the 4th pre-image, in addition to intra-lobe connections, there are strong inter-lobe connections between superior parietal gyrus (28), inferior parietal (30), heschl gyrus (51), posterior cingulate gyrus (63) and other ROIs. These pre-images characterize the variation between Φ-maps of SICE matrices and reveal the underlying structure of SICE matrices. Further exploration of their clinical interpretation will be included in our future work.

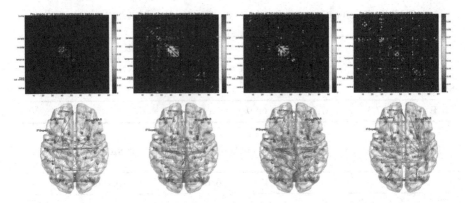

Fig. 1. Pre-images of top 4 eigenvectors extracted in the kernel-induced feature space $\mathcal{F}$ (Best viewed on monitor or in supplementary material. Refer to the supplement for names of ROIs.)

5   Conclusion

Taking advantage of the SPD property of SICE matrices, we use SPD-kernel PCA to extract principal components to obtain a compact representation for classification. The classification results on rs-fMRI data of MCI and NC demonstrate the effectiveness of our proposed method. We also propose a pre-image estimation algorithm, which enables a new perspective to visualize and analyze the extracted principal components in the input space. In this paper, we focus on unsupervised learning to explore compact representation without class label information. Note that our framework can readily be extended to supervised case, such as kernel linear discriminant analysis (KLDA), to explore discriminative representation. This will be studied in our future work.

References

1. Smith, S.M.: The future of fMRI connectivity. Neuroimage 62(2), 1257–1266 (2012)
2. Leonardi, N., Richiardi, J., Gschwind, M., Simioni, S., Annoni, J.M., Schluep, M., Vuilleumier, P., Van De Ville, D.: Principal components of functional connectivity: A new approach to study dynamic brain connectivity during rest. NeuroImage 83, 937–950 (2013)
3. Sporns, O., Honey, C.J., Kötter, R.: Identification and classification of hubs in brain networks. PloS One 2(10), e1049 (2007)
4. Wee, C.-Y., Yap, P.-T., Zhang, D., Wang, L., Shen, D.: Constrained sparse functional connectivity networks for MCI classification. In: Ayache, N., Delingette, H., Golland, P., Mori, K. (eds.) MICCAI 2012, Part II. LNCS, vol. 7511, pp. 212–219. Springer, Heidelberg (2012)
5. Pennec, X., Fillard, P., Ayache, N.: A riemannian framework for tensor computing. International Journal of Computer Vision 66(1), 41–66 (2006)
6. Fletcher, P.T., Lu, C., Pizer, S.M., Joshi, S.: Principal geodesic analysis for the study of nonlinear statistics of shape. IEEE Transactions on Medical Imaging 23(8), 995–1005 (2004)
7. Varoquaux, G., Baronnet, F., Kleinschmidt, A., Fillard, P., Thirion, B.: Detection of brain functional-connectivity difference in post-stroke patients using group-level covariance modeling. In: Jiang, T., Navab, N., Pluim, J.P.W., Viergever, M.A. (eds.) MICCAI 2010, Part I. LNCS, vol. 6361, pp. 200–208. Springer, Heidelberg (2010)

8. Sra, S.: Positive definite matrices and the symmetric stein divergence (2011)
9. Arsigny, V., Fillard, P., Pennec, X., Ayache, N.: Log-euclidean metrics for fast and simple calculus on diffusion tensors. Magnetic Resonance in Medicine 56(2), 411–421 (2006)
10. Kwok, J.Y., Tsang, I.H.: The pre-image problem in kernel methods. IEEE Transactions on Neural Networks 15(6), 1517–1525 (2004)
11. Rathi, Y., Dambreville, S., Tannenbaum, A.: Statistical shape analysis using kernel pca. In: Electronic Imaging 2006, p. 60641B. International Society for Optics and Photonics (2006)
12. Liu, J., Ji, S., Ye, J.: SLEP: Sparse Learning with Efficient Projections. Arizona State University (2009)
13. Chao-Gan, Y., Yu-Feng, Z.: DPARSF: a matlab toolbox for pipeline data analysis of resting-state fmri. Frontiers in Systems Neuroscience 4 (2010)

Deep Learning for Cerebellar Ataxia Classification and Functional Score Regression

Zhen Yang[1], Shenghua Zhong[1], Aaron Carass[1],
Sarah H. Ying[2], and Jerry L. Prince[1]

[1] Johns Hopkins University, Baltimore, USA
[2] Johns Hopkins School of Medicine, Baltimore, USA

Abstract. Cerebellar ataxia is a progressive neuro-degenerative disease that has multiple genetic versions, each with a characteristic pattern of anatomical degeneration that yields distinctive motor and cognitive problems. Studying this pattern of degeneration can help with the diagnosis of disease subtypes, evaluation of disease stage, and treatment planning. In this work, we propose a learning framework using MR image data for discriminating a set of cerebellar ataxia types and predicting a disease related functional score. We address the difficulty in analyzing high-dimensional image data with limited training subjects by: 1) training weak classifiers/regressors on a set of image subdomains separately, and combining the weak classifier/regressor outputs to make the decision; 2) perturbing the image subdomain to increase the training samples; 3) using a deep learning technique called the stacked auto-encoder to develop highly representative feature vectors of the input data. Experiments show that our approach can reliably classify between one of four categories (healthy control and three types of ataxia), and predict the functional staging score for ataxia.

1 Introduction

Cerebellar ataxia is a progressive neuro-degenerative disease that preferentially affects the cerebellum. This relatively rare spectrum of diseases has multiple genetic versions, each with a characteristic pattern of anatomical degenerations that yields distinctive motor and cognitive problems. Despite the significant impact on the lives of patients, the current standard of diagnosis, prognosis, and treatment of ataxia is inadequate. The clinical evaluations are mostly indirect, by use of clinical motor and cognitive testing. There are no accurate methods to predict the character and timing of likely functional losses. MR image analyses provide potentials to improve the evaluation of cerebellar neuro-degeneration by revealing the structural changes of the cerebellum. Fig. 1 shows example coronal sections of the cerebellum from healthy control (HC), spinocerebellar ataxia type 2 (SCA2), spinocerebellar ataxia type 6 (SCA6), and ataxia-telangiectasia (AT). We can see that all of the three ataxia types show cerebellar atrophy compared to the HC. However, SCA2 shows significant atrophy of the corpus medullare (central white matter of the cerebellum and the deep cerebellar nuclei) while

G. Wu et al. (Eds.): MLMI 2014, LNCS 8679, pp. 68–76, 2014.

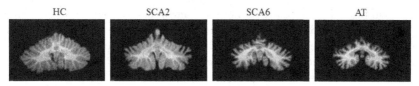

Fig. 1. Example coronal sections of the cerebellum from HC and three ataxia types

SCA6 shows more atrophy in the posterior-inferior regions of the cerebellum. Besides discriminating degeneration patterns, it may be possible to quantitatively study the correlation between the amount of structural change and degree of functional loss.

Various approaches have been proposed for studying the correlation between the structural changes of the brain and the clinical measurements. According to the type of features used to characterize the structural changes, they fall into two categories: 1) using low-dimensional carefully designed features, e.g., volumetric measurement of manually delineated region of interests (ROIs) [1,2]; 2) high dimensional features with the same order as the input images, e.g., brain morphology changes represented by deformation field from a template [3,4]. The latter group of approaches has gained popularity for: 1) less involvement of manual design and delineation and 2) being able to capture the complex patterns of structural changes. However, the high-dimensional input (up to millions) of a typical medical image and the small sample size (often several hundred) that can be acquired makes the problem challenging. Various proposed to encode the high-dimensional input into a relatively small number of features that are both representative of the data and discriminative for classification purposes [5,6].

In this work, we present a learning framework for MR image based classification and regression of cerebellar ataxia degeneration patterns. We address the problem of analyzing high-dimensional data with limited training samples with a series of strategies. Instead of classification/regression directly on the whole image volume, we train weak classifiers/regressors on a set of image subdomains separately, and then learn a classifier/regressor to combine the weak decisions. Based on the local smoothness properties of medical images, we perform a local perturbation to generate more training samples. Stacked auto-encoder (SAE) [7], a deep learning techniques, is used to develop highly representative feature vectors of the input data. Experiments show that our approach can reliably classify four categories, (HC and three types of ataxia), and predict the functional staging score for ataxia (FSFA). This is the first machine learning approach with MR image input for studying the correlation between cerebellar structural change and degeneration patterns of cerebellar diseases.

2   Method

2.1   Pre-processing

Our data consists of T1-weighted MPRAGE images of 168 subjects, 61 HCs and 107 patients with various types of ataxia. 120 of the subjects completed a series of

neurological tests that emphasizes mobility and were assigned a functional staging score for ataxia (FSFA), which provides a score from 0 to 6. The FSFA rating
scale is a subset of the Unified Ataxia Disorders Rating Scale (UADRS) [8]. A
higher FSFA value indicates more functional losses. The MR images were preprocessed with Freesurfer software [9] to generate a masked and intensity-normalized
image that contains only the cerebellum. The masked images are registered to
a template, allowing only rigid and scale transformations. The images are then
cropped to the same bounding box to tightly contain the cerebellum, see Fig. 1.
We use I to denote the MR image after the above processing.

2.2   Method Outline

As shown in Fig. 2(b), we train K weak classifiers/regressors on K image subdomains separately, and then learn a classifier/regressor C to combine the decisions
from weak classifiers. As shown in Fig. 2(a), each of the K image subdomains
is a square plane of the same size, but with different locations and orientations.
The image subdomains are chosen so that they are distributed evenly across the
whole volume. Here we use six coronal planes (three on each hemisphere), and
three sagittal planes, so $K = 9$. Let $\pi_k(u, v), u \in [0, 1], v \in [0, 1]$ be the parametric equation of the square plane at the kth image subdomain, $k = 1, 2, \ldots, K$.

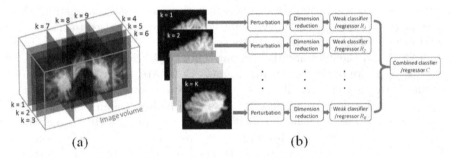

(a)   (b)

Fig. 2. (a) Image subdomains. (b) Method Diagram.

Training Weak Classifier/Regressor R_k: Let I^i be the preprocessed image
for the ith training subject. A 2D image patch $S_k^i(u, v) = I^i(\pi_k(u, v))$ can be
generated by evaluating I^i on $\pi_k(u, v)$. $S_k^i(u, v)$ is discretized to a 32×32 image
and vectorized. We will use S_k^i to represent the vector. In order to increase the
training samples, we perturb π_k by changing its center and orientation by small
amounts, and produces a set of perturbed planes, see Fig. 3. Now each subject
can generate multiple image patches by evaluating I^i on the set of perturbed
planes, resulting in a set of image patches $\Omega_k^i = \left\{ S_{k,m}^i \right\}, m = 1, 2, \ldots, M$.
A stacked autoencoder (SAE) is trained on the image patches thus generated
from all subjects, i.e. $\left\{ S_{k,m}^i \right\}, m = 1, 2, \ldots, M, i = 1, 2, \ldots, N$, and outputs a
low dimensional feature vector s_{k,m_j}^i for each input image patch S_{k,m_j}^i. Finally,

the set of feature vectors $\left\{ s_{k,m}^i \right\}, i = 1, 2, \ldots, N, m = 1, 2, \ldots, M$, is used to train the weak classifier R_k. Let $\mathbf{f}_k(\cdot)$ be the outputs from R_k, which is a vector specifying the class probabilities in the case of classification and the predicted functional score in the case of regression.

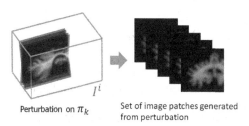

Perturbation on π_k Set of image patches generated from perturbation

Fig. 3. Image patches

Training Combined Classifier/Regressor C: To generate a training sample for C, for each image subdomain k, an image patch S_{k,m_j}^i is randomly selected from Ω_k^i. The selection is carried out independent among different image subdomains. S_{k,m_j}^i is in turn input into SAE to generate a feature vector s_{k,m_j}^i and weak classifier/regressor R_k to generate an output $\mathbf{f}_k(s_{k,m_j}^i)$. The feature vector for a training sample is formed by concatenating the outputs from all R_k, i.e. $[\mathbf{f}_1(S_{1,m_j}^i), \mathbf{f}_2(S_{2,m_j}^i), \ldots, \mathbf{f}_K(S_{K,m_j}^i)]$. We generate multiple training samples from each training subject by repeating the above procedure.

Testing Stage: Given the image of a test subject, multiple samples are generated in a similar way to the process of generating training samples for the combined classifier/regressor C. Each training sample will be assigned by C the class probabilities in the case of classification or a predicted score in the case of regression. For classification, the final output is the class that has the maximum average class probability output by C from the multiple samples. For regression, the final score is the average score predicted by C from the multiple samples.

2.3 Dimensionality Reduction Based on Stacked Autoencoder

In this section, we will describe the stacked autoencoder (SAE) for dimensionality reduction in training R_k. A typical autoencoder proposed by Bengio et al. [7] takes an input vector $\mathbf{x} \in [0, 1]^d$, and maps it to a hidden representation $\mathbf{y} \in [0, 1]^d$ through a mapping function $\mathbf{y} = f_\theta(\mathbf{x}) = sigmoid(\mathbf{W}\mathbf{x} + \mathbf{b})$, parameterized by $\theta = \{\mathbf{W}, \mathbf{b}\}$, the weight matrix and bias, respectively. This latent representation in the hidden layer $\mathbf{y}$ is projected back to reconstruct the input vector $\mathbf{x}$. The reconstructed vector $\mathbf{z} \in [0, 1]^d$ is in the input space, and can be written as $\mathbf{z} = g_{\theta'}(\mathbf{y}) = sigmoid(\mathbf{W}'\mathbf{y} + \mathbf{c}')$ with $\theta' = \{\mathbf{W}', \mathbf{c}'\}$. Often it is constrained in such a way that $\mathbf{W}' = \mathbf{W}^T$, and are referred to as tied weights. Each training sample $\mathbf{x}^{(i)}$ is mapped to a corresponding $\mathbf{y}^{(i)}$ and has a corresponding reconstruction $\mathbf{z}^{(i)}$. The parameter space is optimized to minimize the average reconstruction error:

$$\min_{\theta,\theta'} \frac{1}{n} \sum_{i=1}^{n} L\left(\mathbf{x}^{(i)}, \mathbf{z}^{(i)}\right) = \min_{\theta,\theta'} \frac{1}{n} \sum_{i=1}^{n} L\left(\mathbf{x}^{(i)}, g'_\theta\left(f_\theta(\mathbf{x}^{(i)})\right)\right), \tag{1}$$

where

$$L(\mathbf{x}, \mathbf{z}) = -\sum_{k=1}^{d} \left[\mathbf{x}_k \log \mathbf{z}_k + (1 - \mathbf{x}_k) \log(1 - \mathbf{z}_k)\right], \tag{2}$$

is a loss function based on the reconstruction cross-entropy.

Autoencoders are used as building blocks to build the deep networks, called stacked autoencoder (SAE), and trained in a greedy layer-wise way [7]. In our work, we stacked two autoencoders to form the SAE, see Fig. 4. The input layer has 1024 nodes, with each node corresponding to a pixel in the image patches. The first and second hidden layer have 500 and 100 nodes respectively. After the auto-encoders are constructed and trained, a classification/regression layer is added on top of SAE, and the entire deep network is fine-tuned to find the optimal parameter for the classification/regression purpose. Given a new image patch S, a feature vector s can be computed by feed-forward propagation through the SAE.

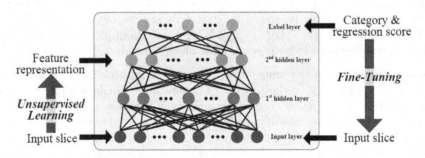

Fig. 4. Stacked auto-encoder

2.4   Classification and Regression

Random forests [10] are used for both the weak classifier/regressor R_k and the combining classfier/regressor C. Random forests are an ensemble learning method for classification and regression. It operates by constructing a set of decision trees at training time and outputting the class that is the mode of the classes output by individual trees. It also assigns the probability $f^t(x)$ that an observation x belongs to a particular class t as the mean predicted class probabilities of the trees in the forest. Random forest have been shown to achieve robust and accurate classification while avoiding over-fitting.

3   Experiments

3.1   Cerebellar Ataxia Classification

In this experiment, we consider the classification problem of classifying four groups: HC, SCA2, SCA6 and AT. We applied a 10-fold cross validation on a dataset of 80 subjects, formed by 31 HC subjects, 4 SCA2 subjects, 27 SCA6 subjects, and 18 AT subjects. The dataset is partitioned into 10 subsets in a way that the proportion of the four groups in each subset are roughly the same. For each trial, one subset is selected for testing and the other nine subsets are used for training. The following classification methods are compared: 1) **ROI volume PCA**: using the relative age-adjusted regional volumes as features [1], PCA for dimensionality reduction and random forest for classification; 2) **Image PCA**: using the whole MR image (masked and intensity normalized) as features, PCA for dimensionality reduction and random forest for classification; 3) **Log-Jacobian PCA**: using the log of the jacobian determinant computed from the deformation field from an template as features [3], PCA for dimension redution and random forest for classification; 4) **Proposed method with PCA**: the proposed method using PCA for dimensionality reduction in R_k; 5) **Proposed method with SAE**: the proposed method using SAE for dimensionality reduction in R_k.

As shown in Table 1 the proposed method produce the best performance, with error rate being 13.75%. It outperforms the ROI volumetric analyses, indicating that high-dimensional data can reveal structural information that is not captured by the low-dimensional volumetric measurement. It also outperforms direct dimensionality reduction on the whole image or jacobian based features, which verifies the effectiveness of the proposed learning framework, and the strategies of dimensionality reduction and feature selection. Within the proposed learning framework, the performance of using SAE for dimensionality reduction is better than using PCA.

Fig. 5 shows the resulting confusion matrix of the proposed method with SAE. There are two major sources of classification errors: 1) Classifying SCA2 as other classes, due to the limited SCA2 subjects in the dataset; 2) Classifying ataxias as HC, because the cerebellum of people with a short disease duration has mild cerebellar atrophy, and it's difficult to distinguish from healthy subjects. The learning framework can be further optimized to discover features that distinguishes the subjects with mild disease from the healthy.

Table 1. Classification error rate

Method	Error rate (%)
ROI volume PCA	16.25 ± 8.44
Image PCA	16.25 ± 11.86
Log-Jacobian PCA	22.50 ± 15.37
Proposed method with PCA	15.00 ± 11.49
Proposed method with SAE	13.75 ± 12.43

True \ Pred	HC	SCA2	SCA6	AT
HC	0.97	0.00	0.03	0.00
SCA2	0.25	0.00	0.50	0.25
SCA6	0.11	0.00	0.89	0.00
AT	0.06	0.00	0.11	0.83

Fig. 5. Average confusion matrix for the proposed method using SAE for dimensionality reduction

3.2 Functional Score Regression

In this experiment, we considered the regression of functional staging score for ataxia (FSFA). We applied a 10-fold cross validation on a dataset of 120 subjects which have FSFA evaluated. As in Sec. 3.1, five methods are compared. Table 2 shows that the proposed method with SAE outperforming the other methods in root mean square error (RMSE), and is compatible with the lobule volume PCA for Pearson's correlation coefficient. Fig. 6 shows the predicted FSFA vs. true FSFA for the test subjects from all 10 trials. Example coronal slices of subjects are plotted against their corresponding points in the plot. The slices from the bottom to the top of the plot show a trend from mild to severe atrophy, which indicates that the proposed method is able to capture the correlation between the degree of cerebellar atrophy and the functional loss. There are several sources for prediction error. Some of the ataxia types, such as AT and SCA3, have profounder sensory changes than other types, which could contribute to a worse FSFA than would be predicted by cerebellar changes alone. Many other factors, such as statue, weight, profession and the amount of exercise can affect their functional performance. Also, as discussed in Section 3.1, there's still room for optimizing the learning framework to discover overlooked features that correlate with FSFA.

Table 2. Root mean square error (RMSE) and Pearson correlation coefficient between the measured functional score and predicted functional score

Method	RMSE	Pearson
Lobule volume PCA	1.187±0.217	0.693± 0.110
Image PCA	1.191±0.274	0.669± 0.153
Log-Jacobian PCA	1.250±0.181	0.635± 0.091
Proposed method with PCA	1.154±0.209	0.687± 0.144
Proposed method with SAE	1.148±0.211	0.685± 0.133

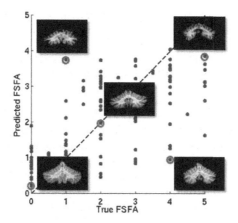

Fig. 6. Predicted FSFA vs. true FSFA, using the proposed method. Typical MR images of the cerebellum are shown.

4   Conclusion

We presented a learning framework for MR image based classification of cerebellar ataxia types and prediction of a disease related functional score. We addressed the difficulty in analyzing high-dimensional image data with limited training subjects by: 1) training weak classifiers/regressors on a set of image subdomains separately, and combining the weak classfier/regressor outputs to make the decision; 2) perturbing the image subdomain to increase the training samples; 3) using stacked auto-encoder (SAE), a deep learning technique, to develop highly representative feature vectors of the input data. Experiments show that our approach can reliably classify between one of four categories (HC and three types of ataxia), and predict the functional staging score for ataxia.

References

1. Jung, B.C., Choi, S.I., Du, A.X., Cuzzocreo, J.L., Geng, Z.Z., Ying, H.S., Perlman, S.L., Toga, A.W., Prince, J.L., Ying, S.H.: Principal component analysis of cerebellar shape on mri separates sca types 2 and 6 into two archetypal modes of degeneration. The Cerebellum 11(4), 887–895 (2012)
2. Jung, B.C., Choi, S.I., Du, A.X., Cuzzocreo, J.L., Ying, H.S., Landman, B.A., Perlman, S.L., Baloh, R.W., Zee, D.S., Toga, A.W., et al.: Mri shows a region-specific pattern of atrophy in spinocerebellar ataxia type 2. The Cerebellum 11(1), 272–279 (2012)
3. Leow, A.D., Klunder, A.D., Jack Jr., C.R., Toga, A.W., Dale, A.M., Bernstein, M.A., Britson, P.J., Gunter, J.L., Ward, C.P., Whitwell, J.L., et al.: Longitudinal stability of mri for mapping brain change using tensor-based morphometry. Neuroimage 31(2), 627–640 (2006)
4. Ashburner, J.: Computational anatomy with the spm software. Magnetic Resonance Imaging 27(8), 1163–1174 (2009)

5. Fan, Y., Shen, D., Gur, R.C., Gur, R.E., Davatzikos, C.: Compare: classification of morphological patterns using adaptive regional elements. IEEE Transactions on Medical Imaging 26(1), 93–105 (2007)
6. Batmanghelich, N.K., Taskar, B., Davatzikos, C.: Generative-discriminative basis learning for medical imaging. IEEE Transactions on Medical Imaging 31(1), 51–69 (2012)
7. Bengio, Y.: Learning deep architectures for AI. Foundations and Trends in Machine Learning 2(1), 1–127 (2009)
8. Subramony, S., May, W., Lynch, D., Gomez, C., Fischbeck, K., Hallett, M., Taylor, P., Wilson, R., Ashizawa, T., et al.: Measuring friedreich ataxia: interrater reliability of a neurologic rating scale. Neurology 64(7), 1261–1262 (2005)
9. Dale, A.M., Fischl, B., Sereno, M.I.: Cortical Surface-Based Analysis I: Segmentation and Surface Reconstruction. NeuroImage 9(2), 179–194 (1999)
10. Breiman, L.: Random forests. Machine Learning 45(1), 5–32 (2001)

Manifold Alignment and Transfer Learning for Classification of Alzheimer's Disease

Ricardo Guerrero, Christian Ledig, and Daniel Rueckert

Biomedical Image Analysis Group, Imperial College London
{reg09,christian.ledig,d.rueckert}@imperial.ac.uk
http://biomedic.doc.ic.ac.uk

Abstract. Magnetic resonance (MR) images acquired at different field strengths have different intensity appearance and thus cannot be easily combined into a single manifold space. A framework to learn a joint low-dimensional representation of brain MR images, acquired either at 1.5 or 3 Tesla, is proposed. In this manifold subspace, knowledge can be shared and transfered between the two distinct but related datasets. The joint manifold subspace is built using an adaptation of Laplacian eigenmaps (LE) from a data-driven region of interest (ROI). The ROI is learned using sparse regression to perform simultaneous variable selection at multiple levels of alignment to the MNI152 template. Additionally, a stability selection re-sampling scheme is used to reduce sampling bias while learning the ROI. Knowledge about the intrinsic embedding coordinates of different instances, common to both feature spaces, is used to constrain their alignment in the joint manifold. Alzheimer's Disease (AD) classification results obtained with the proposed approach are presented using data from more than 1500 subjects from ADNI-1, ADNI-GO and ADNI-2 datasets. Results calculated using the learned joint manifold in general outperform those obtained in each independent manifold. Accuracies calculated on ADNI-1 are comparable to other state-of-the-art approaches. To our knowledge, classification accuracies have not been reported before on the complete ADNI (-1, -GO and -2) cohort combined.

1 Introduction

Imaging biomarkers play an increasingly important role in the early diagnosis of neurodegenerative diseases like Alzheimer's disease (AD), such as assessing or detecting patients with mild cognitive impairment (MCI). The problem of extracting clinically useful biomarkers from MR images can be addressed using machine learning techniques. The curse of dimensionality imposes great challenges on analyzing high-dimensional data, such as medical images. Learning low-dimensional representations of high-dimensional data is thus a central problem of machine learning. Magnetic resonance (MR) imaging is a non-invasive imaging modality with widespread use for clinical disease assessment. As population-based studies that use MR imaging are often conducted at multiple sites, images might be acquired following different protocols, as well as different field strengths (FS).

G. Wu et al. (Eds.): MLMI 2014, LNCS 8679, pp. 77–84, 2014.

Increasing the FS from 1.5 to 3 Tesla (T) during MR image acquisition theoretically doubles the signal-to-noise ratio [1]. However, MR images acquired with different FS lie in different intensity feature spaces.

In [2] regional brain volumes and cortical thickness, derived from MR image data, were used in locally linear embeddings (LLE) to learn a low-dimensional space suitable for AD classification. In [3] 93 predefined brain regions of interest (ROI) are used to learn a multi-modal manifold using the semi-supervised manifold-regularized least squares method for AD prediction. In [4] several features were combined to classify AD subjects. MR image intensities, extracted from a ROI around the hippocampus, were used in Laplacian eigenmaps to find a low-dimensional embedding and the were an AD classifiers was learned. A common problem with using predefined ROI, is that neurodegeneration patterns may not necessarily follow standard definitions of anatomical or functional regions. Hence, limiting the analysis to predefined regions could potentially reduce the power of the biomarker. In [5] this is addressed by using data-driven ROI, which were shown to outperform predefined ROI. However, a common impediment when processing heterogeneous data, e.g. data acquired with different acquisition parameters, is that high-dimensional features should be comparable to allow dimensionality reduction. This usually hampers the joint analysis of multiple cohorts in a common space, where learning using larger, pooled datasets could be beneficial. A popular example of two cohorts residing in different spaces is the ADNI-1 (1.5T) and ADNI-GO/2 (3T) cohorts. It would be desirable to combine image intensity features, independent of field strength, in a single low-dimensional space to transfer complementary information between datasets.

Recently, manifold alignment has been put forward as a dataset alignment technique in computer vision [6,7] and medical image analysis [8]. In the following, a framework is proposed that employs manifold alignment to learn a joint low-dimensional manifold based on 1.5 and 3T MR image intensity features. This embedding allows to share and transfer information between datasets and across field strengths. The joint manifold is learned on a ROI obtained through a novel approach, using sparse regression and multilevel variable selection. Conducted experiments confirmed that our method enables the joint analysis of all publicly available ADNI datasets without sacrificing performance on individual cohorts.

2 Methods

The main objective of the proposed framework is to combine different but related subspaces. Two images acquired at 1.5T and 3T lie in different spaces even if both images have been acquired from the same subject. In the following, it is assumed that images residing in different feature subspaces still follow the same general manifold structure. These different, yet similar, spaces are then combined through manifold alignment [7]. Sparse regression is employed to learn a multilevel 4D ROI in which a distance measure allows to adequately capture the variability associated with the desired variable. In this work, the interest lies in better observing pathological differences in AD subjects. Exploiting corresponding instances from both spaces (1.5/3T) for manifold alignment, a joint manifold

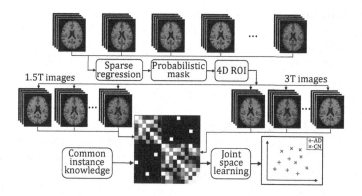

Fig. 1. Overview of the proposed method

is learned based on the learned ROIs. In particular, corresponding instances are forced to be neighbors in the joint manifold, while the local geometry of each input manifold is preserved (see Sec. 2.1). Prior to manifold alignment, multilevel variable selection and manifold learning are performed. An overview diagram of the method's main steps is shown in Fig. 1.

Multilevel Relevant Variable Selection. The goal of variable selection is to reduce the amount of input variables to those that are relevant for a specific task. Sparse regression techniques model the relationship between a dependent variable and a subset of one or more independent variables. Elastic net [9] performs automatic variable selection, encouraging the grouping of correlated variables. For a special case, it can be shown [9] that the elastic net has for each predictor variable a closed-form solution. This problem can be solved for a number of random instance subsets to introduce robustness against sampling errors (stability selection [10]). From the previous step, a probabilistic mask that indicates the likelihood of a variable being selected is obtained. Thresholding the probabilities at τ then yields a binary ROI. In this work, the independent variables are the MR image intensities, while the mini mental state examination (MMSE) score acts as dependent variable. In contrast to commonly used approaches, each of the N subjects (instances) has associated R images that have been created by aligning the original scan to the MNI152 template at R different levels. As disease specific imaging characteristics might manifest at different alignment levels, this allows the selection of the most descriptive variables (voxels) in an unsupervised formulation. A matrix $\mathbf{X}$ is built, where each column represents a spatial location in MNI space at a certain alignment level. Each row in matrix $\mathbf{X}$ represents a subject $n \in N$ and is formed by concatenating vectorized versions of its MR images at multiple levels $r \in R$. The elastic net then selects a subset of D variables from $\mathbf{X}$, that correspond to column indices of $\mathbf{X}$. Finally, this yields a 4D mask, where the first three dimensions are spatial coordinates in MNI space and the fourth is the alignment level of the image to the template.

Manifold Learning. Manifold learning refers to a set of machine learning techniques that aim at finding a low-dimensional representation of high-dimensional data while adequately representing the intrinsic geometry of the data. Given a set of N vectors of length D that represent the most relevant voxels $\mathbf{V} = \{\mathbf{v}_1, \mathbf{v}_2, ..., \mathbf{v}_N\} \in \mathbb{R}^{D \times N}$ from a set of R images at different levels of alignment, the aim is to learn the underlying manifold in $\mathbb{R}^d$ ($d \ll D$) that best represents the population $\mathbf{V}$. Here $\mathbf{v}_k = \{v_1, v_2, ..., v_D\}$ are the D most relevant voxels from subject's k set of R images extracted according to the learned ROI. Laplacian eigenmaps (LE) [11] can then be used to derive a low-dimensional representation of data, $f : \mathbf{V} \to \mathbf{Y} \in \mathbb{R}^d$, $\mathbf{y}_i = f(\mathbf{v}_i)$, while preserving the local geometric properties of the manifold. Local geometry is determined via a similarity graph, using either correlation or the sum of squared differences (SSD). LE aims to place points $\mathbf{y}_i$ and $\mathbf{y}_j$ close together in the low-dimensional space if $\mathbf{v}_i$ and $\mathbf{v}_j$ are close in the original space. This is achieved by minimizing the classical LE cost function $\phi(\mathbf{Y}) = \sum_{i,j} \|\mathbf{y}_i - \mathbf{y}_j\|^2 w_{i,j}$ under the constraint $\mathbf{y}^T \mathbf{M} \mathbf{y} = 1$, where $w_{i,j}$ is an element of the weight matrix $\mathbf{W}$ and $\mathbf{M}$ is a degree matrix.

2.1   Manifold Alignment: Shared and Transfered Knowledge

The key concept behind manifold alignment is the mapping of different feature spaces to a new latent space, simultaneously matching corresponding instances and preserving local geometry of each input space [6]. The new latent space is an augmented space where knowledge from all manifolds is shared and transfered. In this work it is proposed to employ this augmented low-dimensional manifold to map data instances from all feature spaces where the additional information can be leveraged (e.g. in machine learning tasks). Semi-supervised manifold alignment [7] aims to align the underlying manifolds of input datasets $\mathbf{V}_1, ..., \mathbf{V}_m$, where m is the number of independent manifolds. It exploits the additional knowledge about the intrinsic embedding coordinates of some instances, common to one or more feature spaces, to constrain the alignment. This new latent space (of aligned manifolds) is found by optimizing over the joint graph

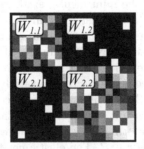

Fig. 2. Construction of the joint weight graph for 1.5T and 3T images. Intra-feature space weights $W_{1,1}$ and $W_{2,2}$, corresponding to the 1.5T and 3T feature spaces, are assigned based on correlation or SSD. Inter-feature space weights $W_{1,2} = W_{2,1}^T$ are assigned only to instances common to the 1.5T and 3T spaces.

Laplacian matrix L, which simultaneously models all input manifolds. Similarity calculations, and hence a neighborhood graph, between instances that belong to different feature spaces cannot be validly calculated using the instances' features. Rather, the joint graph is constructed by concatenating their corresponding weight graphs $\mathbf{W}_{a,b}$ and connecting common instances (i.e. subjects acquired at both field strengths) across manifolds. These additional connections force common instances, belonging to different feature spaces, to be neighbors in the joint manifold. Fig. 2 shows an example of the construction of the joint weight matrix for the 1.5T and 3T MR image intensities manifold alignment problem. Then, the classical LE equation can be re-written as:

$$\phi(\mathbf{Y}_1, ..., \mathbf{Y}_m) = \alpha \sum_{a=1}^{m} \sum_{b \neq a}^{m} \sum_{i=1}^{N_a} \sum_{j=1}^{N_b} \|\mathbf{y}_a^i - \mathbf{y}_b^j\|^2 w_{a,b}^{i,j}$$
$$+ (1 - \alpha) \sum_{a=1}^{m} \sum_{i=1}^{N} \sum_{j=1}^{N} \|\mathbf{y}_a^i - \mathbf{y}_a^j\|^2 w_{a,a}^{i,j} \tag{1}$$

where $w_{a,b}^{i,j}$ refers to the (i,j)th element of the N_a x N_b weight matrix $\mathbf{W}_{a,b}$ that connects instances in manifolds a and b. Accordingly, $w_{a,a}^{i,j}$ is an element of $\mathbf{W}_{a,a}$. N_a and N_b are the number of elements in each dataset. The parameter α trades off the first and second terms of Eq. (1), placing corresponding instances together and preserving the local geometry of each individual manifold, respectively.

3   Data and Results

Data used in this article was obtained from the Alzheimer's Disease Neuroimaging Initiative (ADNI) database (adni.loni.ucla.edu). To date, ADNI in its three studies (ADNI-1, -GO and -2) has recruited over 1500 adults, aged between 55 and 90 years, to participate in the study. Participant subjects consist of cognitive normal (CN), having significant memory concerns (SMC), early MCI (eMCI) or MCI, and with early AD. In this work, a subset of 292 (86 AD, 149 MCI and 57 CN) ADNI-1 subjects with baseline 1.5T MR images and that did not have 1.5T MR images available at 12 or 24 month follow-up, were used for training the multilevel variable selection scheme. The remaining 1.5T and 3T ADNI-1, -GO and -2 baseline images (as of November 2013) were used to evaluate the proposed framework. The number of subjects included in this work is summarized in Tab. 3. In total 1701 images were used, with 1591 unique subjects, from which 292 were used for multilevel variable selection and 1299 for evaluation. Note that a further 63 subjects were discarded, 37 due to classification ambiguities (disease reversion) and 25 due to the brain extraction failing.

All images were brain extracted using "pincram" (pyramidal intra-cranial masking), which is similar to [12]. Intensity normalization was performed using a piecewise linear function [13] that aligned the images' histogram percentiles to the average percentile model from all images. Also, all images were registered to the MNI152 template. From each subject, five different images were generated using different detail levels of deformation to the template: affine, 20mm, 10mm, 5mm and 2.5mm. All images, except the affine case, were generated using free-form-deformations [14] with the mentioned varying control point spacings.

Using sparse regression, as described in Sec. 2, a probabilistic 4D variable relevance mask was obtained that relates to voxel relevance in an MMSE regression model [5]. Higher probability voxels tended to cluster around the hippocampus, which is a well-known marker of AD. Thresholding the probability mask obtained from the described special case of the elastic net at τ yields a binary 4D ROI. An optimal threshold $\tau = 0.2$ was found using classification results of the 292 images used to learn the mask. In order to account for disease manifestation in left- and right-handed populations, selected variables were mirrored between the left and right brain hemisphere. 102, 194, 322, 200 and 42 voxels were selected from the linear, 20, 10, 5 and 2.5 mm deformation levels respectively.

Voxels within the learned ROI were extracted from the unseen images at their corresponding alignment levels and used to learn a low-dimensional representation using classical LE. As similarity metric, both correlation and SSD between the subjects ROIs were used and compared. Low-dimensional space coordinates, for each of the ADNI datasets individually, were learned and used for classification using a linear SVM with a soft-margin constraint $C = 1e^{-6}$. The choice of parameter C was found to have little effect on classification accuracies in [5]. LE parameters were empirically set based on previous experience: $k = 10$ nearest neighbors for the similarity graph, similar results are obtained for values between 10-25; $\sigma = 1$ for heat kernel, if SSD is used. Manifold dimensionality was explored in a range from 1-100, the best values are reported. Tab. 2 shows results of learning a manifold from the extracted ROI on each of the ADNI datasets separately (called: individual manifold).

In order to find a 1.5T and 3T joint low-dimensional embedding, connections between common instances are added (see Fig. 2). The trade-off between placing common instances close and preserving the local geometry of each manifold is controlled by the weight parameter α from Eq. (1). As most classification tasks exhibited robustness against parameter α in the $0.9-0.99$ range, we set $\alpha = 0.95$.

Table 1. Subject groups used for the training and evaluation of the proposed framework. Note that the subset of subjects in ADNI-1 3T are also included in ADNI-1 1.5T and that the subset ADNI-1 1.5T (VS) was only used for multilevel variable selection. MCI subjects where split into those that progressed to AD (pMCI) and and those that remained stable (sMCI), within a 48 month period.

	CN	SMC	eMCI	sMCI	pMCI	AD	Total
ADNI-1 1.5T	170	–	–	113	114	102	499
ADNI-1 1.5T (VS)	57	–	–	103	46	86	292
ADNI-1 3T	40	–	–	23	24	23	110
ADNI-GO 3T	–	–	126	–	–	–	126
ADNI-2 3T	176	73	146	116	39	124	674
Total	443	73	272	355	223	335	1701

Table 2. Classification accuracy (sensitivity/specificity) results after averaging a 100 run leave 10% out cross-validation. Note that since all ADNI-GO baseline subjects are eMCI, classification was done against ADNI-2 CN subjects, which should have the same imaging protocol. C - correlation similarity metric. Best results in terms of accuracy in bold letters. Statistical significance (p<0.05) from a paired t-test between the proposed aligned manifold and other results is indicated by *.

Study	Alignment	Dist	sMCI - pMCI	AD - CN	eMCI - CN	SMC - CN
ALL	No manifold	C	70(73/68)	89(87/91)*	63(55/72)*	53(52/54)*
	alignment	SSD	70(66/74)*	87(79/94)	63(57/70)*	56(47/67)*
	Manifold	C	71(76/67)	87(82/92)	**67(61/73)**	**58(74/43)**
	alignment	SSD	**73(73/73)**	87(81/92)	66(58/73)	56(67/460)
ADNI-1	Individual	C	68(73/69)*	87(88/87)	–	–
	manifold	SSD	69(69/70)*	88(87/90)	–	–
ADNI-GO	Individual	C	–	–	62(57/68)*	–
	manifold	SSD	–	–	63(46/80)*	–
ADNI-2	Individual	C	71(73/69)	87(80/94)	62(58/67)*	53(41/65)*
	manifold	SSD	71(69/74)*	87(79/94)	61(57/66)*	51(42/60)*

Tab. 2 shows classification results on the learned joint manifold (called: manifold alignment), with the remaining LE parameters again set to $\sigma = 1$ and $k = 10$. Additionally, one could treat instances originating from different feature spaces, as equal, calculating similarities between them, building a single neighborhood graph and directly solving classical LE without any manifold alignment. Results on this experiment (called: no manifold alignment) are also shown in Tab. 2.

4   Discussion and Future Work

A framework that learns a joint low-dimensional manifold from two distinct, yet related, feature spaces has been proposed. In this joint manifold knowledge from both spaces is synthesized. In the experiments, the distinct feature spaces consisted of multilevel relevant intensity features extracted from images acquired at different magnetic field strengths. Our analysis confirms that 1.5 and 3T MR brain data shares a significant amount of information, while residing in different feature spaces. By learning their joint manifold representation, we have shown that the additional information can be leveraged in classification/prediction tasks. To our knowledge this is the first time intensity features derived from 1.5T and 3T images from ADNI-1, -GO and -2 have been combined into a single manifold for classification purposes of the whole dataset. Additionally, a multilevel variable selection scheme was presented and independent classification results on ADNI-1, -GO and -2 are shown. Results are comparable to previous studies reported in the literature based on ADNI-1. Our experiments indicate that the proposed method is robust towards the introduced parameter α, for $\alpha > 0.9$. This is related to the fact that there are few common instances, and hence only a small number of connections between the 1.5T and 3T manifolds can be made. A high valued α compensates this by placing more weight on the first term of Eq. (1). One potential limitation relates to the intrinsic geometry of the different individual feature spaces. Assuming that each feature space has its own distinct and optimal low-dimensional embedding, difficulties might arise if these embeddings are significantly different. In this scenario the joint embedding might compromise the individual manifold structures and thus potentially be less descriptive than either one independently. It could be desirable to extend the proposed approach to a more generalizable formulation without the explicit requirement of one-to-one correspondences. Then connections between feature spaces could be modeled using a surrogate variable, such as any type of meta-data or volumetric information extracted from the anatomies under study.

References

1. Ho, A.J., Hua, X., Lee, S., Leow, A.D., Yanovsky, I., Gutman, B., Dinov, I.D., Leporé, N., Stein, J.L., Toga, A.W., Jack, C.R., Bernstein, M.A., Reiman, E.M., Harvey, D.J., Kornak, J., Schuff, N., Alexander, G.E., Weiner, M.W., Thompson, P.M.: Comparing 3 T and 1.5 T MRI for tracking Alzheimer's disease progression with tensor-based morphometry. Human Brain Mapping 31(4), 499–514 (2010)
2. Liu, X., Tosun, D., Weiner, M.W., Schuff, N.: Locally Linear Embedding (LLE) for MRI based Alzheimer's Disease Classification. NeuroImage 83, 148–157 (2013)
3. Cheng, B., Zhang, D., Jie, B., Shen, D.: Sparse Multimodal Manifold-Regularized Transfer Learning for MCI Conversion Prediction. In: Wu, G., Zhang, D., Shen, D., Yan, P., Suzuki, K., Wang, F. (eds.) MLMI 2013. LNCS, vol. 8184, pp. 251–259. Springer, Heidelberg (2013)
4. Wolz, R., Julkunen, V., Koikkalainen, J., Niskanen, E., Zhang, D.P., Rueckert, D., Soininen, H., Lötjönen, J.: Multi-method analysis of MRI images in early diagnostics of Alzheimer's disease. PloS One 6(10), e25446 (2011)
5. Guerrero, R., Wolz, R., Rao, A.W., Rueckert, D.: Manifold population modeling as a neuro-imaging biomarker: Application to ADNI and ADNI-GO. NeuroImage 94C, 275–286 (2014)
6. Wang, C.: A geometric framework for transfer learning using manifold alignment. Ph.D Thesis (2010)
7. Ham, J., Lee, D., Saul, L.: Semi-supervised alignment of manifolds. In: 10th International Workshop on Artificial Intelligence and Statistics (2005)
8. Baumgartner, C.F., Kolbitsch, C., McClelland, J.R., Rueckert, D., King, A.P.: Groupwise simultaneous manifold alignment for high-resolution dynamic MR imaging of respiratory motion. In: Gee, J.C., Joshi, S., Pohl, K.M., Wells, W.M., Zöllei, L. (eds.) IPMI 2013. LNCS, vol. 7917, pp. 232–243. Springer, Heidelberg (2013)
9. Zou, H., Hastie, T.: Regularization and variable selection via the elastic net. Journal of the Royal Statistical Society, Series B 67, 301–320 (2005)
10. Meinshausen, N., Bühlmann, P.: Stability selection. Journal of the Royal Statistical Society: Series B (Statistical Methodology) 72(4), 417–473 (2010)
11. Belkin, M., Niyogi, P.: Laplacian eigenmaps and spectral techniques for embedding and clustering. In: Advances in Neural Information Processing Systems, pp. 585–591 (2002)
12. Heckemann, R.A., Ledig, C., Aljabar, P., Gray, K.R., Rueckert, D., Hajnal, J.V., Hammers, A.: Label propagation using group agreement – DISPATCH. In: MICCAI 2012 Grand Challenge and Workshop on Multi-Atlas Labeling, pp. 75–78 (2012)
13. Nyúl, L.G., Udupa, J.K.: On standardizing the MR image intensity scale. Magnetic Resonance in Medicine 42(6), 1072–1081 (1999)
14. Rueckert, D., Sonoda, L.I., Hayes, C., Hill, D.L.G., Leach, M.O., Hawkes, D.J.: Nonrigid Registration Using Free-Form Deformations: Application to Breast MR Images. IEEE Transactions on Medical Imaging 18(8), 712–721 (1999)

Gleason Grading of Prostate Tumours with Max-Margin Conditional Random Fields

Joseph G. Jacobs, Eleftheria Panagiotaki, and Daniel C. Alexander

Center for Medical Image Computing, Department of Computer Science,
University College London, UK
j.jacobs@cs.ucl.ac.uk

Abstract. Prostate cancer diagnosis involves the highly subjective and time-consuming Gleason grading process. This paper proposes the use of Max-Margin Conditional Random Fields (CRFs) towards the aim of creating an automatic computer-aided diagnosis system. Unlike previous methods, this approach enables us to fuse information from multiple classifiers while leveraging CRFs to model spatial dependencies. We perform grading on superpixels which reduce redundancy and the size of data. Probabilistic outputs from independent classifiers are passed as input to a Max-Margin CRF, which then performs structured prediction on the biopsy core, segmenting the image into regions of benign tissue, Gleason grade 3 adenocarcinoma and Gleason grade 4 adenocarcinoma. The system achieves an accuracy of 83.0% with accuracies of 83.6%, 86.9% and 77.1% reported for benign, grade 3 and grade 4 classes respectively.

1 Introduction

Gleason grading prostate tumour biopsies is a vital part of the prostate cancer diagnostic process. A histopathologist performing Gleason grading first microscopically examines a hematoxylin and eosin (H&E) stained biopsy core at low magnification to indentify regions of interest (ROIs) before inspecting each ROI at a higher magnification to assign it a Gleason grade. Despite being the predominant prostate tumour grading system for nearly 50 years, the Gleason system has its shortcomings. For instance, the method is very subjective with a high degree of intra- and inter-observer variability[9]. Gleason grading is also an incredibly time-consuming process. Considering approximately 60-70% of biopsies are benign, this suggests most of a histopathologist's time is spent sifting through benign tissue[3]. Consequently, there is a need for computer-aided diagnosis (CAD) to improve the accuracy and efficiency of the grading process.

A significant body of research has been dedicated towards this task. Monaco et al.[8] use a probabilistic Markov Random Field (MRF) prior called a Probabilistic Pairwise Markov Model (PPMM) in a gland segmentation framework to enforce spatial dependencies during classification. Doyle et al.[3] and Gorelick et al.[5] both employ AdaBoost to learn meta-classifiers that aggregate

G. Wu et al. (Eds.): MLMI 2014, LNCS 8679, pp. 85–92, 2014.
© Springer International Publishing Switzerland 2014

Table 1. Overview of the proposed method in comparison to closely related work

Method	Classification Algorithm	Meta-classification	Spatial Dependencies	Task
Doyle et al.[3]	AdaBoost	Yes	No	Segment an image into benign and cancerous regions
Gorelick et al.[5]	AdaBoost	Yes	No	Grade images of manually identified ROIs
Monaco et al.[8]	PPMM	No	Yes	Segment and classify glands as benign or cancerous
Proposed method	Max-Margin CRF	Yes	Yes	Segment an image into benign, Gleason 3 and Gleason 4 regions

information from multiple weak 'i.i.d. classifiers'[1] to produce a strong classifier. [3] uses AdaBoost in a multi-resolution pixel-wise framework to segment an image into benign and cancerous regions. On the other hand, [5] uses AdaBoost to (i) classify superpixels as one of nine tissue components and (ii) grade an image based on the distribution of tissue components. Besides these, most studies focus on feature selection, using i.i.d. classifiers such as Support Vector Machines (SVMs) and k-Nearest Neighbours (k-NN) with some combination of colour, texture and morphometric features to segment or classify images[14,11].

This paper presents a method that segments H&E stained biopsy cores into regions of benign tissue, Gleason grade 3 adenocarcinoma and Gleason grade 4 adenocarcinoma. Table 1 compares the proposed method to the closest in previous literature. We use Max-Margin Conditional Random Fields (CRFs) to perform multi-class meta-classification on the outputs of two multi-class i.i.d. classifiers while incorporating spatial dependencies into the process. Like [3] we perform classification on every region in an image (i.e. not just on segmented glands), enabling the algorithm to function even in highly cancerous regions which often have poorly defined glands[4]. However, we use superpixels to over-segment an image prior to performing classification. This significantly reduces redundancy and the size of data.

2   Proposed Method

Our solution uses machine learning and computer vision algorithms to segment and grade H&E stained biopsy cores. The method employs Simple Linear Iterative Clustering (SLIC)[1] to over-segment an image into superpixels. We then extract colour and texture features from each superpixel to perform classification in two stages. In the first stage, we use a k-NN and an SVM to obtain individual class probabilities for each superpixel. A Max-Margin CRF then acts as a meta-classifier, combining information from the first stage classifiers while incor-

---

[1] We define an 'i.i.d. classifier' as a classifier that assumes data points are independent and identically distributed (the i.i.d. assumption).

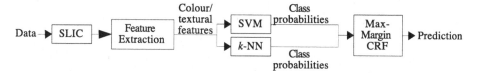

Fig. 1. Overview of the proposed method

porating spatial dependencies into the prediction process. The following sections describe and motivate the selection of each individual algorithm in more detail.

2.1 Pre-Processing

The computational complexity of performing inference on a general CRF increases with the number of vertices and edges in the graph. Our method groups perceptually similar pixels to form superpixels. This reduces the number of vertices in the CRF, thus reducing the computational complexity of inference. We use SLIC[1] to do this as the algorithm is simple, fast and memory efficient. Given a superpixel size S, SLIC clusters an image $\mathcal{I}$ in the colour and spatial domains using an algorithm similar to k-means clustering to form $k = \frac{|\mathcal{I}|}{S^2}$ superpixels.

Next, we extract colour and texture features from each superpixel. A 17-bin histogram of RGB pixel intensities and the mean RGB pixel intensity represent the colour of a superpixel while histograms of Local Binary Patterns (LBP)[12] describe its texture. We use the 'uniform' variant of LBP as it is both greyscale- and rotation-invariant. For each pixel c, we construct a P-bit binary number with the indicator function $\mathbb{I}[g_i \geq g_c]$, $i = 1, \ldots, P$ where g_c is the greyscale pixel intensity of c and g_i are the greyscale pixel intensities of P points at a radius R around c. The LBP label for uniform patterns (i.e. there are, at most, two 0/1 transitions in the P-bit number) is the number of 1s in the P-bit number while the label for non-uniform patterns is $P+1$. We then construct a $(P+2)$-bin histogram of LBP labels to obtain a texture descriptor for each superpixel.

2.2 Classification

At this stage it is possible that some superpixels may not contain enough useful information to distinguish between the three classes. A histopathologist looking at the same region would consider the information in surrounding regions to make a decision. Structured prediction offers the ability to do this by incorporating spatial dependencies between superpixels into the prediction process. We perform structured prediction with a function $f : \mathcal{X} \rightarrow \mathcal{Y}$ from the input domain $\mathcal{X}$ to a structured output domain $\mathcal{Y}$ where

$$f_{\boldsymbol{w}}(X) = \underset{Y \in \mathcal{Y}}{\arg\max} \; g_{\boldsymbol{w}}(X, Y), \quad X \in \mathcal{X} \tag{1}$$

for some cost function $g_{\boldsymbol{w}}(X, Y)$ that describes the compatibility of structured output Y with input X as parameterised by $\boldsymbol{w}$. In our case, the input X is the probabilistic output from our first stage classifiers, a CRF $\mathcal{G}$ encodes the structure of the output and we use max-margin learning to find the optimal $\boldsymbol{w}$.

First Stage Classifiers. The first stage classifiers are a k-NN and an SVM that output class probabilities for each superpixel. The k-NN calculates class probabilities for each data point as the proportion of the k closest points belonging to each class. The SVM uses a modified version of Platt scaling[6] to provide class probabilities given the decision function outputs of a non-linear SVM. The output from this stage is a 6×1 vector of class probabilities for each superpixel.

Conditional Random Fields. The graph $\mathcal{G} = (\mathcal{V}, \mathcal{E})$ is a pairwise CRF that models the conditional probability of a structured output Y as a combination of unary and pairwise terms. We define $\mathcal{G}$ such that each vertex $v \in \mathcal{V}$ represents a superpixel and edges $e_{u,v} \in \mathcal{E}$ connect two adjacent superpixels $u, v \in \mathcal{V}$. The energy or cost of a given labelling $Y \in \mathcal{Y}$ is then expressed as

$$E(Y) = \sum_{v \in \mathcal{V}} U(v) + \sum_{e_{u,v} \in \mathcal{E}} P(u,v) \tag{2}$$

where $U(v)$ is the unary term and $P(u,v)$ is the pairwise term. $U(v)$ encodes the compatibility of a given labelling $y_v \in Y$ with the inputs $\boldsymbol{x}_v \in X$ at vertex v. To use the CRF as a meta-classifier, we model $U(v)$ as a linear combination of the class probabilities from the first stage classifiers $\boldsymbol{x}_v$. This is written as

$$U(v) = \langle \boldsymbol{w}_{y_v}^U, \boldsymbol{x}_v \rangle \tag{3}$$

where $\boldsymbol{w}_{y_v}^U$ are the unary parameters for the class y_v learnt during training. $P(u,v)$ represents the compatibility of the labelling y_u and y_v for the adjacent vertices u and v. This is learnt directly during training and is written as

$$P(u,v) = w_{y_u,y_v}^P \tag{4}$$

where w_{y_u,y_v}^P is the symmetric pairwise parameter for the classes y_u and y_v learnt during training. Performing 'prediction' on the CRF amounts to performing inference on the graph $\mathcal{G}$ to find the optimal solution $Y^\star$ that minimises the energy function E. The general pairwise CRF is usually a loopy graph which renders exact inference intractable. However, good approximations of the solution can be obtained using a variety of methods. Here we use Alternating Directions Dual Composition (AD^3)[7] as it gives us better performance compared to other algorithms such as graph cuts.

Max-Margin Learning. Our method uses the Structured SVM (SSVM) formulation by Tsochantaridis et al.[15] to do max-margin learning. This formulation is particularly appealing as it enables the use of arbitrary loss functions. In this case we have chosen to use per-superpixel 0-1 loss, expressed as

$$\Delta(\hat{Y}, f_{\boldsymbol{w}}(X)) = \sum_{v \in \mathcal{V}} \mathbb{I}[\hat{Y}_v \neq f_{\boldsymbol{w}}(X)_v] \tag{5}$$

where $\mathbb{I}[a]$ is an indicator function and $\hat{Y}$ the ground truth. The SSVM minimises the following empirical risk function to learn the optimal parameters $\boldsymbol{w}^{\star}$:

$$\boldsymbol{w}^{\star} = \arg\min_{\boldsymbol{w}} \frac{1}{2}\|\boldsymbol{w}\|^2 + \frac{C}{|\mathcal{N}|} \sum_{n\in\mathcal{N}} \Delta(\hat{Y}^n, f_{\boldsymbol{w}}(X^n)) - g_{\boldsymbol{w}}(X^n, \hat{Y}^n) + g_{\boldsymbol{w}}(X^n, f_{\boldsymbol{w}}(X^n))$$

$$(6)$$

Here $\mathcal{N}$ is the set of ground truth images.

2.3   Experimental Setup

Our experimental setup uses open source implementations of the above methods [1,2,10,13,16] to make it easily reproducible. The data set contains images of H&E stained biopsy cores collected from 122 patients. These were graded by two experienced histopathologists, each with 10 years experience in genitourinary pathology. We select ten biopsy cores for each of the Gleason scores 3+3, 3+4, 4+3 and 4+4, ensuring each core contains a continuous Gleason pattern at least 0.4mm in length. From these, we extract 146 images of tissue segments at 20× magnification: 90 for training and 56 for testing. We create ground truth by labelling the superpixels in these images. Where there are two or more classes of pixels within a superpixel, we select the higher Gleason grade as the label.

3   Results and Discussion

The Jaccard Index (JI) quantifies the overall performance of the method. We define it as the fraction of superpixels that are correctly labelled, expressed as

$$\mathrm{JI} = \frac{|\hat{\mathcal{L}} \cap \mathcal{L}|}{|\hat{\mathcal{L}} \cup \mathcal{L}|} \qquad (7)$$

where $\hat{\mathcal{L}}$ is the set of predicted superpixel labels and $\mathcal{L}$ is the corresponding ground truth. We compare the performance of i.i.d. classifiers (Table 2) against our method (Figure 2), each using different combinations of normalised input features (i.e. colour/texture features only or both colour and texture features).

Table 2 shows i.i.d. classifiers struggle to perform classification at superpixel level. The two best i.i.d. classifiers are the SVM and k-NN that use both sets of features, achieving JIs of 0.604 and 0.583 respectively. In contrast, the worst variant of our method achieves a JI of 0.666. Figure 3 compares sample output from an SVM against our method, revealing its advantages over i.i.d. classification. The output of our method is a lot smoother and more consistent with the ground truth compared to the SVM. Figure 2 shows the JI of our method as we vary the input features to the first stage classifiers. When the first stage k-NN uses both sets of features, the difference in JI as we vary the features of the SVM is negligible. Similarly, there is an insignificant difference in JI when the SVM uses either texture or both sets of features. This tells us that using the best i.i.d. classifiers does not necessarily lead to better overall performance. Instead,

Table 2. Jaccard Index for i.i.d. classifiers with different combinations of features

Classifier	SVM	SVM	SVM	k-NN	k-NN	k-NN
Input Features	colour	texture	both	colour	texture	both
Jaccard Index	0.562	0.545	0.604	0.547	0.530	0.583

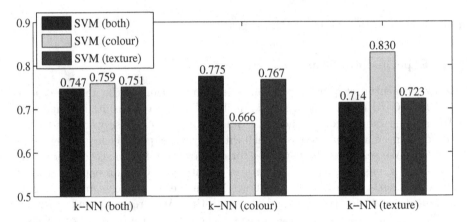

Fig. 2. Comparison of Jaccard Indices for Max-Margin CRFs using different combinations of input features to the first stage classifiers.

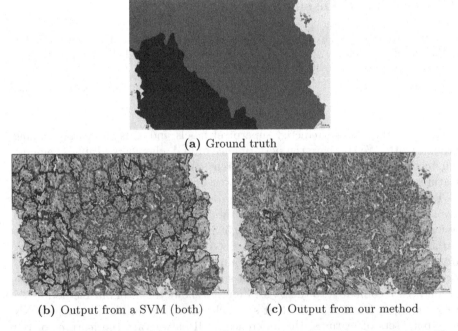

(a) Ground truth

(b) Output from a SVM (both)   (c) Output from our method

Fig. 3. This visualisation demonstrates the advantages of structured prediction. The output of the Max-Margin CRF is clearly a lot smoother and closer to the ground truth data than that of the SVM.

Table 3. Confusion matrix for the max-margin CRF using SVM (colour) and k-NN (texture) as input.

		Predicted			
		Benign	Grade 3	Grade 4	Total
Actual	Benign	1988	301	90	2379
	Grade 3	252	2875	182	3309
	Grade 4	194	370	1902	2466
	Total	2434	3546	2174	8154

Table 4. Confusion matrix to evaluate the performance of the best classifier on the separation between benign and cancerous regions.

		Predicted		
		Cancerous	Benign	Total
Actual	Cancerous	5329	446	5775
	Benign	391	1988	2379
	Total	5720	2434	8154

the method performs best when we use weaker first stage classifiers. The results also indicate that texture features are weighted higher than colour features in an SVM trained on both sets of features. Consequently, dropping colour features and training the SVM with texture features only has little effect on performance. We also notice the method performs best when each of the first stage classifiers use different features. We suggest that this is because each classifier provides the Max-Margin CRF with a different insight into the data.

The confusion matrix of the best performing classifier for the three-class grading problem (Table 3) indicates good grading accuracy for each individual class. The method performs worst on Gleason grade 4 regions, classifying these correctly only 77.1% of the time. These regions were most often misclassified as Gleason grade 3 (15% of the time). While not ideal, this balance of classification error is preferable to the converse. This is more evident when we consider the confusion matrix for the separation between benign and cancerous regions (Table 4). The results indicate that the proposed method has a sensitivity of 92.3% and a specificity of 83.6% for separation between benign and cancerous regions. This balance of misclassification is desirable as we would rather overdiagnose than underdiagnose in a CAD system. Otherwise the system could miss cancerous regions, resulting in the disease being completely undiagnosed in some patients.

4   Conclusion and Future Work

This paper presented a novel approach to grading prostate tumour biopsies for CAD. Max-Margin CRFs were used both as a meta-algorithm and a structured prediction mechanism to provide an accurate segmentation and labelling of prostate tissue images. In this case only colour and texture features were extracted from each superpixel. Using more first stage classifiers on different features (e.g. morphometric features like nuclei density) could improve the system. Specifically, we aim to capture characteristics to distinguish grade 4 from grade 3 tissue. Another weakness to address in future work is the inability to tune the trade-off between sensitivity and specificity for separation between benign and cancerous regions. We also intend to perform pixel-wise evaluation using a larger data set to enable more accurate quantification of performance.

References

1. Achanta, R., Shaji, A., Smith, K., Lucchi, A., Fua, P., Süsstrunk, S.: SLIC Super-pixels Compared to State-of-the-Art Superpixel Methods. IEEE TPAMI 34(11), 2274–2282 (2012)
2. Chang, C.C., Lin, C.J.: LIBSVM: A library for support vector machines. ACM TIST 2(3), 27:1–27:27 (2011)
3. Doyle, S., Feldman, M.D., Tomaszewski, J., Madabhushi, A.: A Boosted Bayesian Multiresolution Classifier for Prostate Cancer Detection From Digitized Needle Biopsies. IEEE TBE 59(5), 1205–1218 (2012)
4. Epstein, J.I.: An Update of the Gleason Grading System. J. Urology 183(2), 433–440 (2010)
5. Gorelick, L., Veksler, O., Gaed, M., Gomez, J.A., Moussa, M., Bauman, G., Fenster, A., Ward, A.D.: Prostate Histopathology: Learning Tissue Component Histograms for Cancer Detection and Classification. IEEE TMI 32(10), 1804–1818 (2013)
6. Lin, H.T., Lin, C.J., Weng, R.C.: A note on Platt's probabilistic outputs for support vector machines. Mach. Learn. 68(3), 267–276 (2007)
7. Martins, A.F.T., Figueiredo, M.A.T., Aguiar, P.M.Q., Smith, N.A., Xing, E.P.: An Augmented Lagrangian Approach to Constrained MAP Inference. In: Getoor, L., Scheffer, T. (eds.) ICML 2011, pp. 169–176. Omnipress (2011)
8. Monaco, J., Tomaszewski, J., Feldman, M.D., Hagemann, I., Moradi, M., Mousavi, P., Boag, A., Davidson, C., Abolmaesumi, P., Madabhushi, A.: High-throughput detection of prostate cancer in histological sections using probabilistic pairwise Markov models. Med. Image Anal. 14(4), 617–629 (2010)
9. Montironi, R., Mazzuccheli, R., Scarpelli, M., Lopez-Beltran, A., Fellegara, G., Al-gaba, F.: Gleason grading of prostate cancer in needle biopsies or radical prostate-ctomy specimens: contemporary approach, current clinical significance and sources of pathology discrepancies. BJU Int. 95(8), 1146–1152 (2005)
10. Müller, A., Behnke, S.: PyStruct-Structured Prediction in Python. JMLR 15, 2055–2060 (2014)
11. Nguyen, K., Sarkar, A., Jain, A.K.: Structure and Context in Prostatic Gland Segmentation and Classification. In: Ayache, N., Delingette, H., Golland, P., Mori, K. (eds.) MICCAI 2012, Part I. LNCS, vol. 7510, pp. 115–123. Springer, Heidelberg (2012)
12. Ojala, T., Pietikäinen, M., Mäenpää, T.: Multiresolution Gray-Scale and Rotation Invariant Texture Classification with Local Binary Patterns. IEEE TPAMI 24(7), 971–987 (2002)
13. Pedregosa, F., Varoquaux, G., Gramfort, A., Michel, V., Thirion, B., Grisel, O., Blondel, M., Prettenhofer, P., Weiss, R., Dubourg, V., VanderPlas, J., Passos, A., Cournapeau, D., Brucher, M., Perrot, M., Duchesnay, E.: scikit-learn: Machine Learning in Python. JMLR 12, 2825–2830 (2011)
14. Tabesh, A., Teverovskiy, M., Pang, H.Y., Kumar, V.P., Verbel, D., Kotsianti, A., Saidi, O.: Multifeature Prostate Cancer Diagnosis and Gleason Grading of Histo-logical Images. IEEE TMI 26(10), 1366–1378 (2007)
15. Tsochantaridis, I., Joachims, T., Hofmann, T., Altun, Y.: Large Margin Methods for Structured and Interdependent Output Variables. JMLR 6, 1453–1484 (2005)
16. van der Walt, S., Schönberger, J.L., Nunez-Iglesias, J., Boulogne, F., Warner, J.D., Yager, N., Gouillart, E., Yu, T., The scikit-image contributors: scikit-image: image processing in Python. PeerJ 2, e453 (2014)

Learning Distance Transform for Boundary Detection and Deformable Segmentation in CT Prostate Images

Yaozong Gao[1,2], Li Wang[1], Yeqin Shao[1,3], and Dinggang Shen[1]

[1] Department of Radiology and BRIC, University of North Carolina at Chapel Hill, USA
[2] Department of Computer Science, University of North Carolina at Chapel Hill, USA
[3] Institution of Image Processing & Pattern Recognition, Shanghai Jiao Tong University, China

Abstract. Segmenting the prostate from CT images is a critical step in the radiotherapy planning for prostate cancer. The segmentation accuracy could largely affect the efficacy of radiation treatment. However, due to the touching boundaries with the bladder and the rectum, the prostate boundary is often ambiguous and hard to recognize, which leads to inconsistent manual delineations across different clinicians. In this paper, we propose a learning-based approach for boundary detection and deformable segmentation of the prostate. Our proposed method aims to learn a boundary distance transform, which maps an intensity image into a boundary distance map. To enforce the spatial consistency on the learned distance transform, we combine our approach with the auto-context model for iteratively refining the estimated distance map. After the refinement, the prostate boundaries can be readily detected by finding the valley in the distance map. In addition, the estimated distance map can also be used as a new external force for guiding the deformable segmentation. Specifically, to automatically segment the prostate, we integrate the estimated boundary distance map into a level set formulation. Experimental results on 73 CT planning images show that the proposed distance transform is more effective than the traditional classification-based method for driving the deformable segmentation. Also, our method can achieve more consistent segmentations than human raters, and more accurate results than the existing methods under comparison.

1 Introduction

CT images are widely used in the image-guided radiotherapy planning (IGRT), as it provides Hounsfield units for all image voxels, which are necessary for dose calculation. In the IGRT for prostate cancer, the prostate and nearby organs (e.g., the bladder and the rectum) need to be segmented in order to optimize the dose plan for precisely targeting the radiation beams on the prostate and minimizing the radiation exposure to the surrounding tissues. The segmentation accuracy of the prostate could largely affect the efficacy of radiation treatment. However, due to the touching boundaries with the bladder and the rectum, the prostate boundary is often indistinct in CT images (Fig. 1), which imposes much difficulty upon the manual delineation. It usually takes an experienced clinician $10 - 12$ minutes to manually delineate the prostate boundary in CT image of each patient. Despite of taking this long delineation time, manual segmentations still vary much among different raters [1,2]. Thus, an automatic and robust segmentation method is highly desired in this context.

G. Wu et al. (Eds.): MLMI 2014, LNCS 8679, pp. 93–100, 2014.

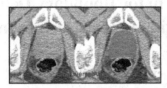 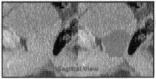

Fig. 1. A typical 3D planning CT image in the transversal view (left panel) and sagittal view (right panel). In each view, the left figure shows the original prostate slice, and the right figure shows the corresponding slice overlaid with the manually segmented prostate (red).

Previous works [3,4] often reply on learning a patient-specific model for addressing the aforementioned challenge, as the prostate appearance and shape variations are small for the image data acquired from the same patient. However, these methods are not applicable for prostate segmentation from the planning CT images, as no segmented CT images of the same patient are available for appearance and shape learning in the radiotherapy planning stage. Consequently, only population information (i.e., CT images of other patients) could be used for guiding the prostate segmentation in the planning CT images. Among the population-based methods, most of them utilize the shape constraint for deriving a robust segmentation. For example, Costa et al. [5] proposed a coupled deformable model for segmenting the prostate by imposing a non-overlapping constraint from the bladder. Chen et al. [6] proposed a Bayesian framework that incorporates anatomical constraints from the surrounding bones for prostate segmentation. However, due to the lack of an effective appearance model for guiding the deformable segmentation, the accuracy of these methods is very limited. Recently, classification-based methods [2,7] have been proposed to segment the prostate from CT images, and achieved significant improvement over the traditional intensity-based methods [5,6,8]. The main idea is to train a classifier for distinguishing prostate voxels from background voxels based on local patch appearance. The learned classifier could be used to label the intensity image into a prostate likelihood map for guiding the deformable segmentation.

In this paper, we propose to learn a distance transform for boundary detection and deformable segmentation of the prostate. The learned distance transform can map a new intensity image into the distance map of the target prostate boundary, which could be further utilized for anatomical boundary detection as well as deformable segmentation. In particular, regression forest is adopted to learn the non-linear relationship between a voxel's local image appearance and its 3D displacement to the nearest point on the target prostate boundary. Once the forest is learned, it can be used to predict the 3D displacement from any voxel in the new testing image to the target prostate boundary. By taking the magnitude of the displacement vector, the distance map of the prostate boundary can be obtained for a new testing image. To enforce the spatial consistency within the obtained distance map, we further combine the high-level context features extracted from the previously obtained distance map with the original image appearance features into the auto-context framework [9] for iterative refinement. Finally, the refined distance map will be integrated into a level set formulation for segmenting the prostate from CT images. Experimental results show that learning a boundary distance transform is more effective than prostate classification for guiding the deformable segmentation.

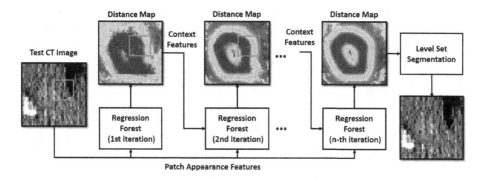

Fig. 2. The flowchart of our method. Green boxes show the local patches where appearance and context features are extracted for the voxel marked as red crosses. Cold and warm colors in the figure indicate voxels with small and large predicted distances to the prostate boundary.

In addition, our method can achieve more consistent segmentations than human raters, and also more accurate results than existing methods under comparison.

2 Method

Our method consists of three components: 1) regression forest for learning boundary distance transform, 2) iterative refinement of the predicted distance map by context features, and 3) distance-map-guided boundary detection and deformable segmentation with level sets. Fig. 2 shows the flowchart of our method.

2.1 Learning Boundary Distance Transform by Regression Forest

Regression forest, as a non-linear regression model, has recently been used for efficient anatomy detection [10], i.e., detecting the bounding box of one specific organ. In this paper, we extend it to learn the distance transform for a specific organ boundary (e.g., prostate boundary). The learned distance transform is used for mapping a new 3D intensity image into the distance map of the target boundary. More specifically, given any voxel in the new testing image, we want to predict its nearest distance to the target boundary. Hence, distance transform learning is essentially a regression problem. In our work, regression forest is particularly used for learning the non-linear relationship between a voxel's local image appearance and its 3D displacement vector to the nearest point on the target boundary. By taking the magnitude of the 3D displacement vector, the distance of this voxel to the target boundary can be obtained. Thus, the learned regression forest can be regarded as a boundary distance transform. In the next paragraphs, we will show how the regression forest is trained for learning boundary distance transform, and how the learned forest could be applied to a new testing image for predicting the distance map.

To learn the distance transform for a specific organ boundary, we first randomly sample voxels near the boundary in every training image according to a Gaussian distribution: $p(\boldsymbol{x}) = 1/(\sqrt{2\pi}\sigma) \times \exp(-d(\boldsymbol{x})^2/2\sigma^2)$, where $p(\boldsymbol{x})$ indicates the probability of voxel $x \in \mathbb{R}^3$ in a training image to be sampled, $d(x)$ is the nearest distance of voxel x to the target boundary in this training image, and σ controls the size of narrowband for sampling. In this way, the majority of sampled voxels will be close to the target boundary, thus making the learned model more specific on detecting the target boundary. This sampling strategy is important for accurate organ segmentation, as boundary voxels are usually the most difficult to characterize. Afterwards, the sampled voxels from all training images are used as our training dataset. For each sampled voxel in one training image, we extract randomized 3D Haar-like features from an intensity patch centered at this voxel for capturing the local image appearance around it. The Haar-like features are defined as follows.

$$ f(I) = \sum_{i=1}^{M} t_i \sum_{\|x - c_i\|_\infty \le s_i} I(x) \tag{1} $$

where $f(I)$ denotes one 3D Haar-like feature extracted from intensity patch I, M is the number of 3D cubic functions used in this Haar-like feature, and $t_i \in \{+1, -1\}$, c_i and s_i are the polarity, the center and the size of the i-th cubic function, respectively. By randomizing the parameters M, t_i, c_i and s_i in Eq. 1, we can generate an unlimited number of 3D Haar-like features for regression forest learning. In this work, M is limited to $\{1, 2\}$, s_i is limited to $\{3, 5\}$, and c_i is not limited as long as the 3D cubic function stays within intensity patch I of size $30 \times 30 \times 30$.

Once the feature representation of each voxel is determined, a regression forest can be trained for predicting the 3D displacement from any image voxel to the nearest point on the target boundary. Given a new testing image, the learned forest can be applied to voxel-wisely estimate the 3D displacement for every image voxel. By taking the magnitude, a boundary distance map can then be obtained.

2.2   Iterative Refinement of Distance Map by Context Features

As the displacement from each image voxel to the target boundary is predicted independently, the estimated distance map for a new testing image is often spatially inconsistent, as shown in the leftmost distance map of Fig. 2. To overcome this limitation, we integrate the proposed distance transform learning with the auto-context model [9] for iteratively refining the estimated distance map. The main idea is to train a sequence of distance transforms, each utilizing both the local image features extracted from the original intensity image, and the high-level context features extracted from the output of the previous distance transform for gradually improving the quality of the estimated distance map.

During the training stage, after the distance transform of the first iteration is learned as described in Section 2.1, it can be used to predict a boundary distance map for every training image. Then, the additional high-level context features can be extracted from the estimated distance map, and further combined with the original image features to form a new feature representation for each voxel. Afterwards, a new distance transform can be learned by using the updated feature representation. This iterative training procedure continues until a specified number N of distance transforms is obtained. In our work, the high-level context features are also the randomized Haar-like features as

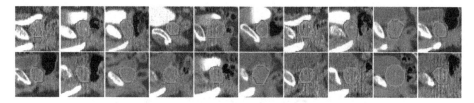

Fig. 3. Typical planning CTs (sagittal view) in our dataset. Green and blue contours indicate the prostate boundaries automatically detected by our boundary detection method and manually delineated by the expert, respectively.

defined in Eq. 1. Different from image appearance features, these context features are extracted from the distance map estimated by the previous distance transform. Since the rough distances of nearby voxels to the target boundary have been encoded in the previously estimated distance map, the new distance transform learning can utilize this valuable information to impose the spatial consistency on the to-be-estimated distance map, thus improving the overall prediction accuracy. In the testing stage, the learned distance transforms can be applied sequentially as shown in Fig. 2 to iteratively refine the estimated distance map for a new testing image.

2.3 Distance-Map-Guided Boundary Detection and Deformable Segmentation (with Level Sets)

Once the boundary distance map is estimated for a new testing image, it can be used for either boundary detection or level set segmentation.

Boundary Detection: In most cases, the estimated distance map of a new testing image will be directly utilized for the final segmentation (e.g., to guide the deformable segmentation). However, sometimes if the organ-specific boundary segments are desired, we can also adopt non-minima suppression and hysteresis thresholding, similar as in the canny edge detector [11], to detect these organ-specific boundaries from the estimated distance map.

Level Set Segmentation: Since the target boundaries are located in the valley of the estimated distance map, the local means in the estimated distance map should be similar for both sides of the zero level set. Based on this assumption, we can design the following evolution flow to segment the prostate from the boundary distance map:

$$\frac{\partial \phi}{\partial t} = \delta(\phi)(u_1(\boldsymbol{x}) - u_2(\boldsymbol{x})) + v\delta(\phi)\text{div}\left(\frac{\bigtriangledown\phi}{\|\bigtriangledown\phi\|}\right) \tag{2}$$

$$u_1(\boldsymbol{x}) = \frac{\int K(\boldsymbol{y} - \boldsymbol{x})H(\phi(\boldsymbol{y}))\Omega(\boldsymbol{y})d\boldsymbol{y}}{\int K(\boldsymbol{y} - \boldsymbol{x})H(\phi(\boldsymbol{y}))d\boldsymbol{y}}, u_2(\boldsymbol{x}) = \frac{\int K(\boldsymbol{y} - \boldsymbol{x})(1 - H(\phi(\boldsymbol{y})))\Omega(\boldsymbol{y})d\boldsymbol{y}}{\int K(\boldsymbol{y} - \boldsymbol{x})(1 - H(\phi(\boldsymbol{y})))d\boldsymbol{y}} \tag{3}$$

where ϕ is the level set function with $\phi > 0$ as the inner part and $\phi < 0$ as the outer part, δ is the Delta function, $u_1(\boldsymbol{x})$ and $u_2(\boldsymbol{x})$ are the local means of the inner and outer parts, respectively, K is a Gaussian kernel function with the standard deviation of 3, H is the Heaviside step function [12], and Ω denotes the estimated boundary distance map. The first data-fitting term attracts the zero level set to the valley of the estimated distance map Ω, and the second regularization term imposes the smoothness constraint on the evolving surface ϕ.

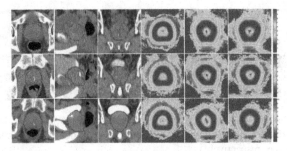

Fig. 4. Qualitative results from three planning CT images with different levels of contrast agent. Each row shows the planning CT images and their corresponding predicted distance maps in transversal, sagittal and coronal views. Red and blue contours indicate our final segmented prostate boundaries and the manually delineated boundaries, respectively.

3 Experiments

Data Descriptions: Our dataset consists of 73 planning CT images, scanned from different patients. The typical image size is $512 \times 512 \times (61 \sim 81)$ with voxel size $0.94 \times 0.94 \times 3.00$ mm^3. The prostate in each planning CT image has been manually delineated by a radiation oncologist, which we use as ground truth. The dataset is of large appearance variability due to the uncertainty on the level of contrast agent that is present. Fig. 3 shows typical planning CT images (sagittal view) in our dataset along with the detected prostate boundaries by our boundary detection method (green) and manual rater (blue).

Parameter Setting: In the regression forest training, the number of trees is 10, the maximum tree depth is 15, the number of randomized Haar-like features is 1000 for both image appearance and context features, and the minimum sample number for each leaf node is 8. σ for controlling the size of narrowband sampling is 8. v in the level set segmentation is set to 0.01. All the parameters of regression forest is typical as adopted in other works [10]. To evaluate our segmentation method, we use four-fold cross-validation with 54 images for training and 19 images for testing. The initialization of the level set function is accomplished by using an affine transformation to transform the mean prostate shape onto the testing image. The affine transformation is estimated between six automatically detected prostate landmarks (i.e., top, base, anterior, posterior, left and right) in the testing image and their counterparts on the mean shape [2].

Qualitative Results: In addition to the boundary detection results in Fig. 3, we also plot the qualitative results for three typical planning CT images (with different levels of contrast agent) in Fig. 4. We can see that, after the proposed distance transform, prostate boundaries can be clearly seen in the predicted distance maps, and are quite consistent with the manually delineated boundaries by radiation oncologist. This demonstrates that our proposed method works very well in various planning CTs with different levels of contrast agent.

Classification versus Distance Transform: Fig. 5 (a) quantitatively compares the classification guided level set method with our proposed method (distance-map-guided level set method) on the same dataset. As aforementioned, the classification-based method

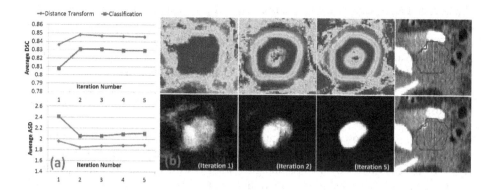

Fig. 5. (a) Quantitative comparison between classification-guided and distance-map-guided level set methods in our dataset. DSC: Dice Similarity Coefficient. ASD: Average Surface Distance. (b) Qualitative comparison between distance-map-based (first row) and classification-based (second row) auto-context refinement on a typical planning CT image. Red and blue contours indicate automatically-segmented and manually-delineated prostates, respectively.

uses a learned classifier to label the new testing image into a prostate likelihood map, which is then utilized for guiding the deformable segmentation with level sets [12]. For fair comparison, we used the classification forest with the same training parameters for the classification-guided level set method. Similarly, we also adopt the auto-context model to iteratively refine the classification response map. From Fig. 5 (a), we can clearly see that our proposed method ("distance transform") outperforms the classification-guided level set method in all iterations (e.g., with higher Dice Similarity Coefficient (DSC) and lower Average Surface Distance (ASD)). In addition, Fig. 5 (b) gives a typical example that compares the classification-based auto-context refinement with our distance-map-based auto-context refinement. We can see that the distance-map-based refinement is able to achieve more accurate segmentation than classification-based refinement. This infers that the context features extracted from the boundary distance map are more helpful to assist the auto-context refinement than the traditional context features extracted from the classification response map.

Comparison with other CT Prostate Segmentation Methods: Our method obtains an average surface distance (ASD) 1.85 ± 0.87 mm on our dataset. Due to the fact that neither the executables nor the datasets of other works are publicly available, it is difficult for us to directly compare our method with other CT prostate segmentation methods. Thus, we only cite the results reported in their publications for reference. The comparison shows that our method achieves more accurate segmentations than [8] (ASD 4.09 ± 0.90 mm), [2] (ASD 3.35 ± 1.40 mm), and the current state-of-the-art method [7] (ASD 2.37 ± 0.89 mm). Besides, it is worth noting that most existing methods were evaluated only on the datasets without contrast agent. It is not clear whether these methods can be applied to the mixed datasets which contain planning CTs with different levels of contrast agent. Actually, this aspect is very important in the clinical application. A desired prostate segmentation method should be able to deal with various kinds of planning CTs obtained with different contrasts and scanning protocols, as it is never pre-known which type of an unseen image would need to be segmented. Clearly, our method wins at this point, since it has been evaluated with good performance on the dataset with planning CTs of different contrasts. Additionally, the comparison with inter-rater variability of manual prostate delineations (ASD $3.03 \pm 1.15mm$ [2]) indicates that our method is also able to obtain more consistent segmentations than the human raters.

4   Conclusion

In this paper, we propose to predict the boundary distance transform for anatomical boundary detection and deformable segmentation. It is applied to segment the prostate from CT images. Validated on 73 planning CT images with various contrasts, our proposed distance transform learning method shows better performance than prostate classification method for guiding the deformable segmentation of the prostate. Moreover, the comparisons with other CT prostate segmentation methods indicate that our method can be more adaptive to different datasets with various contrasts. Also, compared to manual prostate delineations, our method can achieve more consistent segmentations, since there often exists large inter-rater variability for manual delineations.

References

1. Foskey, M., Davis, B., et al.: Large deformation three-dimensional image registration in image-guided radiation therapy. Phy. Med. Biol. 50(24), 5869 (2005)
2. Lay, N., Birkbeck, N., Zhang, J., Zhou, S.K.: Rapid multi-organ segmentation using context integration and discriminative models. In: Gee, J.C., Joshi, S., Pohl, K.M., Wells, W.M., Zöllei, L. (eds.) IPMI 2013. LNCS, vol. 7917, pp. 450–462. Springer, Heidelberg (2013)
3. Feng, Q., Foskey, M., Tang, S., Chen, W., Shen, D.: Segmenting CT prostate images using population and patient-specific statistics for radiotherapy. Med. Phys. 37(8), 4121–4132 (2010)
4. Gao, Y., Liao, S., Shen, D.: Prostate segmentation by sparse representation based classification. Med. Phys. 39(10), 6372–6387 (2012)
5. Costa, M.J., Delingette, H., Novellas, S., Ayache, N.: Automatic segmentation of bladder and prostate using coupled 3D deformable models. In: Ayache, N., Ourselin, S., Maeder, A. (eds.) MICCAI 2007, Part I. LNCS, vol. 4791, pp. 252–260. Springer, Heidelberg (2007)
6. Chen, S., Lovelock, D.M., Radke, R.J.: Segmenting the prostate and rectum in CT imagery using anatomical constraints. Med. Ima. Anal. 15(1), 1–11 (2011)
7. Lu, C., et al.: Precise segmentation of multiple organs in CT volumes using learning-based approach and information theory. In: Ayache, N., Delingette, H., Golland, P., Mori, K. (eds.) MICCAI 2012, Part II. LNCS, vol. 7511, pp. 462–469. Springer, Heidelberg (2012)
8. Rousson, M., Khamene, A., Diallo, M., Celi, J.C., Sauer, F.: Constrained surface evolutions for prostate and bladder segmentation in CT images. In: Liu, Y., Jiang, T.-Z., Zhang, C. (eds.) CVBIA 2005. LNCS, vol. 3765, pp. 251–260. Springer, Heidelberg (2005)
9. Tu, Z., Bai, X.: Auto-context and its application to high-level vision tasks and 3D brain image segmentation. PAMI 32(10), 1744–1757 (2010)
10. Criminisi, A., Shotton, J., Robertson, D., Konukoglu, E.: Regression forests for efficient anatomy detection and localization in CT studies. In: Menze, B., Langs, G., Tu, Z., Criminisi, A. (eds.) MICCAI 2010. LNCS, vol. 6533, pp. 106–117. Springer, Heidelberg (2011)
11. Canny, J.: A computational approach to edge detection. PAMI 8(6), 679–698 (1986)
12. Chan, T., Vese, L.: Active contours without edges. TIP 10, 266–277 (2001)

Geodesic Geometric Mean of Regional Covariance Descriptors as an Image-Level Descriptor for Nuclear Atypia Grading in Breast Histology Images

Adnan Mujahid Khan[1,2,*], Korsuk Sirinukunwattana[1,2,*], and Nasir Rajpoot[1,2]

[1] Department of Computer Science, University of Warwick, UK
[2] College of Engineering & Computer Science, Qatar University, Qatar
a.m.khan@warwick.ac.uk

Abstract. The region covariance descriptors have recently become a popular method for detection and tracking of objects in an image. However, these descriptors are not suitable for classification of images with heterogeneous contents. In this paper, we present an image-level descriptor obtained using an affine-invariant geodesic mean of region covariance descriptors on the Riemannian manifold of symmetric positive definite (SPD) matrices. The resulting image descriptors are also SPD matrices, lending themselves to tractable geodesic distance based k-nearest neighbour classification using efficient kernels. We show that the proposed descriptor yields high classification accuracy on a challenging problem of nuclear pleomorphism scoring in breast cancer histology images.

Keywords: Symmetric positive definite matrices, generalised geometric mean, geodesic nearest neighbourhood, nuclear pleomorphism.

1 Introduction

The Nottingham Grading System is the most widely used standard for grading breast cancer tissue slides recommended by the World Health Organisation [1]. It is based on the assessment of three morphological features: tubule formation, mitotic count and nuclear atypia/pleomorphism. Tubule formation assesses what percentage of the tumour forms normal duct structures. Regular duct structures implies lower grade cancer. Mitotic count assesses the number of dividing cells seen in 10 high power microscope fields. More dividing cells implies high grade cancer. Nuclear Atypia (NA) assesses the deviation in appearance (pleomorphism) of cell nuclei from those in normal breast duct epithelial cells. More deviation implies high grade tumour (see Figure 1).

Previous approaches to NA scoring generally emulate the visual examination by a pathologist. Cosatto *et al.* [2] perform nuclear segmentation using image analysis approach by first detecting seed points using the difference of Gaussian (DoG) operator followed by the Hough transform to delineate the nuclei boundaries. Next, they compute a set of shape, size and texture features to train a classifier for NA scoring. Dalle *et al.* [3] employ a similar approach as well by first performing nuclear segmentation

---

* Joint first authors.

G. Wu et al. (Eds.): MLMI 2014, LNCS 8679, pp. 101–108, 2014.

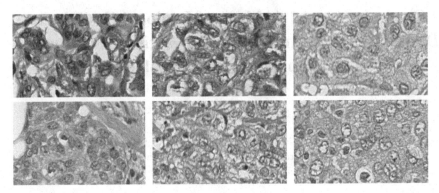

Fig. 1. Visual appearance of different nuclei in breast histological images. Grade-1 (Left Column) , 2 (Middle Column), and 3 (Right Column) nuclear pleomorphism.

followed by fitting a Gaussian mixture model on the features computed from the segmented nuclei. Nuclei segmentation is performed by detecting regions of interest using intensity thresholding followed by fitting a line to the distance transform of this region in polar space where the round nuclei shapes form a curve.

Most existing methods rely heavily on the accurate segmentation of cell nuclei. However, nuclei segmentation in histology images remains a challenging problem in high grade tumours, where nuclei are often hollow inside with broken cell membrane or weakly stained cell membrane and contain unpacked chromatin structures. Moreover, due to occlusion or overlapping nuclei, nuclei segmentation becomes extremely challenging leading to erroneous segmentation which may affect the predicted NA score. Therefore, despite good results obtained on a limited dataset, techniques that rely heavily on the accurate nuclear segmentation run the risk of overfitting on limited training data.

Instead of performing nuclear segmentation, we take a holistic approach and pose the NA scoring as a texture discrimination problem. In literature, a range of texture descriptors (e.g. Haralick, local binary patterns (LBP), Gabor and region covariance (RC) descriptor [4]) have been proposed for performing variety of tasks including histology texture classification [5]. Among these texture descriptors, the RC descriptor is relatively recently proposed and offers some desirable theoretical properties - for instance, RC descriptors are symmetric positive definite (SPD) matrices lending themselves to tractable optimisation. Furthermore, they are also relatively low-dimensional descriptors extracted from several different features computed at the level of regions and consequently reducing the computational cost of classification.

In this paper, we propose an image classification scheme based on the generalised geometric mean of symmetric positive definite matrices (mSPD) computed from features of all regions in a given image (see Figure 2). The regional covariance descriptors computed from sub-image are points lying on the Riemannian manifold of SPD matrices. The image level descriptor given by the mSPD is, therefore, a representative of potentially different covariance matrices calculated from heterogeneous sub-images. The mSPD matrix is calculated using the geodesic connected to affine-invariant Riemannian

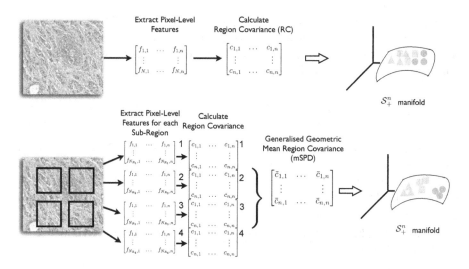

Fig. 2. An illustration of the overall classification framework using (a) the standard region co-variance and (b) generalised geometric mean region covariance. The generalised geometric mean is calculated using equation (1), while the classification is achieved using a geodesic k-nearest neighbour classifier. N is number of pixels in the image, N_{R_K} is number of pixels in sub-image region R_K, n is number of features, $f_{i,j}$ is the feature j at pixel location i, $c_{p,q}$ and $\bar{c}_{p,q}$ are (p, q) elements of RC and mSPD descriptors respectively.

metric [6]. We utilise geodesic k-nearest neighbour (GkNN) approach to assign labels to a test input image. In order to improve the computational efficiency of computing geodesic distances, which cause nontrivial numerical burden, we use the kernel trick that results in comparable accuracy and statistically significant reduction in execution time.

2   The Proposed Scheme for Image Classification

Figure 2 describes the proposed framework for image classification using the mSPD descriptors. An image is divided into small non-overlapping regions. For each region, pixel-level features are collected to form an RC descriptor. RC descriptors of different regions are then summarised into a single mSPD descriptor, by calculating the generalised geometric mean of RC descriptors. A Geodesic k-nearest neighbour classifier, which utilises the known structure of the Riemannian manifold of SPD matrices, is then employed to assign the NA score labels (1, 2 or 3) to test images.

2.1   Generalised Geometric Mean of Symmetric Positive Definite Matrices as an Image-Level Descriptor

An image I can be divided into K small non-overlapping sub-regions $\{R_1, ..., R_K\}$ to calculate the corresponding RC descriptors $\mathbf{C}_{R_k}$, $k = 1, ..., K$. The RC descriptor can be computed simply by calculating n pixel-level features $\mathbf{f}(x,y) = \{f_1(x,y), f_2(x,y), \dots, f_n(x,y)\}$ for all (x,y) image coordinates and then calculating the $n \times n$ covariance matrix $\mathbf{C}_{R_k}$ of $\mathbf{f}(x,y)$ $\forall x, y$. These RC descriptors can then be combined through generalised geometric mean as below:

$$\mathbf{M}(I) = \operatorname{argmin}_{\mathbf{X} \in \mathcal{M}} \sum_{k=1}^{K} \operatorname{dist}^2(\mathbf{X}, \mathbf{C}_{R_k}), \tag{1}$$

where $\operatorname{dist}(\cdot, \cdot)$ is defined based on a metric on the space $\mathcal{M}$ of SPD matrices. In this work, we use geodesic distance (equation (2), (3), and (4)) based on affine-invariant metric due to the Riemannian manifold structure of the space of SPD matrices which will be described in Section 2.2.

2.2 Nearest Neighbour Classification on Riemannian Manifold of Symmetric Positive Definite Matrices

An $n \times n$ mSPD is a member of the space $\mathcal{S}_n^+$ of $n \times n$ symmetric positive definite (SPD) matrices, which is an open convex subset of the Euclidean space. However, $\mathcal{S}_n^+$ is not a vector space with usual addition and scalar multiplication as, for example, it is not closed under negative scalar multiplication. Analysing SPD matrices under usual Euclidean geometry would fail to capture the nonlinearity of $\mathcal{S}_n^+$. In fact, $\mathcal{S}_n^+$ forms a Riemannian manifold with negative curvature when endowed by affine invariant metric [6], and a Riemannian manifold with null curvature when endowed by the log-Euclidean metric [7].

Metrics for SPD Manifolds. We measure the distance between two SPD matrices $\mathbf{X}, \mathbf{Y} \in \mathcal{S}_n^+$ based on geodesic distance of the known Riemannian manifold by using following distance measures.

– **Affine-invariant metric**

$$\operatorname{dist}(\mathbf{X}, \mathbf{Y}) = \| \log(\mathbf{X}^{-1/2} \mathbf{Y} \mathbf{X}^{-1/2}) \|_F = \| \log(\mathbf{Y}^{-1/2} \mathbf{X} \mathbf{Y}^{-1/2}) \|_F \tag{2}$$

where $\| \cdot \|_F$ denotes the Frobenius norm and $\log(\cdot)$ denotes matrix logarithm.
– **Log-Euclidean metric**

$$\operatorname{dist}(\mathbf{X}, \mathbf{Y}) = \| \log(\mathbf{X}) - \log(\mathbf{Y}) \|_F = \| \log(\mathbf{Y}) - \log(\mathbf{X}) \|_F \tag{3}$$

– **Positive Definite kernel** Computation of geodesic distance ((2) and (3)) involves nonlinear log operator which can cause nontrivial numerical burden. Motivated by this, we employ a kernel-based approach which defines an embedding function $\phi : \mathcal{S}_n^+ \to \mathbb{H}$ in order to map the SPD matrices into the high-dimensional reproducing kernel Hilbert space (RKHS) $\mathbb{H}$. Since the RKHS is equipped with inner product, dissimilarity measure between two points $\phi(\mathbf{X}), \phi(\mathbf{Y}) \in \mathbb{H}$ for any $\mathbf{X}, \mathbf{Y} \in \mathcal{S}_n^+$ can simply be calculated by their inner product which is defined in the form of positive definite kernel $k(\mathbf{X}, \mathbf{Y}) : \mathcal{S}_n^+ \times \mathcal{S}_n^+ \to \mathbb{R}$ [8],

$$k(\mathbf{X}, \mathbf{Y}) = e^{-\sigma S(\mathbf{X}, \mathbf{Y})} \tag{4}$$

where $\sigma \in \{\frac{1}{2}, \frac{2}{2}, ..., \frac{n-1}{2}\} \cup \{\tau \in \mathbb{R} : \tau > \frac{n-1}{2}\}$ is a scaling factor, and

$$S(\mathbf{X}, \mathbf{Y}) \equiv \log\left(\det\left(\frac{\mathbf{X} + \mathbf{Y}}{2}\right)\right) - \frac{1}{2}\log\left(\det\left(\mathbf{X}\mathbf{Y}\right)\right) \tag{5}$$

is a symmetric Stein divergence which behaves similarly to geodesic distance (equation 2) induced by affine-invariant metric within a tight bound. Note that $\det(\cdot)$ is determinant operator.

Kernel Geodesic k-Nearest Neighbour Classifiers. The geodesic neighbour (GkNN) classifier explicitly exploits the structure of Riemannian manifold of SPD matrices through the use of geodesic distances (2) and (3). On account of its computational benefits (Table 1), we propose the use of positive-definite kernel distance (4) which behaves similar to the true geodesic distance in the GkNN classifier. The value of the kernel function ranges between 0 and 1, and the higher the value of the kernel function, the smaller the distance between two SPD matrices. Experimental results (Section 3) also confirmed the improvement in classification accuracy of GkNN classifiers over their Euclidean distance-based counterpart.

3   Results and Discussion

3.1   Dataset Description and Preprocessing

We evaluate our method on the publicly available MITOS-Atypia dataset, which comprises of 297 breast histology images extracted from 11 patients, and is part of an ongoing Mitos-Atypia Challenge[1]. The slides are stained with the standard Hematoxylin and Eosin (H&E) dyes and scanned using two slide scanners: Aperio Scanscope XT and Hamamatsu Nanozoomer 2.0-HT. Here, we consider images acquired by the Aperio XT scanner ($\times 20$ magnification), the more widespread and accessible solution among the two. It has a resolution of $0.245\mu m$ per pixel, resulting in a 1376×1539 RGB image for each visual field. Two senior pathologists independently scored the images for NA. The score assigned to each image is a discrete number between 1 and 3. S_1 denotes a low grade NA and S_3 denotes a high grade NA. In approximately 15% of the cases, the two experts disagreed. For these conflicting cases, a third pathologist scored the slides independently and majority vote was used.

All images are stain normalised using [9] to minimise the effect of variation in visual appearance of stains. Histological images may contain stromal regions, where lymphocytes and stromal nuclei are likely to exist. We avoid stromal regions while scoring NA by performing tumour segmentation in order to restrict scoring to tumour areas only [10], [11]. Motivated by the cues used by most to score NA in breast histology images (e.g. the chromatin textures present in the nuclei), we convert RGB images into a blue ratio (BR) image, that the values of BR are positively correlated to the presence of nuclear content in an H&E stained tissue, thus directly revealing spatial distribution of nuclei as follows, $BR = \frac{100B}{1+R+G} \times \frac{256}{1+B+R+G}$ where R, G, B stand for red, green, and blue intensities, respectively. Finally, an average kernel of size 3×3 is applied to smooth the image to remove noise.

---

[1] http://mitos-atypia-14.comicframework.org/

Table 1. Comparative results of $mSPD_{lbp}$, RC_{gabor} and $mSPD_{gabor}$ descriptors using all pixels in the image (columns 2, 4 and 6) and only the tumour pixels (columns 3, 5 and 7) in the image. Last column shows the average execution time over 10 runs. All timings are calculated on an iMac27 machine running Matlab 2013b with 16GB RAM.

Classifier	$mSPD_{lbp}$		RC_{gabor}		$mSPD_{gabor}$		Run Time $\mu \pm \sigma$
	All	Tumour	All	Tumour	All	Tumour	
GkNN-Affine	0.73	0.76	0.71	0.72	0.79	0.83	15.26 ± 6.61
GkNN-logE	0.72	0.73	0.76	0.79	0.80	0.81	120.04 ± 4.67
GkNN-Stein	0.69	0.73	0.74	0.74	0.79	**0.84**	11.64 ± 0.51
kNN	0.71	0.71	0.77	0.75	0.75	0.73	2.15 ± 0.51

Table 2. Performance of a library of texture features when used in conjunction with linear and quadratic discriminant analysis classifiers

Baseline Features	Classifier	Trainin/Test Split	No. of Features	Accuracy
Haralick, LBP, Gabor, Wavelet	LDA	70/30	73	0.75
		50/50	75	0.74
	QDA	70/30	9	0.72
		50/50	13	0.71

3.2 Experimental Setup, Results and Discussion

For computation of the mSPD descriptor, we evaluate LBP and Gabor texture features. As $mSPD_{gabor}$ features perform better (see Table 1), we further compute RC_{gabor} features on whole image level and present a 3-way comparison between whole image level RC_{gabor}, sub-image level $mSPD_{gabor}$ and sub-image level $mSPD_{lbp}$. For computation of $mSPD_{gabor}$ and RC_{gabor} descriptors, SPD matrices of size 29×29 are generated by computing the covariance of 29 channels (BR, gradients and Hessians on BR in horizontal and vertical directions, and Gabor filter responses at 4 scales and 6 orientations) at sub-image level and whole image level respectively. For computation of the $mSPD_{lbp}$ features, a range of options (varying the size and number of filters) were examined and the best results are reported.

In order to establish a baseline performance, an additional experiment was performed on the same dataset where a set texture features (Haralick, LBP, Gabor and wavelet) were computed at image-level, over a range of colour spaces (RGB, Lab, HSV, XYZ, BR and Hematoxylin and Eosine), feature selection was performed using Fisher measure, and classification using linear and quadratic discriminant analysis was performed. In all our experiments, we perform 5-fold cross validation. Each experiment is repeated 10 times and average accuracy results are reported. For fair comparison, the number of nearest neighbours are fixed to 5 for both Euclidean and geodesic nearest neighbour algorithms. For tumour segmentation, a system trained on similar images was used. The choice of all parameters was based on cross-validation experiments on a subset of data.

Tables 1 and 2 show the experimental results for NA subtypes classification. Following important observations can be made from the results: (1) Regional statistics is more effective in small neighbourhoods as compared to on the whole image where the

Table 3. Disagreement between pathologists (*left*); Confusion matrix representing misclassifications using our proposed algorithm in 3 nuclear pleomorphism scores (*right*)

	S_1	S_2	S_3		S_1	S_2	S_3	Misclassifications
No. of Samples	23	222	52	S_1	15	8	0	34.78%
Pathologist-1 Agreed	21	205	52	S_2	4	200	18	9.90%
Pathologist-2 Agreed	22	203	36	S_3	0	16	36	30.76%
Disagreement	3	27	15					
	(13.0%)	(12.1%)	(28.8%)					

heterogeneity in various parts of the image may negatively influence the performance of the descriptor. This can be observed from the results of the RC_{gabor} descriptor which calculates features at the whole image level, and does not perform well as compared to $mSPD_{lpg}$ and $mSPD_{gabor}$ features, which are calculated on sub-image level; (2) Classical texture discrimination approaches do not perform well, even if the feature space is explored in an extensive manner with both linear and quadratic classifiers (as shown in Table 2), and fail to capture subtle differences in the appearance of nuclei. Again, since the texture features are computed at the whole image level, the descriptor does not perform well due to the statistical nature of features; (3) Geodesic kNN mostly outperforms the Euclidean kNN classifier. This essentially refers to the fact that Euclidean kNN is not appropriate for classification of covariance matrices as it does not take into account the structure of manifold while finding the nearest neighbours; (4) Statistically significant improvement (31%) in computational speed, without compromising classification accuracy, is achieved by using kernel trick while calculating geodesic distance between the SPD matrices; (5) Tumour segmentation helps improve the classification accuracy of almost all competing methods in Table 1 (by as high as 6.78%) except kNN, where either marginal improvement ($mSPD_{lbp}$) or an opposite trend (RC_{gabor} and $mSPD_{gabor}$) is seen. Again, this can be attributed to the fact that the Euclidean kNN is not appropriate for classification of covariance matrices.

Table 3 shows the comparison of disagreement, regarding NA scoring, between three expert pathologists and the proposed system. The proposed system performs best on S_2 subtype, where the accuracy of the proposed system is $\approx 2.2\%$ better than the agreement between experts. On the other hand, the proposed system shows worse performance on S_1 NA images, where the accuracy of the proposed system is $\approx 20\%$ lower than the agreement between experts. The best and worse performance of the proposed system correlates positively with the prevalence of the two subtypes in dataset (S_2 - 74%, as compared to S_1 - 7% of the samples). Furthermore, the performance of the proposed system is in line with the agreement between pathologists for S_3 subtype. This indicates the potential of the proposed algorithm to perform even better if provided with more samples from less prevalent NA subtypes.

4   Conclusions

We presented the generalised geometric mean of region covariance descriptors as an image level descriptor along with the geodesic k-nearest neighbour classifier for image classification. Extracting region covariance descriptors locally allows better representation of variability in a region. Generalised geometric mean over all region covariance descriptors of an image offers an effective way to unify several descriptors to represent the whole image. Possible future directions includes incorporation of generalised geometric mean region covariance descriptors in sparse coding and dictionary learning frameworks [12] and hormone receptor scorings [13].

References

1. Elston, C., Ellis, I.: Pathological prognostic factors in breast cancer. I. The value of histological grade in breast cancer: experience from a large study with long-term follow-up. Histopathology 19(5), 403–410 (1991)
2. Cosatto, E., Miller, M., Graf, H.P., Meyer, J.S.: Grading nuclear pleomorphism on histological micrographs. In: International Conference on Pattern Recognition, pp. 1–4. IEEE (2008)
3. Dalle, J.-R., Li, H., Huang, C.-H., Leow, W.K., Racoceanu, D., Putti, T.C.: Nuclear pleomorphism scoring by selective cell nuclei detection. In: Workshop on Applied Computing & Visualization. IEEE (2009)
4. Tuzel, O., Porikli, F., Meer, P.: Region covariance: A fast descriptor for detection and classification. In: Leonardis, A., Bischof, H., Pinz, A. (eds.) ECCV 2006. LNCS, vol. 3952, pp. 589–600. Springer, Heidelberg (2006)
5. Vlachokosta, A.A., Asvestas, P.A., Matsopoulos, G.K., Kondi-Pafiti, A., Vlachos, N.: Classification of histological images of the endometrium using texture features. Analytical and Quantitative Cytology and Histology 35(2), 105–113 (2013)
6. Pennec, X., Fillard, P., Ayache, N.: A Riemannian framework for tensor computing. International Journal of Computer Vision 66(1), 41–66 (2006)
7. Arsigny, V., Fillard, P., Pennec, X., Ayache, N.: Geometric means in a novel vector space structure on symmetric positive-definite matrices. SIAM Journal on Matrix Analysis and Applications 29(1), 328–347 (2007)
8. Sra, S.: A new metric on the manifold of kernel matrices with application to matrix geometric means. In: NIPS, pp. 144–152 (2012)
9. Khan, A.M., Rajpoot, N., Treanor, D., Magee, D.: A non-linear mapping approach to stain normalisation in digital histopathology images using image-specific colour deconvolution. IEEE Transactions on Biomedical Engineering 61(6), 1729–1738 (2014)
10. Khan, A.M., El-Daly, H., Rajpoot, N.: RanPEC: Random projections with ensemble clustering for segmentation of tumor areas in breast histology images. In: Medical Image Understanding and Analysis, pp. 17–23 (2012)
11. Khan, A.M., El-Daly, H., Simmons, E., Rajpoot, N.M.: HyMaP: A hybrid magnitude-phase approach to unsupervised segmentation of tumor areas in breast cancer histology images. Journal of Pathology Informatics 4(2) (2013)
12. Sirinukunwattana, K., Khan, A.M., Rajpoot, N.: Cell Words: Modelling the visual appearance of cells in histopathology images. In: Computerized Medical Imaging and Graphics (2014)
13. Khan, A.M., Mohammed, A.F., Al-Hajri, S.A., Shamari, H.M.A., Qidwai, U., Mujeeb, I., Rajpoot, N.M.: A novel system for scoring of hormone receptors in breast cancer histopathology slides. In: 2014 Middle East Conference on Biomedical Engineering (MECBME), pp. 155–158. IEEE (2014)

A Constrained Regression Forests Solution to 3D Fetal Ultrasound Plane Localization for Longitudinal Analysis of Brain Growth and Maturation

Mohammad Yaqub[1], Anil Kopuri[2,3], Sylvia Rueda[1], Peter B. Sullivan[2], Kenneth McCormick[2,3], and J. Alison Noble[1]

[1] Institute of Biomedical Engineering, Department of Engineering Science, University of Oxford, UK
[2] Department of Paediatrics, University of Oxford, Oxford, UK
[3] Neonatal Unit, John Radcliffe Hospital, Oxford, UK

Abstract. This paper develops a novel approach to find the plane in a 3D fetal ultrasound scan which corresponds to the 2D diagnostic plane used in cranial ultrasound of a neonate to allow image-based biomarkers to be tracked from pre-birth through the first weeks of post-birth life. We propose a method based on regression forests (RF) with important algorithm design considerations taken into account to provide an accurate plane-finding solution. Specifically, the new method constrains the RF method by 1) using informative voxels and voxel informative strength as a weighting within the training stage objective function u, and 2) introducing regularization of the RF by proposing a geometrical feature within the training stage. Results on clinical data indicate that the new automated method is more reproducible than manual plane finding.

Keywords: Ultrasound, Regression Forests, Fetal Brain, Localization.

1 Introduction

Longitudinal analysis of the developing brain is an emerging area of medical image computing and neurology. This may have a potential impact on clinical management of premature infants and neonates with neurological conditions. Most research has considered MRI solutions because of the exquisite level of anatomical detail seen, and possibly the wider availability of MRI from clinical neurology research versus ultrasound. However, ultrasound is the imaging modality most widely used in hospitals to screen for fetal and neonatal neurological abnormalities. The cot-side utility of ultrasound, ease of obtaining imaging, widespread availability of equipment and potential cost benefits combined with advances in medical image computing make it an ideal imaging modality to follow neurodevelopment during early life.

Clinicians are exploring tools to track the changes in image-based biomarkers from womb to the postnatal period [1, 2]. Motivating this paper, a recent study [1] published preliminary findings suggesting a correlation between neonatal gestational age and the thalamic area measured manually on standard 2D cranial ultrasound image of

G. Wu et al. (Eds.): MLMI 2014, LNCS 8679, pp. 109–116, 2014.
© Springer International Publishing Switzerland 2014

the parasagittal plane. Thalamic area measurements were compared with equivalent fetal markers of a normal population as a reference suggesting that this might be a clinically useful way to monitor neuro-development of a premature neonate.

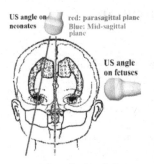 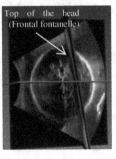 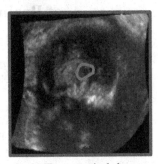

(a) Schematic description   (b) 3D visualization on 3D US   (c) The parasagittal plane

Fig. 1. Parasagittal plane from a brain. (a) Schematic of the mid-sagittal plane (*blue*), parasagittal plane (*red*), and the typical angle of acquisition in fetuses and neonates. (b) 3D visualization of the fetal brain from the coronal ultrasound view where the *red* slice corresponds to the parasagittal plane. (c) Parasagittal plane with the thalamus manually segmented (*green* contour).

For ultrasound-based longitudinal analysis across the perinatal period correlating clinical scans taken before and after birth is a challenge. Antenatal scans (for the basic examination at mid-pregnancy) are acquired in utero with either a 2D or a 3D transducer positioned to take axial slices of the fetal brain; see Fig. 1. Scans of neonates and infants are taken ex utero, with a different and normally 2D transducer positioned to image through the anterior fontanelle (AF) to provide angled coronal and sagittal planes. The question is therefore how can you correlate the two? The approach we have developed is to automatically find in a 3D fetal scan the equivalent (and non-conventional) 2D plane, called the parasagittal plane, used in neonatal neurosonography via a machine-learning approach. Detecting such a plane reliably would allow neurological information to be correlated in theory from around 14 weeks GA up to at least 8 weeks post birth or potentially 6 months depending on when the AF closes.

3D ultrasound plane finding has received some recent interest with machine learning methods proving popular and successful. A supervised learning method based on marginal space learning was developed in [3] to detect several planes in 3D echocardiography. [4] and [5] used respectively a boosting framework and regression forests (RF) to find 2, 3 and 4 chamber views in 3D echocardiography. Finally, [6] developed a machine learning method based on the Integrated Detection Network (IDN) to detect several fetal brain planes in 3D ultrasound and estimate standard clinical 2D fetal biometry parameters.

In this paper, we propose a method based on RF with important algorithm design considerations taken into account to provide an accurate parasagittal plane-finding solution. Specifically, the new technique constrains the RF method by 1) forcing the model to use informative voxels and voxel informative strength as a weight when optimizing the objective function used in the training stage, and 2) introducing regularization of the RF by proposing a geometrical feature within the training stage. The new feature uses the distance between each training point and a common reference plane (the mid-sagittal plane). We demonstrate that our approach leads to plane detection accuracies which are as good as manual plane finding and which show promise for their intended use of standardizing parasagittal plane acquisition.

2   Constrained Regression Forests for Plane Localization

2.1   Regression Forests for Plane Localization

In the training stage, a set of 3D training images with their manual planes are used to build the forest. A plane is represented as 3 parameters normal vector and 3 parameters to represent a point on the plane.   Each voxel in each 3D image is used as a training example. The perpendicular distance $d = (dx, dy, dz)$ between a voxel and the manual plane is computed [5] and used as a continuous label for each training example. Appearance features are computed within a neighborhood around each voxel. We use appearance features like voxel intensity, mean intensity within a cuboid and difference of mean intensity of two cuboids. These types of features have been successfully used in related classification and regression forest applications and showed promising results [5, 7, 8].

2.2   Constrained RF via the Use of Informative Examples

During RF training on image volumes, millions of features need to be computed on typically millions of examples (voxels in our case). RF is responsible for finding the best set of features to build each tree. Although many of the training examples are non-informative, RF treats all training examples equally during training. Here we propose a technique which locates the informative voxels within a 3D image and uses their strength to weight their contribution during tree training. We present a solution to overcome a common problem observed in machine learning in ultrasound of otherwise generating a sub-optimal RF because of the existence of many non-informative voxels.

An informative voxel is a voxel which is discriminative within its neighborhood. Here we use Feature Asymmetry (FA) to highlight informative voxels motivated by its successful application to 3D echo feature enhancement and detection, e.g. [9, 10]. FA computes the step edge strength at a specific voxel and provides a value in the range [0, 1], thus providing directly a measure of strength at a specific voxel. The region-of-interest (ROI) highlighted in red in Fig. 2 shows an area with speckle texture while the ROI highlighted in green shows an area containing fetal brain structures (part of the falx). Most importantly, even within areas of apparent weak image appearance (red ROI in Fig. 2), FA identifies the voxels which may be discriminative. Fig. 2 motivates the choice of using FA measure to represent voxels informative strength.

How do we use FA in our solution? We use FA to create stronger trees during training by (1) masking out all voxels which has FA measure below a specific threshold and (2) using the FA value to weight the importance of each training example when finding a splitting score in a tree node.

The traditional function that is optimized is

$$\arg\min \; error = \sum_{p \in S}(z - \bar{z})^2 - \sum_{i \in \{L,R\}} \sum_{p \in S^i}(z - \bar{z})^2, \qquad (1)$$

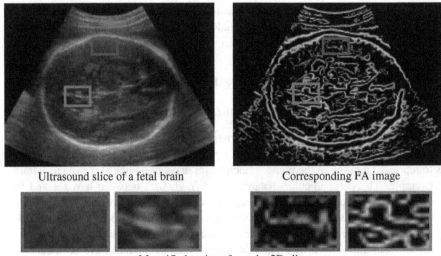

Ultrasound slice of a fetal brain   Corresponding FA image

Magnified regions from the 2D slices

Fig. 2. Localization of informative voxels. Red is a region with little informative voxels while green is a region with highly informative voxels

where z is the variable that defines the optimal split of a training set. Instead we normalize the traditional variable by the FA measure i.e. $z' = \frac{z}{FA}$. Note that we divide rather than multiple since we are minimizing an objective function. We find the best split of a training set S (p is a training point) to left (L) and right (R), denoted (S_L and S_R). $\bar{z}$ is the mean value of z for all training points reaching a specific tree node.

2.3   Constrained RF via Distance to Mid-Sagittal Plane

The use of appearance features within RF creates a learner which works well if image appearance is clear and not ambiguous. However, in ultrasound imaging this is not always the case as previously discussed. To address this issue we introduce a geometric constraint expressed as a distance feature to help constrain RF training. This feature type imbeds the perpendicular distance between the voxel of interest and the mid-sagittal plane. Given the mid-sagittal plane normal $n=(n_x, n_y, n_z)$, a point on the plane $p = (p_x, p_y, p_z)$ and a point in space $v = (v_x, v_y, v_z)$, the perpendicular distance D between v and the plane parameterized by n and p can be expressed as:

$$D = \frac{|n \cdot w|}{|n|} \qquad where \qquad w = v - p. \tag{2}$$

This feature clusters training examples depending on their distance from the mid-sagittal plane. However, this distance feature alone is not sufficient to capture the variability of plane appearance in different fetuses especially when dealing with different gestational ages. Therefore, it is important to incorporate both appearance and distance features inside the RF and to let the optimization of the objective function choose a feature at a specific depth depending on its ability to split the training points properly.

2.4   Localizing the Parasagittal Plane

In the testing stage, the informative voxels in a test image traverse the trees until each voxel ends up in a leaf. Only voxels that reach confident leaves are allowed to vote for the output plane parameters. The confidence level is measured using the variance of the training examples that reached a specific leaf during training. The mean parameters of all informative voxels reaching confident leaves are used to output the final plane parameters by fitting a mean plane which represents the estimated parasagittal plane position.

3   Experiments

3.1   Dataset

87 3D ultrasounds of the fetal brain between 23 and 27 weeks of gestation were acquired on a Philips HD9 ultrasound machine from 45 normal fetuses[1]. These fetal brain volumes were not acquired specifically for our study but for biometry so were not optimized by any means to our application.

For each volume, the parasagittal plane was manually identified twice by an experienced clinician. To minimize bias, the two manual measurements were performed a month apart. The mid-sagittal planes were also manually located by the clinician to help build the constrained RF. The Thalamic Area (TA) was measured manually on the second manual plane which was the one also used in training, and on automatically detected planes to investigate TA measurement accuracy.

3.2   Validation

To validate the accuracy of parasagittal plane-finding, two validation metrics were used. The first is the angular distance between the manual and the detected planes defined as

$$\theta = cos^{-1} \frac{n_m . n_d}{|n_m||n_d|} \tag{3}$$

where n_m is the normal to the manually defined plane and n_d is the normal to the automatically found plane. The angular distance provides insight into how close two planes are in 3D space but does not take into consideration their line of intersection - two planes may have a small angle between them but their intersection be far outside the brain which means the error in diagnostic plane finding is large. To circumvent this problem, we include, as a second validation metric, the Euclidian distance

---

[1] Fetal images are from the Intergrowth-21st study (http://www.intergrowth21.org.uk/)

between the centers of the manual and the automatic planes. Since the fetal brain will appear approximately in the middle of the volume in most cases (given this requirement is part of the scanning protocol), the distance metric expresses how far the middle of the two planes are from each other. The smaller the distance and angle the better the accuracy.

We report 5 comparisons: 1) manual-to-manual plane agreement; 2) manual-to-automatic plane agreement with the RF trained on appearance features only; 3) manual-to-automatic plane agreement using the RF trained on appearance features only but constrained by the use of informative voxels (CRF-FA); 4) manual-to-semi-automatic plane agreement using RF trained on all examples but constrained by distance features (CRF-Dist); and 5) manual-to-semi-automatic plane agreement using RF constrained by the use of informative voxels and distance features (CRF-FA-Dist).

3.3   Implementation Details

We split the 87 volumes into 44 for training and 43 for testing such that no two volumes of the same fetus exist in both sets. In all experiments we optimized the method parameters on the classic RF and fixed them for the proposed RFs to allow a fair comparison. We used 10 trees with a maximum depth 18. We optimized 300 candidate features during node creation. The FA threshold we used is 0.1 to allow as much as possible informative voxels during the training stage. In addition, when comparing multiple thresholds, visual inspection showed that the chosen threshold provides a suitable spread of voxels in different images. This implies informative voxels from all over the volume are selected during the training and testing stages. We used the 3D Gaussian derivative as a filter to compute FA and we experimentally set its Sigma to 4. Finally, we used the C# language to build the methods in a parallel fashion.

4   Results

In our parallel implementation, training time was approximately 6 days while testing a new volume took under 3 seconds. However, optimizing the technique was performed on a smaller set of training examples to tune the different parameters. Visual demonstration of the detected plane on a typical volume using the different proposed variation of the method is shown in Fig. 3. We found that the distance constraint feature is more discriminating towards the top of the tree and was found to be used in approximately 30% of all feature decisions. In Table 1 we report distances (mm) and angles (degree) for the different planes. The results shown are separated by gestational age where we also report the number of volumes used at each gestation. Note how distance and angles in 24 weeks are higher. This is possibly because of the existence of a small number of images; notice the second row in in Table 1 which represents the number of training / testing images in each gestational age. The classic RF has larger errors (distance & angle) than the manual agreement. However, using the informative voxels in RF (CRF-FA) slightly improves the agreement with the manual reference. The use of the mid-sagittal plane constraint (CRF-Dist) allows RF to provide errors smaller than in the manual agreement. Ultimately, RF with the use of informative voxels constrained by the mid-sagittal plane (CRF-FA-Dist) provides better agreement with manual than manual-manual agreement. Additionally, by looking at the standard deviation of the distances and angles in Table 1, the parasagittal plane found manually or using the classic RF is highly inconsistent. However, the three proposed RFs offer a more consistent and reproducible planes than those obtained manually.

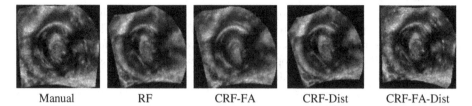

| Manual | RF | CRF-FA | CRF-Dist | CRF-FA-Dist |

Fig. 3. Visual comparisons of the detected plane from all methods for the same volume.

Table 1. Mean ± standard deviation of angles and distances between two planes. We report these between the two manual planes, manual and the detected planes using RF, manual and the detected planes using CRF-FA, manual and the detected planes using the CRF-Dist, and manual and the detected planes using the CRF-FA-Dist.

	GA Weeks	23	24	25	26	27	All
	# training/testing	9 / 9	5 / 5	8 / 8	11 / 11	11 / 10	44 / 43
Angles (degree)	Manual vs Manual	12.1°± 9.6	13.2°±12.4	11.7°±9.8	13.7°±9.4	12.2°±9.3	12.6°±9.8
	Manual vs RF	12.7°±2.9	17.0°±9.9	15.5°±7.2	15.3°±8.7	16.3°±5.1	15.2°±6.5
	Manual vs CRF-FA	10.2°±5.7	14.5°±8.9	11.8°±8.1	12.1°±7.2	12.4°±6.0	12.0°±6.9
	Manual vs CRF-Dist	6.4°±3.7	15.9°±5.9	10.8°±6.0	10.1°±5.2	11.9°±4.8	10.6°±5.0
	Manual vs CRF-FA-Dist	**6.1°±3.4**	**12.4°±4.7**	**9.0°±5.6**	**8.1°±3.9**	**10.6°±4.2**	**9.0°±4.3**
Distance (mm)	Manual vs Manual	8.3±7	8.2±6.2	9.6±7.2	10.3±8.4	10.7±9.1	9.6±7.8
	Manual vs RF	10.1±1.9	10±2.1	9.5±2.1	11.5±2.6	12±2.4	10.8±2.3
	Manual vs CRF-FA	8.9±1.7	10.5±2.7	9.6±2.5	10.7±2.3	11.9±2.9	10.4±2.4
	Manual vs CRF-Dist	8.2±1.8	9.3±1.8	9±1.8	10.2±1.3	11.5±3.1	9.8±2.0
	Manual vs CRF-FA-Dist	**6.0±2.5**	**8.5±5.1**	**7.5±3.0**	**9.3±2.6**	**9.7±3.2**	**8.3±3.1**

5   Discussion and Conclusion

In this paper, we have developed a novel plane-finding solution for 3D fetal brain ultrasound. The plane is clinically important to locate because the TA measurement on this plane showed to correlate well with gestational age which could also help monitor neuro-development of a neonate, especially in preterm infants [1]. The clinical validation of this tool for estimating TA is an ongoing work. The solution we proposed constrains the RF technique by the use of informative voxels during training and with a new feature which regularizes RF through the use of distance to a reference plane. Although the CRF-Dist and CRF-FA-Dist methods provide a better agreement with a manual reference than manual-manual agreement, they are semi-automatic approaches requiring the mid-sagittal plane as an input. However, the mid-sagittal plane is a much easier plane to find within a 3D ultrasound of a fetal brain and will be automated in future work. On the other hand, the RF and CRF-FA methods are fully automatic. It turns out that the CRF-FA-Dist provides the best agreement with the manual reference.

Although this technique is developed to solve a specific plane finding problem, it is applicable to other plane finding problems which suffer from a significant amount of non-informative training examples and possibly have a common reference plane or even a structure of interest. The proposed technique was developed for 3D ultrasound images but it is also applicable to other medical imaging modalities.

References

[1] Kopuri, A., Yaqub, M., Rueda, S., Sullivan, P., McCormick, K., Noble, A.: Cranial Ultrasound derived 'Thalamic Area' as a marker for brain growth in premature infants and comparison with similar markers from a normal fetal population. PAS ASPR (2014)

[2] Ball, G., Boardman, J.P., Rueckert, D., Aljabar, P., Arichi, T., Merchant, N., Gousias, I.S., Edwards, A.D., Counsell, S.J.: The Effect of Preterm Birth on Thalamic and Cortical Development. Cerebral Cortex 22, 1016–1024 (2012)

[3] Xiaoguang, L., Georgescu, B., Yefeng, Z., Otsuki, J., Comaniciu, D.: AutoMPR: Automatic detection of standard planes in 3D echocardiography. In: ISBI, pp. 1279–1282 (2008)

[4] Domingos, J., Lima, E., Leeson, P., Noble, J.A.: Local Phase-Based Fast Ray Features for Automatic Left Ventricle Apical View Detectionin 3D Echocardiograph. In: Menze, B., Langs, G., Montillo, A., Kelm, M., Müller, H., Tu, Z. (eds.) MCV 2013. LNCS, vol. 8331, pp. 119–129. Springer, Heidelberg (2013)

[5] Chykeyuk, K., Yaqub, M., Noble, J.A.: Class-specific regression random forest for accurate extraction of standard planes from 3D echocardiography. In: Menze, B., Langs, G., Montillo, A., Kelm, M., Müller, H., Tu, Z. (eds.) MCV 2013. LNCS, vol. 8331, pp. 53–62. Springer, Heidelberg (2013)

[6] Sofka, M., Zhang, J., Good, S., Zhou, S., Comaniciu, D.: Automatic Detection and Measurement of Structures in Fetal Head Ultrasound Volumes Using Sequential Estimation and Integrated Detection Network (IDN). IEEE Transactions on Medical Imaging 33(5), 1054–1070 (2014)

[7] Criminisi, A., Shotton, J., Robertson, D., Konukoglu, E.: Regression Forests for Efficient Anatomy Detection and Localization in CT Studies. In: Menze, B., Langs, G., Tu, Z., Criminisi, A. (eds.) MICCAI 2010 Workshop MCV. LNCS, vol. 6533, pp. 106–117. Springer, Heidelberg (2011)

[8] Yaqub, M., Javaid, M.K., Cooper, C., Noble, J.A.: Investigation of the Role of Feature Selection and Weighted Voting in Random Forests for 3-D Volumetric Segmentation. IEEE Transactions on Medical Imaging 33(2), 258–271 (2014)

[9] Grau, V., Becher, H., Noble, J.A.: Phase-based registration of multi-view real-time three-dimensional echocardiographic sequences. In: Larsen, R., Nielsen, M., Sporring, J. (eds.) MICCAI 2006. LNCS, vol. 4190, pp. 612–619. Springer, Heidelberg (2006)

[10] Rajpoot, K., Noble, A., Grau, V., Rajpoot, N.: Feature detection from echocardiographic images using local phase information. In: Medical Image Understanding and Analysis (2008)

Deep Learning of Image Features from Unlabeled Data for Multiple Sclerosis Lesion Segmentation

Youngjin Yoo[1,2,3], Tom Brosch[1,2,3], Anthony Traboulsee[3],
David K.B. Li[3,4], and Roger Tam[2,3,4]

[1] Department of Electrical and Computer Engineering
[2] Biomedical Engineering Program
[3] Division of Neurology
[4] Department of Radiology,
University of British Columbia, Vancouver, BC, Canada

Abstract. A new automatic method for multiple sclerosis (MS) lesion segmentation in multi-channel 3D MR images is presented. The main novelty of the method is that it learns the spatial image features needed for training a supervised classifier entirely from unlabeled data. This is in contrast to other current supervised methods, which typically require the user to preselect or design the features to be used. Our method can learn an extensive set of image features with minimal user effort and bias. In addition, by separating the feature learning from the classifier training that uses labeled (pre-segmented data), the feature learning can take advantage of the typically much more available unlabeled data. Our method uses deep learning for feature learning and a random forest for supervised classification, but potentially any supervised classifier can be used. Quantitative validation is carried out using 1450 T2-weighted and PD-weighted pairs of MRIs of MS patients, with 1400 pairs used for feature learning (100 of those for labeled training), and 50 for testing. The results demonstrate that the learned features are highly competitive with hand-crafted features in terms of segmentation accuracy, and that segmentation performance increases with the amount of unlabeled data used, even when the number of labeled images is fixed.

Keywords: Multiple sclerosis lesions, MRI, machine learning, segmentation, deep learning, random forests.

1 Introduction

Multiple sclerosis (MS) is a chronic, inflammatory and demyelinating disease of the brain and spinal cord. Lesions are a hallmark of MS pathology, and are primarily visible in white matter (WM) on conventional magnetic resonance imaging (MRI) scans. Manual segmentation by expert users is a common way to determine the extent of MS lesions, which is a time-consuming task and can suffer from intra- and inter-expert variability. Automatic segmentation is an attractive alternative, but it is a challenging task and remains an open problem [1].

G. Wu et al. (Eds.): MLMI 2014, LNCS 8679, pp. 117–124, 2014.
© Springer International Publishing Switzerland 2014

Many automatic approaches have been proposed over the last two decades and they have two main categories: supervised and unsupervised. Supervised methods learn from training images previously segmented, and use user-selected image features to discriminate between lesions and healthy tissue (e.g. [2]). The availability of representative labeled images and the choice of image features are important considerations and may be difficult to optimize. Some methods use a very large starting set of features and select the more discriminative ones through labeled training (e.g. [3]). Unsupervised methods do not require labeled training data, but instead typically use an intensity clustering method to model tissue distributions and rely on expert's a priori knowledge of MRI and anatomy to reduce false positives (e.g. [4]). While both supervised and unsupervised approaches have had some success, supervised methods that can automatically learn useful spatial features from unlabeled images are an attractive alternative that remains under-investigated. The amount of unlabeled data typically far exceeds that of labeled data, and using a large database to build a feature set has the potential to improve robustness and generalizability over current supervised methods.

We present a new method for automatic learning, from unlabeled images, image features for MS lesion segmentation. We train our model on a large batch of unlabeled images to identify common patterns, then add labels to a subset of the training images so that the features and labels can be used in a supervised learning method to perform the segmentation. To our knowledge, this is the first attempt to automatically learn discriminative 3D image features from unlabeled images for MS lesion segmentation. Previous papers have proposed advanced feature selection methods, such as those based on modifications of random forests [5,6], but the features were still pre-determined and filtered using relatively small sets of labeled data to identify the more discriminative features. The main difference is that our method automatically learns data-driven features from unlabeled images without the potential bias of predefined features or those learned from labeled data. This allows large data sets to be used to generate broadly representative feature sets. We show that the learned features enable segmentation performance that is competitive with hand-crafted features, and that increasing the amount of unlabeled data improves segmentation performance, even when the amount of labeled data is fixed.

2   Materials and Methods

Our data set consists of the image data from 581 MS patients scanned at multiple time points. The total number of cases, where a case consists of a pair of T2-weighted and proton density (PD) weighted scans, is 1450. Each T2/PD pair was acquired using a dual-echo MR sequence so they are inherently co-registered. The data set was collected from 48 sites, each using a different scanner, as part of a clinical trial in MS. All the images have the same resolution, $256 \times 256 \times 50$, and the same voxel size, $0.936 \times 0.936 \times 3.000$ mm^3. We divided the data set into independent training and test sets. The training set consists of 1400 cases

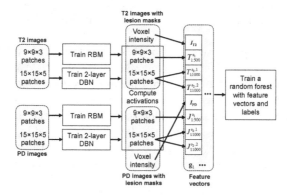

Fig. 1. A training algorithm for our MS lesion segmentation framework. A large number of unlabeled images and a smaller number of labeled images are used in a deep learning framework to generate the feature vectors used to train a random forest classifier.

from 531 patients and the test set contains 50 cases from 50 patients. Within the training set, 100 cases from 100 patients have expert segmentations that we used for supervised training. For preprocessing, N3 inhomogeneity correction [7] is first applied. Then, the entire set of T2-weighted (and independently, PD-weighted) images are intensity-normalized to produce a mean of 0 and a standard deviation of 1. Skull-stripping is then performed with the brain extraction tool [8].

2.1   Algorithm Overview

Our algorithm for learning image features from unlabeled data is built using restricted Boltzmann machines (RBMs), which are two-layer, undirected networks each consisting of a visible layer and a hidden layer, where the activations of the hidden units capture patterns in the visible units. RBMs can be stacked to form a deep belief network (DBN) for learning more abstract features. Our model (Fig. 1) consists of two RBMs, one for the T2 images, the other for the PD images, that learn smaller-scale features. In addition, two DBNs are used, again separately for the T2 and PD images, to learn larger-scale features. After training with unlabeled data, the model can be used to identify, in a probabilistic sense, the learned features in any given image. The model is then applied to a subset of the training data that has lesion labels. Any of the learned features found are then fed, along with the labels, into a random forest, which is used to build a voxel-wise probabilistic classifier to find lesion voxels in unseen images.

2.2   Unsupervised Feature Learning Using RBMs and Deep Learning

To target features at different scales, we extract image patches of two different sizes at the same locations from each image. To make feature learning on large batches of data feasible, we extract 100 uniformly spaced and non-overlapping patches at each scale, and set those patches as a mini-batch. The spacing and patch sizes allow complete coverage of the whole brain in most images. For the smaller scale, we use a patch size of $9 \times 9 \times 3$, and convert the image values to one-dimensional vectors $\mathbf{v}_1, \ldots, \mathbf{v}_{100} \in \mathbb{R}^D$ with $D = 243$. For the larger scale features, we use a 3D patch size of $15 \times 15 \times 5$ for $D = 1125$. We learn features from each 3D image patch using a Gaussian-Bernoulli RBM model [9] with a set of binary hidden random units $\mathbf{h}$ of dimension K ($K = 500$ for the smaller scale, 1000 for the larger scale), a set of real-valued visible random units $\mathbf{v}$ of dimension D ($D = 243$ for the smaller scale, 1125 for the larger scale), and symmetric connections between these two layers represented by a weight matrix $W \in \mathbb{R}^{D \times K}$. We follow a published guide [10] for choosing the number of hidden units to avoid severe overfitting. We minimize the energy function [9]:

$$E(\mathbf{v}, \mathbf{h}) = \frac{1}{2} \sum_{i=1}^{D} (v_i - c_i)^2 - \sum_{j=1}^{K} b_j h_j - \sum_{i=1}^{D} \sum_{j=1}^{K} v_i W_{ij} h_j, \qquad (1)$$

where b_j are hidden unit biases ($\mathbf{b} \in \mathbb{R}^K$) and c_i are visible unit biases ($\mathbf{c} \in \mathbb{R}^D$). The units of a binary hidden layer (conditioned on the visible layer) are independent Bernoulli random variables $P(h_j = 1 | \mathbf{v}) = \sigma\left(\sum_i W_{ij} v_i + b_j\right)$, where $\sigma(s) = \frac{1}{1+\exp(-s)}$ is the sigmoid function. The visible units (conditioned on the hidden layer) are independent Gaussians with diagonal covariance $P(v_i | \mathbf{h}) = \mathcal{N}\left(\sum_j W_{ij} h_j + c_i, 1\right)$. We perform the contrast divergence approximation [11] to update the weights and biases during training. In order to capture a higher-level representation of local brain structures, another layer of hidden units is stacked on top of the larger scale RBM to form a deep belief network. Hinton *et al.* [11] showed that greedily training each pair of layers (from lowest to highest) as an individual RBM using the previous layer's activations as input is an efficient approach for training DBNs. Our DBN has a layer of real-valued visible units $\mathbf{v}$ of dimension $D = 1125$ and two layers of $K = 1000$ binary hidden units $\mathbf{h}$.

2.3   Feature Vector Construction for Supervised Learning

To train a random forest, we use the labeled set of training images and construct feature vectors computed by applying our trained RBM/DBN model to 200 image patches within the lesion mask and 3800 image patches from normal-appearing tissue in each T2 and PD image. The patches are extracted in the same way described above. The activations of the RBM/DBN model represent the strength of the learned features present in the labeled images. We define $\mathbf{x}$ as a voxel location and let $\mathbf{v}_{s_1}(\mathbf{x})$ represent a one-dimensional vector reformatted from a 3D image patch of size $9 \times 9 \times 3$ centered at $\mathbf{x}$. We define $\mathbf{v}_{s_2}(\mathbf{x})$ as an one-dimensional vector reformatted from a 3D image patch of size $15 \times 15 \times 5$ centered at $\mathbf{x}$. We let $I_{\text{T2}}(\mathbf{x})$ and $I_{\text{PD}}(\mathbf{x})$ represent intensity values at a voxel position $\mathbf{x}$ of a T2 image and a PD image, respectively. A feature vector $\mathbf{g} \in \mathbb{R}^L$ with $L = 5002$ is constructed for a given voxel in a pair of T2/PD images by concatenating the intensity values and activations of the learned features:

$$\mathbf{g}(\mathbf{x}) = \{I_{\text{T2}}(\mathbf{x}), T_{1:500}^{s_1}(\mathbf{v}_{s_1}(\mathbf{x})), T_{1:1000}^{s_2,1}(\mathbf{v}_{s_2}(\mathbf{x})), T_{1:1000}^{s_2,2}(\mathbf{v}_{s_2}(\mathbf{x})),$$
$$I_{\text{PD}}(\mathbf{x}), J_{1:500}^{s_1}(\mathbf{v}_{s_1}(\mathbf{x})), J_{1:1000}^{s_2,1}(\mathbf{v}_{s_2}(\mathbf{x})), J_{1:1000}^{s_2,2}(\mathbf{v}_{s_2}(\mathbf{x}))\}, \tag{2}$$

where $T_k^{s_1}$ is an activation of the k-th hidden unit from the trained RBM when the image patch $\mathbf{v}_{s_1}(\mathbf{x})$ from the T2 image is used as input. Similarly, $T_k^{s_2,n}$ is an activation of the k-th hidden unit of the n-th layer from the trained DBN when the image patch $\mathbf{v}_{s_2}(\mathbf{x})$ from the T2 image is used as input. $J_k^{s_1}$ and $J_k^{s_2,n}$ are the analogous activations calculated from the PD image.

2.4   Random Forest Training and Prediction

We have chosen to use a random forest [12] for supervised classification because random forests have been successfully used for MS lesion segmentation using hand-crafted features [2], and because random forests are able to provide information on the relative importance of the features used. We construct a random forest consisting of 30 randomized binary decision trees with a maximum depth of 20. We use the same structure for the random forest as used for previous work [2] in MS lesion segmentation, which may not necessarily be optimal for our learned features, but should be sufficient for a proof-of-concept. As described above, we collect feature vectors from image patches inside and outside of the lesion mask of each labeled image. The information gain is used to measure the quality of a split. To segment the lesions in a new image, a feature vector for each voxel is computed using (2) and voxel-wise classification is performed by propagating the computed feature vectors through all the trees by successive application of the relevant binary tests. The final posterior probability is estimated by averaging the posteriors from every leaf node in all trees.

3   Experiments and Results

To evaluate the segmentation performance using the automatically learned features, we used a validation procedure in which we varied the amount of unlabeled data (100, 400, 700, 1000, and 1400 cases) used for training the RBMs and DBNs, while keeping the labeled (100 cases) and test images (50 cases) the same, and compared the automatic probabilistic segmentations to the binary segmentations by the experts. The parameters for training the RBMs and DBNs were kept consistent for all experiments. We used three measures for comparing segmentations: the Dice similarity coefficient (DSC), the true positive rate (TPR) and the positive predictive value (PPV) [1,13]. To produce binary segmentations, we thresholded the probabilistic segmentations using a visually derived value of 0.4. Since relative segmentation accuracy generally increases with lesion load, we stratified the cases into 5 lesion load categories for interpreting the results. An example of a segmentation result with a larger lesion load is shown in Fig. 2.

Table 1 summarizes the segmentation performance as measured by the DSC. For all of the lesion load categories, there is an apparent trend toward greater accuracy with an increase in the number of unlabeled training images. The improvement is monotonic up to 700 cases, except for a slight aberration in the

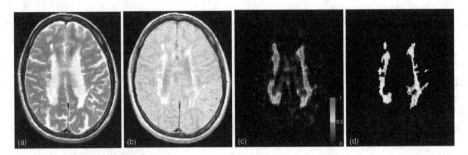

Fig. 2. Probabilistic segmentation example. (a) T2 input image, (b) PD input image, (c) probabilistic segmentation result, (d) ground truth. DSC = 73.15%.

Table 1. DSC results (%) calculated on 50 T2/PD test pairs. Ten T2/PD pairs were used for each lesion load range and average scores were computed. The number of unlabeled images used for feature learning was varied, while the supervised training set was fixed at 100 T2/PD pairs. There is an apparent trend toward improved accuracy with a greater number of unlabeled training images.

Number of cases (number of patients)	Lesion load ($1000 \times mm^3$)				
	0.0-4.0	4.0-7.8	7.8-14.7	14.7-28.5	28.5+
100 (45)	12.8	32.7	45.2	51.2	51.4
400 (152)	12.1	34.2	48.1	54.8	55.3
700 (264)	12.8	35.5	49.0	**56.3**	**56.5**
1000 (384)	12.2	34.2	47.8	55.1	55.8
1400 (532)	**14.0**	**36.2**	**49.6**	55.7	55.4

lowest lesion load category. However, in all categories, the DSC decreased slightly when using 1000 cases as compared to 700 cases. This may be a problem arising from some unusual similarities between some of the 700 unlabeled cases, the labeled cases, and test images, leading to over-fitting, which may be determined by further experiments with multiple randomizations.

To compare fairly with other state-of-the-art methods [2,13,14], we selected 38 cases from our test set so that the range in lesion load (128 mm^3 to 20695 mm^3) is similar to that of the data set used for evaluation in [2,13,14] (105 mm^3 to 22542 mm^3). Table 2 shows the performance statistics for the other methods and our own, using the features learned from 1400 cases, and demonstrates that our method is highly competitive in accuracy, although the use of different data sets only allows for an indirect comparison. The lower PPV value suggests that our model appears to under-segment the lesions compared to the other methods.

Finally, we examined the training results of the random forest to determine which sets of features (intensity, RBM, DBN first layer, DBN second layer), and which MR channel were the most important. Table 3 shows the relative discriminative power of each category of features as represented by the percentage of nodes in which the category of features was selected by the random forest. These results suggest that spatial features were much more important (96.9%) than intensity features (3.1%) for distinguishing between lesion and non-lesion

Table 2. Average TPR/PPV/DSC results (%). Our method is compared to three state-of-the-art methods (2008: Souplet [14], 2011: Geremia [2], 2013: Weiss [13]). Note that DSC measures were not available in [14,2], and our data set was different which only allows for an indirect comparison.

Souplet [14]		Geremia [2]		Weiss [13]			Our Method		
TPR	PPV	TPR	PPV	TPR	PPV	DSC	TPR	PPV	DSC
19 ± 14	30 ± 16	39 ± 18	40 ± 20	33 ± 18	37 ± 19	29 ± 13	58 ± 17	35 ± 24	38 ± 19

Table 3. Relative discriminative power (%) of the features used for voxel-wise classification as determined by the random forest. The percentages indicate the relative frequency each category of features was selected when training the random forest using the features learned from 1400 unlabeled cases.

T2 intensity	T2 RBM	T2 DBN Layer 1	T2 DBN Layer 2	PD intensity	PD RBM	PD DBN Layer 1	PD DBN Layer 2
1.3	14.9	17.7	19.0	1.9	14.3	15.0	16.0

voxels. The spatial features computed from the second layer of DBNs were selected slightly more often (35.0%) than those from the first layer (32.7%) and the RBMs (29.2%), but the RBM contribution still seems significant. The features learned from T2 images were selected slightly more often (51.6%) than the features learned from PD images (45.3%).

4   Conclusion and Future Work

We have presented a new MS lesion segmentation method based on automatic feature learning from unlabeled images. Using a multi-scale RBM/DBN framework, we showed that the automatically learned features can be highly competitive to hand-crafted features for subsequent use in the supervised training of random forests, and that adding more unlabeled images generally increases segmentation performance, with the main advantage that minimal manual effort is involved. The main current limitation is the high dimensionality of the feature vectors used for training the random forest, which is the reason we only used 4000 patches per labeled image. This limitation is more critical than the small number of patches used for RBM and DBN training, because much fewer labeled images are typically available. Future work would include improvements in training efficiency for the RBMs, DBNs, and random forests in order to use a greater number of sample patches for both the unsupervised and supervised stages. Another limitation is that although we have shown that increasing the amount of unlabeled training data generally increases segmentation performance, the interactions between the unlabeled, labeled, and test data are poorly characterized and deserve further investigation (for example, by varying the amount of labeled data). In addition, our model can likely be further optimized, for instance by tuning the deep learning and random forest parameters, and adding more layers to the network. Despite the limitations, we believe we have demonstrated the potential for unsupervised feature learning in MS lesion segmentation.

Acknowledgements. This work was supported by the MS/MRI Research Group at the University of British Columbia, the Natural Sciences and Engineering Research Council of Canada, the MS Society of Canada, and the Milan and Maureen Ilich Foundation.

References

1. García-Lorenzo, et al.: Review of automatic segmentation methods of multiple sclerosis white matter lesions on conventional magnetic resonance imaging. Med. Image Anal. 17(1), 1–18 (2013)
2. Geremia, E., et al.: Spatial decision forests for MS lesion segmentation in multichannel magnetic resonance images. NeuroImage 57(2), 378–390 (2011)
3. Morra, J., et al.: Automatic segmentation of MS lesions using a contextual model for the MICCAI grand challenge. In: MS Lesion Segmentation Challenge (MICCAI Workshop), pp. 1–7 (2008)
4. Shiee, N., et al.: A topology-preserving approach to the segmentation of brain images with multiple sclerosis lesions. NeuroImage 49(2), 1524–1535 (2010)
5. Montillo, A., Shotton, J., Winn, J., Iglesias, J.E., Metaxas, D., Criminisi, A.: Entangled decision forests and their application for semantic segmentation of CT images. In: Székely, G., Hahn, H.K. (eds.) IPMI 2011. LNCS, vol. 6801, pp. 184–196. Springer, Heidelberg (2011)
6. Yaqub, M., Javaid, M.K., Cooper, C., Noble, J.A.: Improving the classification accuracy of the classic RF method by intelligent feature selection and weighted voting of trees with application to medical image segmentation. In: Suzuki, K., Wang, F., Shen, D., Yan, P. (eds.) MLMI 2011. LNCS, vol. 7009, pp. 184–192. Springer, Heidelberg (2011)
7. Sled, J.G., et al.: A nonparametric method for automatic correction of intensity nonuniformity in MRI data. IEEE T. Med. Imaging 17(1), 87–97 (1998)
8. Smith, S.M.: Fast robust automated brain extraction. Human Brain Mapping 17(3), 143–155 (2002)
9. Krizhevsky, A., Hinton, G.: Learning multiple layers of features from tiny images. University of Toronto, Tech. Rep. (2009)
10. Hinton, G.: A practical guide to training restricted Boltzmann machines. University of Toronto, Tech. Rep. (2010)
11. Hinton, G., Osindero, S., Teh, Y.W.: A fast learning algorithm for deep belief nets. Neural Computation 18(7), 1527–1554 (2006)
12. Breiman, L.: Random forests. Machine Learning 45(1), 5–32 (2001)
13. Weiss, N., Rueckert, D., Rao, A.: Multiple sclerosis lesion segmentation using dictionary learning and sparse coding. In: Mori, K., Sakuma, I., Sato, Y., Barillot, C., Navab, N. (eds.) MICCAI 2013, Part I. LNCS, vol. 8149, pp. 735–742. Springer, Heidelberg (2013)
14. Souplet, J.C., et al.: An automatic segmentation of T2-FLAIR multiple sclerosis lesions. In: MS Lesion Segmentation Challenge, MICCAI Workshop (2008)

Fetal Abdominal Standard Plane Localization through Representation Learning with Knowledge Transfer

Hao Chen[1], Dong Ni[2,1,*], Xin Yang[2], Shengli Li[3], and Pheng Ann Heng[1,4]

[1] Department of Computer Science and Engineering,
The Chinese University of Hong Kong, Hong Kong SAR, China
[2] National-Regional Key Technology Engineering Laboratory for Medical
Ultrasound, School of Medicine, Shenzhen University, China
[3] Department of Ultrasound, Affiliated Shenzhen Maternal and Child Healthcare
Hospital of Nanfang Medical University, China
[4] Human Computer Interaction Research Center,
Shenzhen Institutes of Advanced Technology, Chinese Academy of Sciences, China
nidong@szu.edu.cn

Abstract. Acquisition of the fetal abdominal standard plane (FASP) is crucial for prenatal ultrasound diagnosis. However, it requires a thorough knowledge of human anatomy and substantial experience. In this paper, we propose an automatic method to localize the FASP from US images. Unlike the previous methods that consider simple low-level features such as Haar features, we exploited the deep convolutional neural network to automatically learn the latent representation. In addition, we adopted the novel knowledge transfer method to enhance the learning performance by making use of the knowledge obtained in other domain. Experimental results on 219 fetal abdomen videos showed that the classification accuracy of our method was above 90%, outperforming other methods by a significant margin.

1 Introduction

Acquisition of the fetal abdominal standard plane (FASP) is crucial for the biometric measurements and ultrasound (US) diagnosis. In clinical practice, the FASP is manually acquired in the presence of three key anatomical structures (KASs): stomach bubble (SB), umbilical vein (UV), and spine (SP) located in the region of interest (ROI) by experienced clinicians [1]. However, this process requires a thorough knowledge of human anatomy, which makes it challenging for novices and time-consuming for experts. Hence, the development of automatic methods for localizing the FASP would enhance the ability of non-experts to operate US devices and improve the examination efficiency for experts. However, this task is very challenging for several reasons. First, the FASP often has high intra-class variations due to the artifacts, deformations, different fetal postures

---

* Corresponding author.

G. Wu et al. (Eds.): MLMI 2014, LNCS 8679, pp. 125–132, 2014.

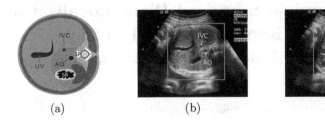

(a)   (b)   (c)

Fig. 1. (a) Fetal abdominal anatomy, (b) True FASP, (c) False FASP with similar anatomical structure GB and IC (ROI marked with green rectangle)

and scanning orientations. Second, as shown in Fig. 1, large numbers of regions, e.g. shadows, abdominal aorta (AO), gall bladder(GB), intestinal canal(IC) and inferior vena cava (IVC), often carry similar appearance to the KASs.

A few recent studies have contributed to the automatic localization of standard planes from 2D US images. Zhang et al. [2] proposed to select standard planes of gestational sac from US videos based on cascade AdaBoost classifier. Kwitt et al. [3] presented a kernel dynamic texture (KDT) model to localize target structures from US videos acquired from phantoms. Yang et al. [4] proposed a radial component-based detection (RCD) framework to identify FASP by incorporating the prior geometric knowledge into the detection procedure.

Although previous researchers presented their efficacy in localizing standard planes from 2D US images, the main limitation of previous works was that they considered only simple low-level features such as Haar features by observation and experiences. Recently, there was a surge interest of deep neural networks which achieved great success in object recognition with expressive power for feature representation [5]. Instead of manually designing a feature detector according to different task-specific problems, the latent representation learned from deep neural networks can better re-apply to generic tasks across different domains [6]. Another limitation of previous works was that the relatively insufficient training data sets in medical domain may lead to the overfitting problem and degrade the learning performance. Knowledge transfer has been proved to address this problem and improve the performance of learning in one domain of interest by making use of the knowledge obtained in another domain [7].

Motivated by the recent works [5,6], we exploited the deep learning method to learn the powerful and discriminative features automatically. Specifically, the supervised deep convolutional neural network (DCNN) implemented by the Caffe framework [8] was utilized to train a robust classifier for the localization of FASP from 2D US images. DCNN trained on large auxiliary data could disentangle various factors accounting for recognition and help to initialize the parameters of fine tuning, we combined the knowledge transfer into our framework. To our best knowledge, this is the first work that considers deep learning for the localization of standard planes from US images. Our experimental results on 219 videos prove the effectiveness of the proposed methods.

2   Methods

The pipeline of the proposed method is shown in Fig. 2. First, the DCNN classifier was trained on the labelled ROIs extracted from the training images. Second, given a test image, the probability map p was produced by the model averaging technique. The probability map was further smoothed by bilateral filter for outlier elimination. Finally, the test image was classified as a FASP when the score generated by performing the non-max suppression on the smoothed probability map is larger than one threshold value.

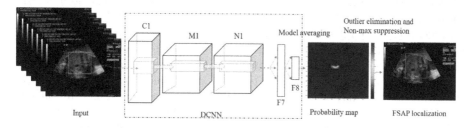

Fig. 2. The pipeline of the proposed method

2.1   The Architecture of DCNN

A DCNN is a feed-forward neural network comprised of several pairs of convolutional, max-pooling and normalization layers, followed by several fully connected layers. Due to the limited number of medical training data, we first transferred the model trained on ImageNet [8] into our DCNN architecture and subsequently refined this model according to our specific task. The DCNN architecture used in this paper is shown in Table 1 (activation, padding and dropout layers are

Table 1. Architecture of the deep neural network

Layer	Feature maps	Kernel size	Stride	Group
input	227x227x3	-	-	-
C1	55x55x96	11	4	-
M1	27x27x96	3	2	-
N1	27x27x96	5	-	-
C2	27x27x256	5	-	2
M2	13x13x256	3	2	-
N2	13x13x256	5	-	-
C3	13x13x384	3	-	-
C4	13x13x384	3	-	2
C5	13x13x256	3	-	2
M5	6x6x256	3	2	-
F6	1024	-	-	-
F7	256	-	-	-
F8	2	-	-	-

not shown). The convolution layers (C) connect the local receptive field of the former layer, the max-pooling layers (M) partition the reception field into non-overlapping regions and output the maximum value, and the response normalization layers (N) prevent the neurons from saturating. F represents the fully connected layer. The final layer is the output layer with softmax function for classifying.

2.2   DCNN Fine Tuning with Knowledge Transfer

Although the deep neural network has the advantages of learning the powerful feature representations, with limited training data in medical domain, fully-supervised deep architectures will generally overfit the training data and thus degrade the learning performance. Previous studies [6,9] have indicated that the pre-trained model in other domain could well initialize the training of the DCNN in one domain of interest. But how to adapt it into medical applications with knowledge transfer hasn't been well exploited. In this paper, we first initialized the parameters of the DCNN layers using the pre-trained model. This process can be seen as a supervised pre-training prior, which disentangled variation factors for our specific task of FASP localization. Then the DCNN was further fine tuned on the training data in a supervised way using the softmax regression method defined in Eq.(1).

$$p(r = j|f) = \frac{e^{o(f_j)}}{\sum_{c=1}^{k} e^{o(f_c)}} \tag{1}$$

Where $o(f_j)$ is the output of neural network, and $p(r = j|f)$ is the predicted probability result for the jth class given the input feature vector f. Note that such fine tuning process converged much faster than the randomly initialized DCNN.

2.3   FASP Localization with Pre-trained DCNN

Given the input test image I, the probability map p was produced by the trained DCNN classifier in a sliding window way. Specifically, each sliding window was augmented by cropping the center and corners of the sliding window as well as its mirrored versions, resulting in 10 inputs to the DCNN. The final score of the sliding window was obtained by averaging the scores of these 10 inputs. Ideally, we want p to be zero everywhere except at the center of the true ROI of the FASP, but it could be noisy in practice. In this regard, p was further smoothed with a bilateral filter. Then the maximum probability value at the position C_m was calculated by performing the non-max suppression on the smoothed probability map p_s, defined in Eq.(2). If $p_s(C_m)$ was larger than the threshold value T obtained by the cross validation ($T = 0.68$ in our experiments), the test image was regarded as FASP, or non-FASP if smaller.

$$p_s(x, y) = \frac{\sum_{x_i, y_i \in \Omega} p(x_i, y_i) w_i}{\sum_{x_i, y_i \in \Omega} w_i}$$
$$w_i = f_r(||p(x_i, y_i) - p(x, y)||^2) g_s(||x_i - x||^2 + ||y_i - y||^2) \qquad (2)$$
$$C_m = \underset{x,y}{\mathrm{argmax}}\, p_s(x, y)$$

Where (x, y) is the pixel coordinate, Ω is the window centered at (x, y), f_r is the range smoothing kernel, g_s is the spatial smoothing kernel.

3 Experimental Results and Discussion

Dataset In order to train the DCNN classifier, we first generated the training samples (1911 positive and 3160 negative samples) by manually extracting the ROI of fetal abdomen from the expert-annotated US images. Note that some of the training samples were further rotated and mirrored to augment the training database. In addition, 219 videos with total 8718 US images were obtained for test by performing the conventional US sweep on the pregnant women(fetal gestational age from 18 to 40 weeks). The testing images were also manually labeled to obtain 1588 FASPs and 7130 nonFASPs for the performance evaluation by a clinical radiologist with more than five years of experience in obstetrics US. All the images and videos used in our experiments were acquired using a Siemens Acuson Sequoia 512 US scanner.

Qualitative Performance Evaluation. In order to show the feature representation power of the DCNN, we first illustrate the automatically learned features of the intermediate layers by reducing the dimensions of the features utilizing the Barnes-Hut Stochastic Neighbor Embedding(BH-SNE) method [10]. As shown in Fig. 3 (a) and (b), the low inter-class difference between FASP and non-FASP makes the classification very challenging. However, Fig. 3 (c) and (d) show that the automatically learned features with high level information make it easier to classify the FASP and nonFASP. This result visually certified our hypothesis that extracted features encoding high level information could disentangle the variation factors and benefit more to our task than using the original data. Fig. 4(a) and (b) show two typical FASPs correctly classified by our method, where the KASs including UV, SB and SP are contained. Fig. 4(e) and (f) are the corresponding probability maps of Fig. 4(a) and (b), respectively. Fig. 4(c) shows one false FASP classified by our method, due to its similar appearance with the true FASP.

Comparison of Quantitative Performance. We then compared the performance of our method on the US images and videos with the state-of-the-art method [4]. For the localization of FASP from one video, the US image of the highest score is selected as the FASP. In [4], three Random Forests Classifiers trained on Haar features were used to detect the KASs: UV, SB and SP separately. A novel radial component-based model (RCM) was incorporated in the detection procedure to improve the performance. In order to show the efficacy of

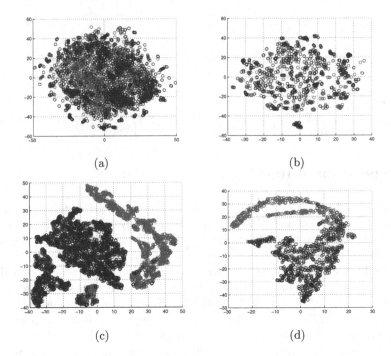

Fig. 3. Feature embedding and visualization (red and blue points represent FASP and non-FASP respectively). (a) raw training data (b) raw testing data (c) F7 layer of training data (d) F7 layer of testing data.

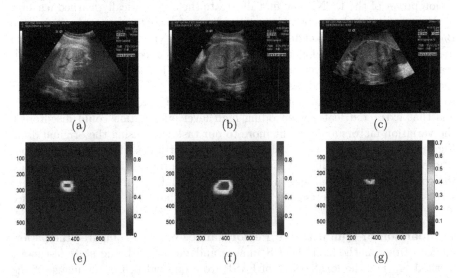

Fig. 4. Examples of FASP localization: the first row is original US images, the second row is the corresponding probability maps(the color bar indicates the probability value). (a)-(b) are the true FASPs, (c) is the false FASP.

Table 2. Results of FASP Localization in US Videos and Images

Method	Accuracy (images)	Accuracy (videos)
DCNN with pre-train	**0.910**	**0.904**
DCNN without pre-train	0.857	0.822
RCD[4]	0.775	0.762

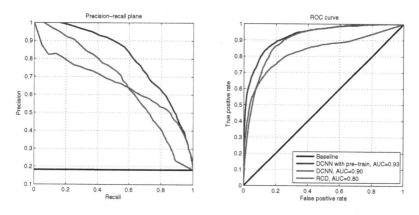

Fig. 5. Precision-recall plane (left) and ROC curve (right) of different methods

the knowledge transfer strategy employed in our method, we further compared the performance of our method with the DCNN method without using the pre-trained parameters. We computed the following performance measures: recall ($R = N_{TP}/(N_{TP} + N_{FN})$), precision ($P = N_{TP}/(N_{TP} + N_{FP})$) and accuracy ($A = (N_{TP} + N_{TN})/N$), where N_{TP}, N_{TN}, N_{FP} and N_{FN} are the number of true positives, true negatives, false positives and false negatives, respectively; N is the number of total test samples. The Precision-Recall (PR) and Receiver Operating Characteristic (ROC) curves are shown in Fig.5. Our proposed method (pre-trained DCNN) achieved the best performance and the result of the DCNN method without pre-training is better than the RCD method, which proved the efficacy of both the deep learning algorithm and the knowledge transfer method. As shown in Table 2, the classification accuracies of the pre-trained DCNN on testing images and videos are 0.910 and 0.904, respectively, which significantly outperformed the state-of-the-art method [4]. In addition, the results shown in Table 2 further demonstrated that the pre-trained DCNN with knowledge transfer outperformed the DCNN without pre-training by a large margin. It also indicates that the knowledge transferred from related domain can benefit our specific task when limited data is available.

4   Conclusions

In this paper, we proposed a deep learning based method to automatically localize the FASP from US images. This method can automatically learn the latent representation information instead of using the low-level features by observations or experiences. We further adopted the knowledge transfer method to enhance the learning performance by making use of the knowledge learned from other domain. Experimental results showed the efficacy of our method. In the future, we will apply this framework to the automatic localization of other ultrasonic standard planes.

Acknowledgement. The work described in this paper was supported in part by the National Science Foundation of China (No. 61101026 and 81270707), in part by the Shenzhen Key Basic Research Project (No. JCYJ20130329105033277 and 201101013), in part by the Shenzhen-Hong Kong Innovation Circle Funding Program (No. JSE201109150013A), in part by the Hong Kong Innovation and Technology Fund (Project No. GHP/003/11SZ), in part by Foshan and The Chinese Academy of Sciences Collaborative Project (Project No. 2012HY100631).

References

1. Ni, D., et al.: Selective search and sequential detection for standard plane localization in ultrasound. In: Yoshida, H., Warfield, S., Vannier, M.W. (eds.) Abdominal Imaging 2013. LNCS, vol. 8198, pp. 203–211. Springer, Heidelberg (2013)
2. Zhang, L., Chen, S., Chin, C.T., Wang, T., Li, S.: Intelligent scanning: Automated standard plane selection and biometric measurement of early gestational sac in routine ultrasound examination. Medical Physics 39(8), 5015–5027 (2012)
3. Kwitt, R., Vasconcelos, N., Razzaque, S., Aylward, S.: Localizing target structures in ultrasound video–a phantom study. Medical Image Analysis 17(7), 712–722 (2013)
4. Yang, X., Ni, D., Qin, J., Li, S., Wang, T., Chen, S., Heng, P.A.: Standard plane localization in ultrasound by radial component. In: ISBI (2014)
5. Krizhevsky, A., Sutskever, I., Hinton, G.E.: Imagenet classification with deep convolutional neural networks. In: NIPS, vol. 1, p. 4 (2012)
6. Donahue, J., Jia, Y., Vinyals, O., Hoffman, J., Zhang, N., Tzeng, E., Darrell, T.: Decaf: A deep convolutional activation feature for generic visual recognition. arXiv preprint arXiv:1310.1531 (2013)
7. Pan, S.J., Yang, Q.: A survey on transfer learning. IEEE Transactions on Knowledge and Data Engineering 22(10), 1345–1359 (2010)
8. Jia, Y.: Caffe: An open source convolutional architecture for fast feature embedding (2013), http://caffe.berkeleyvision.org
9. Sharif Razavian, A., Azizpour, H., Sullivan, J., Carlsson, S.: Cnn features off-the-shelf: an astounding baseline for recognition. arXiv preprint arXiv:1403.6382 (2014)
10. Maaten, L.: Barnes-hut-sne. In: Proceedings of the International Conference on Learning Representations (2013)

Searching for Structures of Interest in an Ultrasound Video Sequence

Mohammad Ali Maraci[1], Raffaele Napolitano[2],
Aris Papageorghiou[2], and J. Alison Noble[1]

[1] Institute of Biomedical Engineering, Dep. of Engineering Science,
Center for Doctoral Training, University of Oxford UK
[2] Nuffield Department of Obstetrics and Gynaecology, University of Oxford UK

Abstract. Ultrasound diagnosis and therapy is typically protocol driven but often criticized for requiring highly-skilled sonographers. However there is a shortage of highly trained sonographers worldwide, which is limiting the wider adoption of this cost-effective technology. The challenge therefore is to make the technology easier to use. We consider this problem in this paper. Our approach combines simple standardized clinical US scanning protocols (defined by our clinical partners) with machine learning driven image analysis solutions to enable a non-expert to perform ultrasound-based diagnostic tasks with minimal training. Motivated by recent work on dynamic texture analysis within the computer vision community, we have developed, and evaluated on clinical data, a framework that given a training set of Ultrasound Sweep Videos (USV), models the temporal evolution of objects of interest as a kernel dynamic texture which can form the basis of a metric for detecting structures of interest in new unseen videos. We describe the full original method, and demonstrate that it outperforms a simpler recently proposed approach on phantom data, and is significantly superior in performance on real clinical data.

1 Introduction

Compared with other imaging modalities, current advantages of ultrasound (US) including absence of adverse effects, lower cost, real-time acquisition and portability, have encouraged wide use of the technology for diagnostic and therapeutic purposes. Skilled operators are adept at both guiding the transducer to the correct diagnostic plane as well at interpreting often complex sonographic patterns. A non-expert finds both tasks hard. The medical image analysis field has worked hard to develop automated solutions to the second step (quantification). To address the former, 3D ultrasound helps to some extent in that it simplifies acquisition, but shifts the burden of finding the diagnostic plane to finding a plane in an ultrasound volume and a number of recent papers have looked at this problem e.g. [1]. Image analysis to assist in the acquisition stage for 2D scanning is a largely unexplored area, other than the recent work [2] which was developed in parallel to our own (we compare with this work later in this paper). Here the

G. Wu et al. (Eds.): MLMI 2014, LNCS 8679, pp. 133–140, 2014.
© Springer International Publishing Switzerland 2014

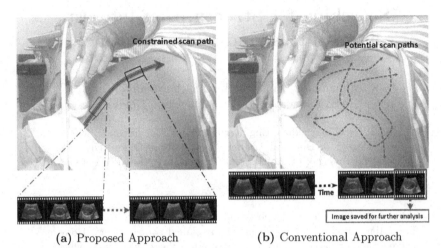

(a) Proposed Approach   (b) Conventional Approach

Fig. 1. User follows a simple scanning protocol for automated analysis to find the SOI (a). Conventional ultrasound scanning protocol where user scans over multiple paths to locate the best visual representation of the SOI where it is saved for further analysis (b).

general problem can be posed as, given an ultrasound video sweep (USV), defined by a standardized clinical protocol, identify video segments which contain the structure of interest (SOI). This approach is illustrated schematically in Fig. 1a for obstetrics scanning and compared with conventional scanning in Fig. 1b.

While this is a special case of general ultrasound use, many clinical applications in ultrasound, of which fetal biometry analysis is just one, can be defined by simplified scanning protocols which can be readily learnt by a non-expert sonographer. While the work of Kwitt et al. [2] considered a related technical approach to the one we present, it was only applied to phantom data, and was not taken through to consideration of real clinical use or evaluation. The latter is one of the contributions of our work and to our knowledge we are the first to demonstrate clinical applicability. Compared to [2], the technical contributions of this paper are to employ an extended image processing pipeline which includes a pre-processing filtering stage and a more robust distance metric, both of which turn out to be critical for good performance on clinical data.

2   Method

The steps are illustrated schematically in Fig. 2. First, the user acquires a USV following a simple and repeatable protocol, such as in Fig. 1a. The protocol used is application dependent in general (see Experimental section for the ones used in our work). USVs are then pre-processed as explained in section 2.1 to enhance acoustically significant images. Dynamic Texture model parameters are then estimated for segments of the enhanced video and a distance metric is computed to compare video segments. A classifier is then trained on the distance metric and evaluated on unseen data (we used SVM but other classifiers could have equally been used). Details of each step are given below.

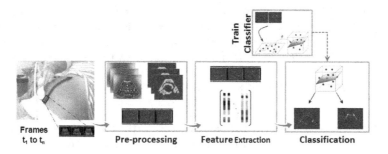

Fig. 2. First the video is filtered and divided into overlapping sub-sequences. Dynamic texture model parameters are then learnt based on appropriate features (pixel values in this case) followed by classification.

2.1 Pre-processing

Pre-processing involves masking the USV frames followed by downsapling using a Gaussian pyramid reduction method for computational efficiency. Furthermore as simple edge detection methods are too sensitive to speckle in ultrasound images, local phase based filters are used for detecting intensity invariant features as initially described in [3], to enhance discrimination between frames with and without SOI. This filtering process produces a feature symmetry map of locations with high amplitude as a result of the product of the local phase symmetry and the local energy. For the clinical application considered in this paper, this combination can nicely discriminate between the fetal skull and the soft tissue objects as indicated in Fig.3. Thus an isotropic Gaussian derivative filter was used with it's parameter σ in a range of 10, 14 and 18 pixels, and local phase symmetry and local energy are both calculated using the monogenic signal [4]. It is important to note that the values for σ were chosen to correspond to the size of the features of interest, in pixels, and may require tuning for other applications.

2.2 Detecting Sections of Interest in an USV

To model the statistical properties of sequences of multivariate observations, it is generally assumed that each observation is correlated to some underlying latent variable, $\mathbf{x}$, that evolves over the duration of the sequence. Following the system identification of the dynamic texture (DT) model in [5], pixel intensities in each frame are modeled as the output of a linear dynamical system (LDS). In this model the appearance of each video frame is determined through the observed variable denoted as $\mathbf{y}$, and the motion and dynamics in the video over a given time is determined through the hidden-state variables denoted as $\mathbf{x}$ which are sampled from a Gauss-Markov process. In such a model the observed frame at any given time can be constructed from a linear combination of the hidden state variables. Therefor given an ultrasound sequence $\mathbf{S}$ of T video frames, let $\mathbf{S} = [\mathbf{y}_1, ..., \mathbf{y}_T]$, where $\mathbf{y}_t \in \mathbb{R}^d$ is the frame observed at time t. It is assumed that at each time instance t, a noisy version of the image can be measured, $\mathbf{y}(t) = \mathbf{S}(t) + \mathbf{w}(t)$, where $\mathbf{w}(t) \in \mathbb{R}^d$ is an independent and identically distributed (i.i.d.) sequence drawn from a known distribution, resulting in a positive measured sequence $\mathbf{y}(t) \in \mathbb{R}^d$ for $t = 1, ..., T$. The evolution of an LDS can be modelled as:

$$\begin{cases} \mathbf{x}_{t+1} = \mathbf{A}\mathbf{x}_t + \mathbf{v}_t \\ \mathbf{y}_t = \mathbf{C}\mathbf{x}_t + \mathbf{w}_t \end{cases} \tag{1}$$

Here $\mathbf{x}_t \in \mathbb{R}^T$ is the state of the LDS and $\mathbf{y}_t \in \mathbb{R}^d$ is the observed pixel intensities at time t. Matrix $\mathbf{A} \in \mathbb{R}^{T \times T}$ is the state transition matrix that describes the dynamics of the state evolution and $\mathbf{C} \in \mathbb{R}^{d \times T}$ is the output matrix. We assume $\mathbf{v}_t \sim N(\mathbf{0}, \mathbf{I})$ and $\mathbf{w}_t \sim N(\mathbf{0}, \mathbf{R})$ are the state and observation noise which we argue to be a valid assumption due to our Gaussian pyramid reduction approach.

In a linear system such as (1), the output matrix $\mathbf{C}$ can be estimated via singular value decomposition of observation matrix $\mathbf{y}$, where $\mathbf{C}$ can be restricted to the N largest eigenvalues. However here a kernelized version of the DT model known as KDT is used where the evolution of the hidden states of the model are kept linear but in order to capture the dynamics of the video the output matrix $\mathbf{C}$ is replaced by a non-linear observation function $C : \mathbb{R}^T \to \mathbb{R}^d$. Therefore given the same ordered US sequence $\mathbf{S} = [\mathbf{y}_1, ..., \mathbf{y}_T]$ and a kernel function $k(y_1, y_2)$ with associated feature transformation $< \phi(y_1), \phi(y_2) >$, the c-th eigenvector $\mathbf{v}_c$ can be used to obtain the c-th kernel principal component in the feature space:

$$\mathbf{v}_c = \sum_{i=1}^{T} \alpha_{i,c} \phi(\mathbf{y}_i) \tag{2}$$

where $\alpha_{i,c}$ represents the i-th component of the c-th weight vector and $\alpha_c = \frac{1}{\sqrt{\lambda_c}} \mathbf{v}_c$, assuming the eigenvectors are sorted in descending order of the eigenvalues $\{\lambda_c\}_{c=1}^{T}$. Here λ_c and $\mathbf{v}_c$ are the c-th largest eigenvalue and eigenvector of the kernel matrix $\mathbf{K}$. Finally the sequence of hidden states $\mathbf{X}$ and the state transition matrix $\mathbf{A}$ can be estimated as

$$\begin{aligned} \mathbf{X} &= \alpha^\mathsf{T} \mathbf{K} \\ \mathbf{A} &= [\mathbf{x}_1, ..., \mathbf{x}_{T-1}][\mathbf{x}_0, ..., \mathbf{x}_{T-2}]^\dagger \end{aligned} \tag{3}$$

The reader is referred to [6] and [2] for a more detailed explanation of the method as well as the estimation of the state and observation noise.

2.3   Distance Metrics

Given a KDT model estimate for each sub-sequence, a suitable metric now needs to be defined to assess similarity between any two sub-sequence models. For this we deviate from [2] in using the Binet-Cauchy (BC) singular value kernel [7], which empirically we have found performs significantly better than the Martin Distance (MD) used in [2] as shown in the next section. A technical report on various metrics that could be utilized can be found in [8]. BC kernels were introduced in [7] as a class of metrics for LDSs. It has been shown that trace

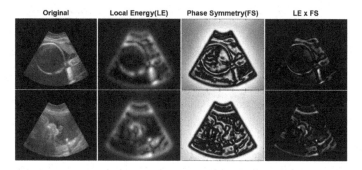

Fig. 3. Filtered positive (top row) and negative (bottom row) frames. The Local Energy, Phase Symmetry and the product of the two filters are shown.

kernel can be used for comparing two LDS models $\mathbf{M_1}$ and $\mathbf{M_2}$ (represented by their model parameters), with corresponding sequences $\{y_t^{M_i}\}_{t=1}^T$ which have the same underlying noise process. This was later extended for Non-Linear Dynamical Systems (NLDS) as follows;

$$K_{NLDS}(\mathbf{M_1}, \mathbf{M_2}) := \mathbb{E}_{v,w}\left[\sum_{t=0}^{\infty} \lambda_t k(\mathbf{y_t^1}, \mathbf{y_t^2})\right], \tag{4}$$

where λ is a weight factor between 0 and 1 and $\mathbb{E}$ is expected value of the infinite sum of inner products with respect to the joint probability distribution of v_t and w_t. Thus the BC trace kernel for NLDS is defined as

$$K_{NLDS}(\mathbf{M_1}, \mathbf{M_2}) = \mathbf{x_0^\mathsf{T}}\bar{\mathbf{P}}\mathbf{x_0^\mathsf{T}} + \frac{\lambda}{1-\lambda}trace(\mathbf{Q}\bar{\mathbf{P}} + \mathbf{R}) \tag{5}$$

where $\mathbf{x_0}$ is the initial state of the system, $\bar{\mathbf{P}} = \sum_{t=0}^{\infty} \lambda_t (\mathbf{A_t^1})^\mathsf{T}\mathbf{FA_t^2}$, $\mathbf{F}$ is the inner product matrix between all the KPCA components and $\mathbf{Q}$ and $\mathbf{R}$ are the state and output covariance matrices. To remove the dependency on the initial state and the noise process, [9] also proposed the BC maximum singular value kernel for NLDSs as $K_{NLDS}^\sigma = \max \sigma(\bar{\mathbf{P}})$, where σ represents the singular values kernel, to take into account only the dynamics of the NDLS. Thus a normalized kernel of the similarity values can be constructed such that $K(\mathbf{M_1}, \mathbf{M_2}) = 1$ if $\mathbf{M_1} = \mathbf{M_2}$ as

$$K(\mathbf{M_1}, \mathbf{M_2}) = \frac{K(\mathbf{M_1}, \mathbf{M_2})}{\sqrt{K(\mathbf{M_1}, \mathbf{M_1}), K(\mathbf{M_2}, \mathbf{M_2})}} \tag{6}$$

A distance can now be computed as $d(\mathbf{M_1}, \mathbf{M_2}) = 2(1 - K(\mathbf{M_1}, \mathbf{M_2}))$ and classification is then carried out using these values. For further detail regarding this metric the reader is referred to [7, 8].

3   Experiments

Experiments have been designed to illustrate the capabilities of the proposed method; one on phantom data, and one on clinical data. The phantom data used

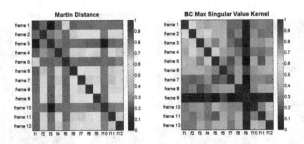

Fig. 4. Distance matrices comparing the 12 videos (sequences 1 ot 6 contain fetal head structures) with each other where 1 indicates perfect match. Martin distance (left) and Binet-Cauchy singular value kernel (right).

in this study for comparison purposes is kindly provided by the authors of [2] and enables direct comparison with that work. The clinical data was generated specifically for this paper and consisted of two 2D fetal USVs each acquired from 35 subjects. Clinical data acquisition was carried out using a mid-range US machine (Philips HD9 with a V7-3 transducer) by an experienced obstetrician who was asked to follow a simple scanning protocol of moving the ultrasound probe from bottom to top of the abdomen in approximately 6 seconds.

Phantom Study Comparison: This experiment allowed to systematically compare the Martin distance (MD) used in [2] with the BC trace kernel distance proposed in our work on phantom data. We re-implemented the method described in [2] without applying our pre-processing step to learn the MD model parameters and to carry out classification. As in [2], the experiment was repeated to vary the number of LDS states. Average Precision (AP), mean AP and mini/max AP are reported with the best threshold for the precision/recall value. Furthermore to visually demonstrate the performance of the two metrics on our dataset, 12 sub-sequences of which the fist 6 contain a fetal skull were selected and their system parameters were estimated following the procedures outlined in section 2. Fig. 4 illustrates the similarity kernels calculated between these sequences using the two metrics. Values are normalised from 0-1 where 1(red) indicates exact match. As it can be seen, MD incorrectly indicates relatively high similarity between sequences of different kind. Please refer to the electronic copy for color encoding.

Clinical Data Comparison: A similar experimental protocol to the phantom study comparison was followed for the clinical data evaluation with the following changes. The goal here was to find the position of the fetal head. Clinically it is important to know if the fetal head is upwards facing (breach) or downwards facing (not) and the idea of this protocol was to define a simple way to determine this from a single ultrasound sweep. In this case the SVM classifier was trained to identify sequences of frames that contained the fetal skull. For the purposes of measuring the performance of the classifier, the average precision (AP) value was calculated for each classification outcome as before, and

Table 1. Classification on the phantom dataset(a) and the raw(b) and pre-processed(c) clinical datasets using 10-fold cross validation.

<table>
<tr><td colspan="5" align="center">(a) Phantom Study Comparison</td><td colspan="2" align="center">Table Keys</td></tr>
<tr><td>State</td><td>mAP</td><td>min/max AP</td><td colspan="2">P/R, α=0.05</td><td>Precision</td><td>TP/(TP+FP)</td></tr>
<tr><td>(n)</td><td>(%)</td><td>(%)</td><td colspan="2">(%)</td><td>Recall</td><td>TP/(TP+FN)</td></tr>
<tr><td>D_m 2</td><td>45.24</td><td>08.50/72.92</td><td colspan="2">53.35/45.25</td><td>AP</td><td>Average Precision</td></tr>
<tr><td>5</td><td>51.14</td><td>18.21/84.49</td><td colspan="2">45.62/50.39</td><td>mAP</td><td>Mean Average Precision</td></tr>
<tr><td>8</td><td>31.99</td><td>01.19/72.41</td><td colspan="2">61.89/34.04</td><td>P/R</td><td>Precision/Recall</td></tr>
<tr><td></td><td></td><td></td><td colspan="2"></td><td>D_m</td><td>Martin Distance Metric</td></tr>
<tr><td>D_b 2</td><td>62.18</td><td>24.86/80.76</td><td colspan="2">67.42/59.87</td><td>D_b</td><td>Binet-Cauchy</td></tr>
<tr><td>5</td><td>67.98</td><td>27.70/88.32</td><td colspan="2">69.85/68.30</td><td></td><td>Singular Value Metric</td></tr>
<tr><td>8</td><td>70.14</td><td>26.77/90.44</td><td colspan="2">77.43/51.79</td><td>mCA</td><td>mClassification Accuracy</td></tr>
</table>

<table>
<tr><td colspan="4" align="center">(b) Clinical Data (no preprocessing)</td><td colspan="4" align="center">(c) Clinical Data (preprocessed)</td></tr>
<tr><td>State</td><td>mAP</td><td>min/max AP</td><td>mCA</td><td>State</td><td>mAP</td><td>min/max AP</td><td>mCA</td></tr>
<tr><td>(n)</td><td>(%)</td><td>(%)</td><td>(%)</td><td>(n)</td><td>(%)</td><td>(%)</td><td>(%)</td></tr>
<tr><td>D_m 2</td><td>23.90</td><td>20.29/25.90</td><td>65.82</td><td>D_m 2</td><td>17.28</td><td>13.95/19.57</td><td>61.79</td></tr>
<tr><td>5</td><td>21.47</td><td>20.33/22.86</td><td>67.53</td><td>5</td><td>29.51</td><td>26.90/33.35</td><td>44.72</td></tr>
<tr><td>8</td><td>23.84</td><td>22.68/26.32</td><td>63.56</td><td>8</td><td>20.70</td><td>19.03/21.95</td><td>62.72</td></tr>
<tr><td>D_b 2</td><td>87.26</td><td>79.60/91.37</td><td>82.80</td><td>D_b 2</td><td>**95.85**</td><td>94.14/96.80</td><td>**90.21**</td></tr>
<tr><td>5</td><td>90.56</td><td>86.96/93.91</td><td>85.03</td><td>5</td><td>86.64</td><td>79.15/95.14</td><td>78.55</td></tr>
<tr><td>8</td><td>76.31</td><td>57.70/87.89</td><td>77.02</td><td>8</td><td>72.81</td><td>49.78/94.61</td><td>81.24</td></tr>
</table>

to summarise this statistics, the mean average precision (mAP), and the mean classification accuracy (mCA) are calculated over a 10-fold cross-validation.

4   Results

Phantom Study: Results from the phantom study experiment are summarised in Table 1a. Consistent with [2] for the Martin distance, a 5-state KDT model yielded the best performance. The highest mAP achieved on the phantom dataset using the Martin Distance was 51.14% (5-state KDT model). In general, results obtained using the BC similarity metric were much higher compared to those of the Martin distance. The highest mAP achieved using the BC metric was 70.14% (8-state KDT model).

Clinical Study: Tables 1b and 1c summarise classification results for sub-sequences of 20 frames long. As shown in table 1b without the pre-processing step, the best results were achieved with a 5-sate KDT model (mAP 90.56%, mCA 85.03%) in comparison to when the frames are pre-processed where the motion in the video is best described with a 2-state KDT model (mAP 95.85%, mCA 90.21%) using the BC singular value kernel. Generally when filtering is not applied, increasing the number of states from 2 to 5 increases the classification accuracy however a further increase to 8 states leads to a decrease in performance. This can be explained by the fact that when KPCA is used, the main dynamics of the video are best described using the first 2/5 eigenvalues for the filtered/raw frames respectively, therefore additional eigenvalues capture a very small portion of the variation in the feature space, thus resulting in noisier KDT model parameter estimates.

5   Discussion and Conclusion

Ultrasound image acquisition and interpretation can be a challenging task for non-experts. We have tackled this obstacle and as the results demonstrate our proposed method outperforms previous work on structure detection in ultrasound videos. In summary, we have proposed a general framework for ultrasound video analysis, motivated by our interest in ultrasound in pregnancy and perinatal care, which couples standardised, and possibly non-conventional scanning protocols, with image analysis methods designed to extract predefined useful information from ultrasound videos. We emphasise that the accuracy achievable in other applications will be dependent on both the choice of scanning protocol and to a lesser extent (in our experience at least) on the ultrasound equipment. Our technical interest is extending this work to detect other structures. In collaboration with clinicians in Africa, we are exploring the role of methodology of this kind in supporting medical training and roll out of ultrasound services in rural areas.

Acknowledgments. The authors acknowledge RCUK Digital Economy Programme grant number EP/G036861/1 (Oxford Centre for Doctoral Training in Healthcare Innovation).

References

[1] Chykeyuk, K., Yaqub, M., Noble, J.A.: Class-specific regression random forest for accurate extraction of standard planes from 3d echocardiography. In: Menze, B., Langs, G., Montillo, A., Kelm, M., Müller, H., Tu, Z. (eds.) MCV 2013. LNCS, vol. 8331, pp. 53–62. Springer, Heidelberg (2013)

[2] Kwitt, R., Vasconcelos, N., Razzaque, S., Aylward, S.: Localizing target structures in ultrasound video - a phantom study. Medical Image Analysis 17(7) (2013)

[3] Kovesi, P.: Symmetry and asymmetry from local phase. In: Tenth Australian Joint Conference on Artificial Intelligence, pp. 185–190. Citeseer (1997)

[4] Felsberg, M., Sommer, G.: The monogenic signal. IEEE Transactions on Signal Processing 49(12), 3136–3144 (2001)

[5] Doretto, G., Chiuso, A., Wu, Y.N., Soatto, S.: Dynamic textures. International Journal of Computer Vision 51(2), 91–109 (2003)

[6] Chan, A.B., Vasconcelos, N.: Classifying video with kernel dynamic textures. In: CVPR, pp. 1–6. IEEE (2007)

[7] Vishwanathan, S.V., Smola, A.J., Vidal, R.: Binet-cauchy kernels on dynamical systems and its application to the analysis of dynamic scenes. Int. J. Comput. Vision 73(1), 95–119 (2007)

[8] Chaudhry, R., Vidal, R.: Recognition of visual dynamical processes: Theory, kernels and experimental evaluation. Department of Computer Science, John Hopkins University, Technical Report, 09–01 (2009)

[9] Chaudhry, R., Ravichandran, A., Hager, G., Vidal, R.: Histograms of oriented optical flow and binet-cauchy kernels on nonlinear dynamical systems for the recognition of human actions. In: CVPR 2009, pp. 1932–1939. IEEE (2009)

Anatomically Constrained Weak Classifier Fusion for Early Detection of Alzheimer's Disease

Mawulawoé Komlagan[1,2], Vinh-Thong Ta[1,2,3], Xingyu Pan[1,2],
Jean-Philippe Domenger[1,2], D. Louis Collins[4],
Pierrick Coupé[1,2], and the Alzheimer's Disease Neuroimaging Initiative[*]

[1] Univ. Bordeaux, LaBRI, UMR 5800, PICTURA, F-33400 Talence, France
[2] CNRS, LaBRI, UMR 5800, PICTURA, F-33400 Talence, France
[3] IPB, LaBRI, UMR 5800, PICTURA, F-33600 Pessac, France
[4] McConnell Brain Imaging Centre, Montreal Neurological Institute,
McGill University, Montreal, Canada

Abstract. The early detection of Alzheimer's disease (AD) is a key step to accelerate the development of new therapies and to diminish the associated socio-economic burden. To address this challenging problem, several biomarkers based on MRI have been proposed. Although numerous efforts have been devoted to improve MRI-based feature quality or to increase machine learning methods accuracy, the current AD prognosis accuracy remains limited. In this paper, we propose to combine both high quality biomarkers and advanced learning method. Our approach is based on a robust ensemble learning strategy using gray matter grading. The estimated weak classifiers are then fused into high informative anatomical sub-ensembles. Through a sparse logistic regression, the most relevant anatomical sub-ensembles are selected, weighted and used as input to a global classifier. Validation on the full ADNI1 dataset demonstrates that the proposed method obtains competitive results of prediction of conversion to AD in the Mild Cognitive Impairment group with an accuracy of 75.6%.

Keywords: Ensemble learning, Weak classifier, Sparse logistic regression.

1 Introduction

Alzheimer's disease (AD) and its prodromal phase, Mild Cognitive Impairment (MCI), are the most common neurodegenerative diseases affecting elderly people. In the early stage of the disease, neural degeneration is subtle making it

---

[*] Data used in the preparation of this article were obtained from the Alzheimer's Disease Neuroimaging Initiative (ADNI) database (www.loni.ucla.edu/ADNI). Hence, the investigators within the ADNI contributed to the design and implementation of ADNI and/or provided data, but did not participate in analysis or writing of this report. ADNI investigators include (complete listing available at www.loni.ucla.edu/ADNI/Collaboration/ADNI Author ship list.pdf).

G. Wu et al. (Eds.): MLMI 2014, LNCS 8679, pp. 141–148, 2014.
© Springer International Publishing Switzerland 2014

difficult to predict which MCI subjects will progress to AD (pMCI) and which MCI subjects will remain stable (sMCI) during the follow up. Hereon, AD prediction, *i.e.*, AD early detection will address the classification of MCI subjects into pMCI and sMCI subjects.

Several biomarkers have been proposed to achieve early AD diagnosis [1]. Among them, it has been established that measurements of brain atrophy extracted from structural MRI are valid markers of early stages of AD [2]. Therefore, automatic frameworks using MRI-based features have been developed to achieve computer-aided prognosis [3–5]. One part of these works focused on advanced machine learning techniques [6] while another part aimed to enhance the biomarker quality [4, 7]. Among them, patch-based methods [8, 9] demonstrated competitive AD prediction results. Despite these efforts, the current AD prognosis accuracy remains around 70%, that suggests the limitation of using (i) traditional features with advanced learning processes or (ii) high quality features with basic machine learning methods. In this paper, we propose to combine high quality biomarkers with advanced learning method to improve AD prediction accuracy.

To this end, we first propose to extend the patch-based scoring method proposed in [8]. In this approach, the anatomical pattern similarity is estimated between the MCI test subject and two training populations (*i.e.*, Cognitively Normal (CN) and AD) using a non-local patch-based scoring method. For each voxel, a score (*i.e.*, a grade) that measures the proximity to both training populations is computed. In [8], the *a priori* ROI-based strategy focused mainly on hippocampus and may discard other possible informative anatomical regions. To overcome this limitation, we propose to score the whole gray matter (GM). Moreover, to be more robust to intensity normalization discrepancies between MRI, probabilities are used in place of intensities during patch comparison. Finally, while a local patch-based strategy is used in [9], a non-local approach is privileged to better handle inter-subject variability and registration error [8].

Afterwards, an ensemble learning method [10] is considered to efficiently use the estimated advanced biomarkers. Since the scoring value, assigned to each voxel of the GM, estimates the proximity to AD and CN, it can be viewed as the posterior probability of a weak classifier. Combined together, these weak classifiers form an ensemble that can be used to classify subjects [11]. As noticed in [2], it appears that AD-related brain alterations are mainly a region-by-region process. Hence, we propose to further use this clinical knowledge to create atlas-based anatomical sub-ensembles of weak classifiers before fusing them into intermediate classifiers. Finally, to discard brain areas that may not be related to AD, we propose to select the most relevant anatomical sub-ensembles using a Sparse Logistic Regression (SLR).

In this work, the contributions are threefold: (i) unlike ROI-based approach, non-local scoring values are estimated over the whole GM and considered as weak classifiers; (ii) an advanced ensemble learning technique is used to fuse these weak classifiers into anatomical sub-ensembles; and (iii) a sparse approx-

Table 1. Demographic information about the considered study subjects

Pathological group	Size	Gender (% Female)	Age ± SD	MMSE± SD
AD	192	48%	75.7±7.6	22.9±3.0
CN	220	49%	76.1±4.9	29.1±0.9
pMCI	166	39%	74.5±7.2	26.4±2.0
sMCI	236	33%	74.9±7.8	27.2±2.5

imation is used to efficiently select and weight the most relevant anatomical sub-ensembles.

2 Materials and Methods

2.1 The ADNI Dataset and Image Processing

To evaluate the performance of the proposed method, all the subjects with an available baseline ADNI preprocessed 1.5T MRI scan are used. The considered dataset is composed of 814 subjects divided into 4 groups AD, CN, pMCI and sMCI. AD and CN groups are used exclusively as training population during GM grading step (see 2.3). The size, the genders, the average ages and the average MMSE (Minimal Mental State Examination) are summarized in Table 1. These groups are similar to the ones used in [4,7–9]. All 814 MRI were first segmented, normalized, modulated (correction of volume changes due to the normalization), and registered into a common space. These processing steps were performed with the VBM8 toolbox[1] added to the SPM8 software[2]. The resulting images correspond to tissue-class probability maps in the MNI space. The obtained GM probability maps are then used as inputs of our GM grading process.

2.2 Method Overview

The framework of the proposed method is summarized here and in Fig. 1. First, the grading method is applied to all the MCI subjects GM maps using the AD and CN populations. Second, the grading values obtained over the whole GM are fused into anatomical sub-ensembles to form intermediate classifiers. Third, the age-effect is corrected using a control population. Afterwards, SLR feature selection is applied to select and weight the most relevant intermediate classifiers. Finally, the selected intermediate classifiers are used to train a global linear SVM classifier. The methods are detailed in the following sections.

2.3 Weak Classifier Estimation via Whole GM Grading

This work is based on the Scoring by Non-local Image Patch Estimator (SNIPE) method [8] where a non-local patch-based estimator is used to perform anatomical structure grading. The patch surrounding each voxel of a test subject is

---

[1] http://dbm.neuro.uni-jena.de/vbm.html

[2] http://www.fil.ion.ucl.ac.uk/spm

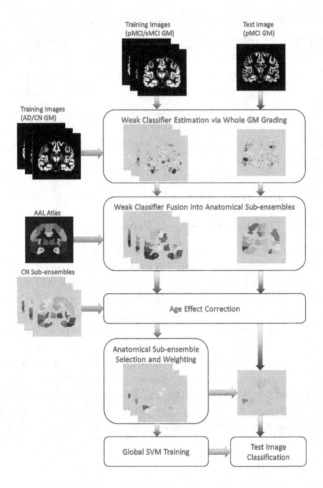

Fig. 1. Overview of the proposed method

involved to estimate the anatomical pattern similarity between the considered patch and the most similar patches extracted from AD and CN training populations. This pattern similarity is quantified with L_2-norm between the patch intensities. The resulting grading value indicates if the considered anatomical pattern is typical of AD (AD-like) or CN (CN-like) populations. Such values can be viewed as the posterior probabilities of a weak classifier. In the proposed method, the grade of each GM voxel is calculated using probability of GM tissue instead of voxel intensities. By using GM tissue probability, our method is more robust to multi-site MR image acquisition. In addition, in our approach the grading is performed on the whole GM, and not only in the hippocampal area. This prevents discarding any relevant information that could be found in other brain regions.

2.4   Weak Classifier Fusion into Anatomical Sub-Ensembles

After the grading step, the dimensionality of the weak classifiers space is too high to be directly used for classification. A straightforward solution is to fuse the weak classifiers into a global classifier [11]. However, this may lead to a sub-optimal result since local relevant information may be lost in a high level global fusion. Additionally, as noticed in [2], AD affects specific regions of the brain in a typical progressive manner. Therefore, we propose to group the weak classifiers into anatomical sub-ensembles using an atlas-based strategy. An ensemble learning principle fuses them into intermediate classifiers [10]. The intermediate classifiers, $c_i = \frac{1}{K} \sum_k c_w(k)$, are constructed by an un-weighted vote of the K weak classifiers c_w included in each anatomical sub-ensemble. In this work, the whole GM is divided into the 116 segmented anatomical regions corresponding to the Automatic Anatomical Labeling (AAL) atlas [12]. Thus, the grades are averaged within each anatomical structure and their mean values considered as predictor values of the 116 c_i intermediate classifiers. Since the grades estimate the AD-related brain anatomical changes, it could be interesting to remove the normal aging effect from the features used. Moreover, it has been shown that SNIPE grades are correlated to age [8]. Therefore, as in [13], we used the CN population to correct the age effect on the MCI populations. For each intermediate classifier, we estimated the age-related effect on the CN population using linear regression. Intermediate classifiers in the MCI populations were then corrected using the estimated linear regression coefficients (see [14]).

2.5   Anatomical Sub-Ensemble Selection and Weighting

As shown in [1], anatomical regions may not be similarly impacted by the progression from MCI stage to the moderate stage of AD. Therefore, using all the intermediate classifiers could be suboptimal. Moreover, beyond classification efficiency reasons and for clinical considerations, it could also be interesting to know the most impacted brain regions. In this work, we selected the most relevant anatomical sub-ensembles by using SLR with L_1/L_2-norm regularization [15, 16]. It has been established that combining the two norms take into account possible inter-feature correlation while imposing sparsity [17]. Additionally, SLR provides a coefficient for each intermediate classifier that represents its relative importance in the sparse approximation. In our method, these coefficients are used to weight each corresponding intermediate classifier before global classification. We used the SLEP package[3] to solve SLR. The selected weighted intermediate classifiers are then used to train a linear SVM as implemented in LIBSVM[4].

2.6   Validation Framework

As is done in [7–9], the classification process is performed using a leave-one-out cross-validation procedure to avoid bias. To validate the efficiency of our frame-

---

[3] http://www.public.asu.edu/~jye02/Software/SLEP/
[4] http://www.csie.ntu.edu.tw/~cjlin/libsvm/

Table 2. Methods comparison. The used features were corrected for age-effect.

Methods	Accuracy (%)	Sensitivity (%)	Specificity (%)
GM Volume	59.7	47.6	68.2
GM Volume + SLR	70.1	56.0	80.0
GM Grading	67.7	57.8	74.8
GM Grading + SLR	75.6	61.5	85.6

Table 3. Comparison with recently published methods using similar dataset

Method	Acc. (%)	Sen. (%)	Spe. (%)
GM Grading + SLR	75.6	61.5	85.6
GM Volume + SLR	70.1	56.0	80.0
ROI-based SNIPE (hippocampal grading) [8]	71	70	71
Multi-instance learning [9]	70.4	66.5	73.1
Multi-methods [4]	68	67	69
Cortical thickness [7]	67.8	64.6	70.0

work, we conducted several experiments. First, to highlight the relevance of using high quality features, we compared the efficiency of our framework using volume-based and grading-based features. For the volume-based approach, we computed the volumes of each AAL region performing the sum of its corresponding GM probability values. Second, to measure the contribution of SLR sub-ensemble selection, we tested our framework while removing this step for both volume-based and grading-based approaches. For the grading step, we used the default parameters proposed in [8]. In each experiment, the L_1/L_2 regularization parameters for solving SLR were set by searching their optimal values while the penalization parameter of the SVM was estimated by a grid search and a nested 10-fold cross validation over the training set.

3   Results and Discussion

The results are summarized in Table 2. First, we notice that using grading-based features improves the result of the classification compared to volume-based features with an increase of about 5pp (percentage points). This confirms the relevance of using high quality features in our method. Second, we observe an improved accuracy of at least 8pp when performing an SLR feature selection with both volume and grading. Moreover, compared to hippocampal scoring [8], we improve the accuracy of 4.6pp using our framework (see Table 3). It is interesting to note that directly using all the anatomical sub-ensembles (*i.e.*, without SLR) provided worst results than using only hippocampal grading. However, when selecting the most relevant anatomical sub-ensembles an important increase is observed. This indicates that areas other than hippocampus seem to be impacted at MCI stage. Thus, automatic *a posteriori* selection of these areas instead of using predefined ROIs leads to higher accuracy.

Table 4. 10 first AAL regions selected by SLR and ordered by decreasing weight

AAL-based gyrus:	
1. Right middle temporal	6. Left cerebelum
2. Left hippocampus	7. Right inferior frontal
3. Left superior frontal	8. Left medial orbital frontal
4. Right middle cingulum	9. Right hippocampus
5. Left posterior cingulum	10. Left para-hippocampal

As shown in Table 3, our method achieves better accuracy than other state-of-the-art methods validated on the same ADNI database and with the same unbiased leave-one-out cross-validation process [7–9]. This establishes the robustness and the efficiency of the proposed framework that combines high quality features with an advanced learning method, *i.e.*, sub-ensemble learning based on constrained weak-classifier-fusion combined with SLR. Additionally, it should also be noted that even using usual GM volumes as features in our framework leads to similar or even competitive accuracy as compared to other methods.

Finally, we can note that even though our method is based on one imaging modality it performs similarly or even better than recent multi-modality methods [6, 18, 19]. Furthermore, for clinical reasons, it could be interesting to analyze the anatomical regions selected via SLR. Table 4 presents, on average, the first selected AAL regions at each run of the leave-one-out cross-validation process. It appears that some anatomical regions like middle temporal gyrus, hippocampus and parahippocampal gyrus are included in the presented list. Such structures are known to be impacted by AD [20]. They are also among the most selected regions in [7] using cortical thickness features.

4   Conclusion

In this study, we proposed an anatomically constrained weak classifier fusion classification procedure extending the grading technique presented by [8]. This work aimed to combine high quality biomarkers with advanced learning method to improve AD detection at its prodromal stage. We demonstrated through our experiments that the contributions made to the method proposed by [8] lead to high classification accuracy for the early detection of AD. Compared to recently proposed MRI-based prediction techniques, we obtained a very competitive accuracy result of 75.6% for the prediction of AD.

Acknowledgments. This study has been carried out with financial support from the French State, managed by the French National Research Agency (ANR) in the frame of the Investments for the future Programme IdEx Bordeaux (ANR-10-IDEX-03-02), Cluster of excellence CPU and TRAIL (HR-DTI ANR-10-LABX-57). We also acknowledge funding from the Fonds de Recherche Québec - Santé (FRQS-Pfizer).

References

1. Jack Jr., C.R., et al.: Tracking pathophysiological processes in Alzheimer's disease: an updated hypothetical model of dynamic biomarkers. The Lancet Neurology 12(2), 207–216 (2013)
2. Frisoni, G.B., et al.: The clinical use of structural MRI in Alzheimer disease. Nature Reviews Neurology 6(2), 67–77 (2010)
3. Cuingnet, R., et al.: Automatic classification of patients with Alzheimer's disease from structural MRI: a comparison of ten methods using the ADNI database. Neuroimage 56(2), 766–781 (2011)
4. Wolz, R., et al.: Multi-method analysis of MRI images in early diagnostics of Alzheimer's disease. PloS One 6(10), e25446 (2011)
5. Davatzikos, C., et al.: Prediction of MCI to AD conversion, via MRI, CSF biomarkers, and pattern classification. Neurobiology of Aging 32(12), 2322–e19 (2011)
6. Suk, H.-I., Shen, D.: Deep learning-based feature representation for AD/MCI classification. In: Mori, K., Sakuma, I., Sato, Y., Barillot, C., Navab, N. (eds.) MICCAI 2013, Part II. LNCS, vol. 8150, pp. 583–590. Springer, Heidelberg (2013)
7. Eskildsen, S.F., et al.: Prediction of Alzheimer's disease in subjects with mild cognitive impairment from the ADNI cohort using patterns of cortical thinning. NeuroImage 65, 511–521 (2013)
8. Coupé, P., et al.: Scoring by nonlocal image patch estimator for early detection of Alzheimer's disease. NeuroImage: Clinical 1(1), 141–152 (2012)
9. Tong, T., et al.: Multiple instance learning for classification of dementia in brain MRI. Medical Image Analysis 18(5), 808–818 (2014)
10. Dietterich, T.G.: Ensemble methods in machine learning. In: Kittler, J., Roli, F. (eds.) MCS 2000. LNCS, vol. 1857, pp. 1–15. Springer, Heidelberg (2000)
11. Liu, M., et al.: Ensemble sparse classification of Alzheimer's disease. NeuroImage 60(2), 1106–1116 (2012)
12. Tzourio-Mazoyer, N., et al.: Automated anatomical labeling of activations in SPM using a macroscopic anatomical parcellation of the MNI MRI single-subject brain. Neuroimage 15(1), 273–289 (2002)
13. Koikkalainen, J., et al.: Improved classification of Alzheimer's disease data via removal of nuisance variability. PloS One 7(2), e31112 (2012)
14. Dukart, J., et al.: Age correction in dementia – matching to a healthy brain. PLoS ONE 6(7) (July 2011)
15. Dubey, R., et al.: Analysis of sampling techniques for imbalanced data: An n= 648 ADNI study. NeuroImage 87, 220–241 (2014)
16. Ye, J., et al.: Sparse learning and stability selection for predicting MCI to AD conversion using baseline ADNI data. BMC Neurology 12(1), 46 (2012)
17. Zou, H., Hastie, T.: Regularization and variable selection via the elastic net. Journal of the Royal Statistical Society: Series B 67(2), 301–320 (2005)
18. Zhang, D., Shen, D.: Multi-modal multi-task learning for joint prediction of multiple regression and classification variables in Alzheimer's disease. Neuroimage 59(2), 895–907 (2012)
19. Cheng, B., Zhang, D., Shen, D.: Domain transfer learning for MCI conversion prediction. In: Ayache, N., Delingette, H., Golland, P., Mori, K. (eds.) MICCAI 2012, Part I. LNCS, vol. 7510, pp. 82–90. Springer, Heidelberg (2012)
20. Braak, H., Braak, E.: Neuropathological stageing of Alzheimer-related changes. Acta Neuropathologica 82(4), 239–259 (1991)

Automatic Bone and Marrow Extraction from Dual Energy CT through SVM Margin-Based Multi-Material Decomposition Model Selection

Harini Veeraraghavan[1], Duc Fehr[1,*], Ross Schmidtlein[1],
Sinchun Hwang[2], and Joseph O. Deasy[1]

[1] Medical Physics, Memorial Sloan Kettering Cancer Center, NY, USA
[2] Radiology, Memorial Sloan Kettering Cancer Center, NY, USA
{veerarah,fehrd,schmidtr,hwangs1,DeasyJ}@mskcc.org

Abstract. In this work, we present a fully-automatic approach for segmenting bone and marrow structures from dual energy CT (DECT) images. The images are represented using a multi-material decomposition model (MMD) computed from a triplet of physical materials at two different energy attenuation levels. We employ support vector machine learning to select the most relevant MMD model for the anatomical structure of interest so that highly accurate segmentation of the said structures can be achieved. We evaluated our approach for segmenting bone and marrow structures with varying amounts of metastatic bone disease on multiple longitudinal follow up patient scans. Our approach shows consistent and robust segmentation despite changes in bone density due to disease progression, high-density contrast material uptake in neighboring tissue, and significant metal artifacts.

1 Introduction

Computed tomography (CT) is the frequently used modality for routine diagnosis and evaluation of disease progression in patients with metastatic bone cancers. Accurate extraction of bone and marrow structures is an important first step for the analysis of abnormalities in the marrow. Although, bony structures can be detected from single energy CT scans, obtaining highly accurate automatic segmentation of the same structures [1] is difficult. Dual energy CT (DECT) on the other hand has been shown to provide good differentiation of bone marrow and structures in the marrow such as bone edema and bone bruise lesions [1]. In [2], manually selected multi-material decomposition models (MMD) were used for removing contrast from CT images and for organ segmentation. Our work automates the MMD model selection and tunes the selected models specific to the structure of interest such that accurate segmentation can be achieved in the presence of confounding structures.

Concretely, our approach computes several candidate MMD models from the DECT image pair. SVM classifiers are trained using the coefficient images obtained from the models and the SVM-MMD model that maximizes the SVM

---

* Equal contributing.

G. Wu et al. (Eds.): MLMI 2014, LNCS 8679, pp. 149–156, 2014.
© Springer International Publishing Switzerland 2014

margin is selected for generating segmentations on novel images. Previously, SVM margins were employed for feature selection and disease classification in [3, 4]. Our work extends this concept to DECT images. Unlike [3,4], in our work, feature selection refers to selecting a candidate model from among multiple models where the cardinality of features in all the models is the same, albeit with different combination of features. Our approach requires training on utmost a single patient scan and can then be used on scans with varying amounts of disease and metal artifacts. Finally, our approach makes use of physical materials such as bone, fat, contrast agent, etc at different energy levels to formulate the candidate models and therefore, yields intuitively meaningful models for interpreting the images. For example, the best model selected using our approach for the bone and marrow segmentation consists of $bone - mix1(gastrografin + water) - mix2(hydroxylapatite + water)$, where gastrografin is the contrast agent typically used for imaging the patients, and hydroxylapatite is an important constituent of the bones.

Fully automatic methods based on intensity thresholding such as in [5, 6] are adversely affected by the presence of high density materials such as contrast in the bowel. On the other hand, user interaction based methods including [7–9] require significant user interaction to achieve reasonably accurate segmentation. Apriori learning-based methods for bone segmentation [10] have been applied only to single energy CT. Fig. 1 shows example segmentations generated using robust statistics [8], interactive Grow Cut [9], and our approach SVM-MMD for a typical case. As seen, our approach generates more accurate segmentation compared to the other two methods.

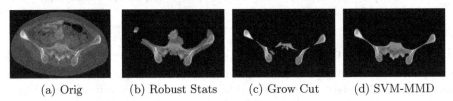

    (a) Orig   (b) Robust Stats   (c) Grow Cut   (d) SVM-MMD

Fig. 1. Segmentation results with different methods

2 Background

2.1 Dual Energy Computed Tomography

Material differentiation in standard CT is based on the X-ray attenuation caused by absorption and Compton scattering of radiation by the material in a region of interest. The attenuation and the resulting CT number (HU) depend on the material and its density. DECT on the other hand uses two scans at two different energy levels to achieve material differentiation. Two physical properties that DECT depends on are the mass attenuation coefficient ($\mu_M(E)$) of a material M at a particular energy E and the density ρ_M of the material. The product of these quantities is the *linear attenuation coefficient* $\mu_L(E) = \rho_M\mu_M(E)$. Linear attenuation images at arbitrary energy levels can be computed from a pair of images (ρ_1, ρ_2) which result in better separation of anatomical structures than when using the DECT image pairs [11].

2.2   Multi Material Decomposition Model

While DECT can help to differentiate two elements, it is not sufficient to obtain a good separation of the materials in the human body. This is because, materials in the human body are often a mixture of more than two elements. Multi-material decomposition methods have been successfully applied for bone composition determination [12], and liver fat quantification in [2]. In this work we use the volume conservation based multi-material decomposition in [2].

The central assumption used in [2] for computing the multi-material decomposition is that the mixture of materials in the human body behaves as an ideal solution at a given temperature and pressure, for which volume preservation applies. In other words, volume of a material mixture equals the sum of the volumes of its constituent parts. Given this, the linear attenuation coefficient of a mixture $\mu_L(E)$ can be expressed as: $\mu_L(E) = \sum_{i=1}^{S} \alpha_i \mu_{L,i}(E)$, where, $\mu_{L,i}(E)$ is the attenuation coefficient of the individual materials at a nominal density ρ_i which is available from standard tables [13]. α_i is the volume fraction of the constituent materials in the mix and S is the number of materials used, which in our case is 3. [2] shows that the solution to the above equation when subject to the constraint $\sum_i \alpha_i = 1$ gives the mixing coefficients of the set of materials.

Geometrically, the volume fractions can be interpreted as the *barycentric coordinates* of a point $\mu_L = (\mu_L(E_l), \mu_L(E_h))$ in two dimensional linear attenuation coefficient space Λ with respect to a triangle whose vertices are formed by the coordinates of three materials. We call this triangle, *material basis triplet*. Given a material basis triplet, each point in the DECT image can be expressed in the coordinates of the same triplet using their volume fractions. The triplet, together with the energy pair form a multi-material decomposition model (MMD).

3   Method

3.1   Support Vector Machine Margin Based Multi-Material Decomposition (SVM-MMD)

Given a set of examples $X = \{x_1, x_2, \ldots, x_n\}$ which are vectors in some d dimensional space, $X \subseteq R^d$ and their labels $\{y_1, \ldots, y_n\}$, SVM projects the data into a higher dimensional space and finds the best separating hyper-plane classifier with the largest sample margin. Margin is a geometric measure for evaluating the confidence of a classifier. Margins have previously been employed to evaluate the "goodness" of a classifier in the context of active learning-based segmentation in [14] and for feature selection [15]. Our work complements [15] by extracting the best combination of a fixed number of features (three for the material basis and two for the energy pairs).

3.2   Algorithm Description

The algorithm for the SVM margin-based MMD model selection is shown in Alg. 1. As shown, the inputs to the algorithm are the DECT material density image pair ρ_1, ρ_2, the set of J materials $M = \{s_1, \ldots, s_J\}$, P energy levels

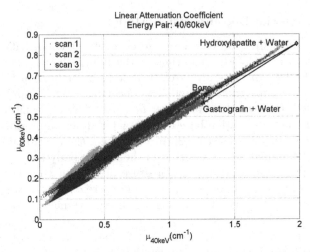

Fig. 2. Points μ_L in linear attenuation coefficient space $\Lambda(40, 60)$ for three different patients. One basis triplet is given in black.

$E = \{E_1, \ldots, E_P\}$ and the labeled voxels $Y = \{y_1, \ldots, y_\lambda\}$. The output of the algorithm is the SVM model m_i with the maximum margin e_i and the corresponding multi-material decomposition model $B_i = \{\{s_x, s_y, s_z\}, (E_u, E_v)\}_i$, containing the material triplet $\{s_x, s_y, s_z\} \subset M$ and the energy pair $(E_u, E_v) \in E^2$. Initially, all possible material and energy models are constructed by combining materials and energy pairs from which the individual linear attenuation coefficient images are computed [line 3]. Fig. 2 shows the distribution of voxels obtained at energy levels $(40, 60)keV$ and the basis triplet $(bone, mix1, mix2)$. From these coefficient voxels the volume fractions α_i are computed for each voxel [line 4] and they constitute the input to the SVM classifier. The SVM classifier is trained on the volume fractions α_i to produce the model m_i and margin e_i [line 5]. The model with the largest margin is chosen as the best model whose MMD basis is retained for analysis of novel data [line 7].

Algorithm 1. Multi-material Decomposition Model Selection

---

    input : DECT density pair (ρ_1, ρ_2), materials $M = \{s_1, \ldots, s_J\}$, energy levels
          $E = \{E_1, \ldots, E_P\}$, labeled voxels $Y = \{y_1, \ldots, y_\lambda\}$
    output: maximum margin SVM model m_i, MMD basis model
          $B_i = \{\{s_x, s_y, s_z\}, (E_u, E_v)\}_i$

1 Construct all feasible MMD basis models $\mathcal{B} = \{B_1, \ldots, B_N\}$
2 **for** *Basis model* $B_i \in \mathcal{B}$ **do**
3   Compute linear attenuation coefficient space $\Lambda_i = \Lambda(E_u, E_v)_i$
4   Transform voxels to volume fractions α_i using basis $\{s_x, s_y, s_z\}_i$
5     $\{m_i, e_i\} \leftarrow SVMTrain(\alpha_i, Y)$
6 **end**
7 Choose MMD basis model $B_i = \arg\max_i(e_i)$

3.3   Segmentation

The selected MMD model together with the corresponding SVM is used to perform voxelwise classification. The result of the classification is refined using morphological opening and closing operations followed by active contour segmentation available in Matlab [16] applied to the $70keV$ image to produce the final result. The $70keV$ image was chosen as the best contrast is obtained in this energy and is also used in clinic. Although, we chose the active contour segmentation, note that any segmentation technique can be employed. We have experimented with the geodesic active contour [17] method available in ITK [18] and obtained similar results. Currently, we are investigating the use of our technique with other segmentation methods including Grow Cut. The use of the SVM output as a likelihood in the segmentation is potential future work.

4   Results and Discussion

4.1   Experimental Setup

DECT imaging was performed with a GE Discovery CT750HD scanner. Eight patients with multiple follow up scans were used for analysis. Patients had varying number of follow up scans ranging from one to five resulting in a total of 30 image volumes. All the patients had one or two artificial metal hip prosthesis. While some of the scans in the patients were subjected to metal artifact reduction technique to eliminate metal artifacts, others retained metal artifacts. This increased the complexity and variability in the scans. The ground truth segmentation of the bone and marrow regions were drawn manually and validated by a radiologist with several years of experience. We used the following materials for the analysis: air, cortical bone, adipose tissue, hydroxylapatite, mix1 and mix2, which are respectively hydroxylapatite mixed with water (ratio: 0.6/0.4) and gastrografin mixed with water (ratio: 0.3/0.7). The energies used for analysis ranged from $40keV$ to $140keV$.

4.2   Multi-Material Decomposition Selection

Our approach was trained using data from a single patient scan. In order to validate the MMD selection, the SVM training was repeated for all the patient scans individually using $K = 10$ fold cross-validation. Our approach always selected the material basis triplet $(bone, mix1, mix2)$ and the energy pair $(40, 60)\,keV$. This model selection confirms the observation that the scatter plot distribution of the image voxels in the linear attenuation space is very similar across multiple patients, as can be observed in Fig. 2. Furthermore, our result suggests that it is sufficient to train the model from one patient to achieve highly accurate segmentation from multiple patients. The SVM training achieved a cross-validation accuracy of 92.6% (for just the bone voxels). The SVM parameters $\gamma = 0.05$ used in the RBF kernel, and $C = 1$ have been set empirically.

4.3   Segmentation

The segmentation results obtained from the postprocessed classification were validated by comparing against ground truth masks. The dice overlap scores shown

Table 1. Dice overlap scores

Scan	SVM MMD	Region Growing	Robust Statistics	Grow Cut	Scan	SVM MMD	Region Growing	Robust Statistics	Grow Cut
1	**0.87**	0.71	0.61	0.67	16	**0.68**	0.13	0.48	0.52
2	**0.88**	0.64	0.56	0.66	17	**0.69**	0.09	0.44	0.57
3	**0.87**	0.59	0.54	0.76	18	**0.68**	0.07	0.49	0.56
4	**0.86**	0.11	0.60	0.71	19	**0.59**	0.19	0.50	0.51
5	**0.85**	0.57	0.55	0.70	20	**0.84**	0.03	0.45	0.56
6	**0.87**	0.62	0.60	0.69	21	**0.84**	0.01	0.58	0.61
7	**0.83**	0.06	0.52	0.56	22	**0.86**	0.04	0.65	0.70
8	**0.79**	0.20	0.58	0.45	23	**0.85**	0.14	0.63	0.68
9	**0.84**	0.02	0.59	0.54	24	0.48	0.15	0.43	**0.52**
10	**0.84**	0.58	0.57	0.53	25	0.50	0.14	0.43	**0.58**
11	**0.86**	0.46	0.70	0.59	26	0.55	0.10	0.40	**0.61**
12	**0.79**	0.06	0.45	0.57	27	**0.52**	0.12	0.45	0.48
13	**0.75**	0.09	0.50	0.57	28	**0.68**	0.16	0.46	0.53
14	**0.82**	0.46	0.57	0.59	29	**0.73**	0.15	0.45	0.52
15	**0.80**	0.44	0.59	0.64	30	**0.70**	0.12	0.44	0.60

in Table 1 were obtained by generating segmentations using the SVM model trained on the first scan of patient 1. We only report the results for patient 1 as the segmentation accuracies obtained using the other patients were very similar. Since the training was performed on a small subset of voxels from patient 1's first scan, we also report the this scan's segmentation. We compared the results of our segmentation approach with region growing available in 3DSlicer [19], robust statistics segmentation [8], and Grow Cut segmentation [9]. The parameters for the afore-mentioned approaches were optimized empirically to achieve the best possible segmentation on patient 1's first scan at $70keV$. Despite subjecting the results generated using the other methods to the postprocessing, the accuracies in segmentation were very similar to when not using such postprocessing. Additionally, we also compared our segmentation with the Graph Cuts method [6] using the opensource implementation [20]. However, as the method is only for 2D images and required significant fine tuning to achieve reasonable segmentation even for individual slices (parameters needed to be changed for each slice), we do not report the dice overlap scores and instead show qualitative results.

Fig. 3 shows snapshots of segmentations using the aforementioned methods including Graph Cuts. As shown, our approach obtains very good segmentation of the structures for different scans. In addition, it is also fairly robust to the presence of metal artifacts.

The SVM-MMD approach is a method for selecting the "best" model using the material basis and attenuation energies for representing the DECT images. Once the model is learned, any segmentation method can be used either using the vectorized image representation or the classifier result with its probabilities applied to a 70KeV image. We have successfully combined the classification result and the probabilities with both active contours and geodesic active contours and obtained reasonably accurate segmentation.

Original	Region Growing	Robust Statistics	Grow Cut	Graph Cut	SVM-MMD

(a) Scan1

(b) Scan2

(c) Scan3

(d) Scan4

(e) Scan5

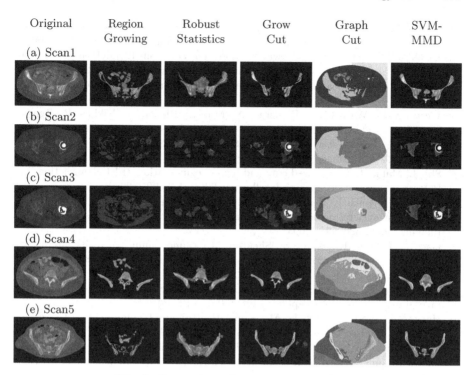

Fig. 3. Comparison of segmentation methods

5   Conclusions

In this work, we presented a SVM margin maximization-based approach for automatically selecting the "best" multi-material decomposition model from dual energy CT for structure specific segmentation and combined the SVM learning based classification with an active contour segmentation to achieve reasonably accurate segmentations. We evaluated our approach to segment bone and marrow structures in multiple patients with more than one follow up scan. We have shown that our approach achieves consistently reasonable segmentation and obtains more robust segmentation compared to multiple segmentation methods.

References

1. Pache, G., Krauss, B., Strohm, P., Saueressig, U., Blanke, P., Bulla, S., Schäfer, O., Helwig, P., Kotter, E., Langer, M., et al.: Dual-energy CT virtual noncalcium technique: Detecting posttraumatic bone marrow lesions–feasibility study. Radiology 256(2), 617–624 (2010)
2. Mendonca, P., Lamb, P., Sahani, D.: A flexible method for multi-material decomposition of dual-energy CT images. IEEE Trans. on Medical Imaging 33(1), 99–116 (2014)

3. Guyon, I., Weston, J., Barnhill, S., Vapnik, V.: Gene selection for cancer classification using support vector machines. Machine Learning 46(1-3), 389–422 (2002)
4. Zacharaki, E.I., Wang, S., Chawla, S., Soo Yoo, D., Wolf, R., Melhem, E.R., Davatzikos, C.: Classification of brain tumor type and grade using MRI texture and shape in a machine learning scheme. Magnetic Resonance in Medicine 62(6), 1609–1618 (2009)
5. Westin, C.F., Warfield, S., Bhalerao, A., Mui, L., Richolt, J., Kikinis, R.: Tensor controlled local structure enhancement of CT images for bone segmentation. In: Wells, W.M., Colchester, A.C.F., Delp, S.L. (eds.) MICCAI 1998. LNCS, vol. 1496, pp. 1205–1212. Springer, Heidelberg (1998)
6. Shi, J., Malik, J.: Normalized cuts and image segmentation. IEEE Transactions on Pattern Analysis and Machine Intelligence 22(8), 888–905 (2000)
7. Kang, Y., Engelke, K., Kalender, W.: A new accurate and precise 3D segmentation method for skeletal structures in volumetric CT data. IEEE Trans. on Medical Imaging 22(5), 586–598 (2003)
8. Gao, Y., Kikinis, R., Bouix, S., Shenton, M., Tannenbaum, A.: A 3D interactive multi-object segmentation tool using local robust statistics driven active contours. Medical Image Analysis 16(6), 1216–1227 (2012)
9. Vezhnevets, V., Konouchine, V.: GrowCut - Interative multi-label N-D image segmentation. In: Proc. of Graphicon, pp. 150–156 (2005)
10. Haas, B., Coradi, T., Scholz, M., Kunz, P., Huber, M., Oppitz, U., Andre, L., Lengkeek, V., Huyskens, D., van Esch, A., Reddick, R.: Automatic segmentation of thoracic and pelvic CT images for radiotherapy planning using implicit anatomic knowledge and organ-specific segmentation strategies. Phys. Med. Biol. 53(6), 1751 (2008)
11. Alvarez, R., Seppi, E.: A comparison of noise and dose in conventional and energy selective computed tomography. IEEE Transactions on Nuclear Science 26(2), 2853–2856 (1979)
12. Goodsitt, M.M., Rosenthal, D.I., Reinus, W.R., Coumas, J.: Two postprocessing CT techniques for determining the composition of trabecular bone. Investigative Radiology 22(3), 209–215 (1987)
13. Hubbell, J., Seltzer, S.: NISTIR 5632, National Institute of Standards and Technology, Gaithersburg, MD (1995), http://physics.nist.gov/xaamdi
14. Veeraraghavan, H., Miller, J.V.: Active learning guided interactions for consistent image segmentation with reduced user interactions. In: Intl. Symposium on Biomedical Imaging (2011)
15. Bachrach, R.G., Navot, A., Tishby, N.: Margin based feature selection - Theory and algorithms. In: Proc. of Intl. Conf. on Machine Learning (2004)
16. Chan, T.F., Vese, L.A.: Active contours without edges. IEEE Transactions on Image Processing 10(2), 266–277 (2001)
17. Caselles, V., Kimmel, R., Sapiro, G.: Geodesic active contours. International Journal of Computer Vision 22(1), 61–79 (1997)
18. Johnson, H.J., McCormick, M., Ibáñez, L., The Insight Software Consortium: The ITK Software Guide, 3rd edn. Kitware, Inc. (2013) (in press)
19. Fedorov, A., Beichel, R., Kalpathy-Cramer, J., Finet, J., Fillion-Robin, J., Pujol, S., Bauer, C., Jennings, D., Fennessy, F., Sonka, M., Buatti, J., Aylward, S., Miller, J., Pieper, S., Kikinis, R.: 3D Slicer as an image computing platform for the quantitative imaging network. Magn. Reson. Imaging 30(9), 1323–1341 (2012)
20. Cour, T., Yu, S., Shi, J.: Normalized cut segmentation code, http://www.cis.upenn.edu/~jshi/software/

Sparse Discriminative Feature Selection for Multi-class Alzheimer's Disease Classification

Xiaofeng Zhu, Heung-Il Suk, and Dinggang Shen*

Department of Radiology and BRIC,
University of North Carolina at Chapel Hill, USA
dgshen@med.unc.edu

Abstract. In neuroimaging studies, high dimensionality and small sample size have been always an issue, and it is common to apply a dimension reduction method to avoid the over-fitting problem. Broadly, there are two different approaches in reducing the feature dimensionality: feature selection and subspace learning. When it comes to the feature interpretability, the feature selection approach such as the sparse regularized linear regression method is preferable to the subspace learning methods, especially in Alzheimer's Disease (AD) diagnosis. However, based on recent machine learning researches, the subspace learning methods presented promising results in various applications. To this end, in this work, we propose a novel method for discriminative feature selection by combining two conceptually different methodologies of feature selection and subspace learning in a unified framework. Specifically, we integrate the ideas of Fisher's linear discriminant analysis and locality preserving projection, which consider, respectively, the global and local information inherent in observations, in a regularized least square regression model. With the help of global and local information in data, we select class-discriminative and noise-resistant features that thus help enhance classification performance. Furthermore, unlike the previous methods that mostly considered only a binary classification, in this paper, we consider a multi-class classification problem in AD diagnosis. Our experiments on the Alzheimer's Disease Neuroimaging Initiative dataset showed the efficacy of the proposed method by enhancing the performances in multi-class AD classification.

1 Introduction

Previous studies of the computer-aided Alzheimer's Disease (AD) diagnosis usually applied the sequential processes of feature extraction, feature dimensionality reduction, and classifier learning, to make a decision on the clinical status of a subject, *e.g.*, AD, Mild Cognitive Impairment (MCI), and Normal Control (NC) [4,14,16,17,20]. In this paper, we focus on the feature selection, which has the effect of lowering feature dimensionality. Furthermore, unlike the previous methods that mostly considered only binary classification of either AD vs. NC or MCI

---

* Corresponding author.

G. Wu et al. (Eds.): MLMI 2014, LNCS 8679, pp. 157–164, 2014.
© Springer International Publishing Switzerland 2014

vs. NC, we consider a multi-class classification problem, *e.g.*, AD vs. MCI vs. NC, for practical applications. Based on the observation that there are three or four different clinical status related to AD, *i.e.*, AD, MCI (MCI-Converter: MCI-C, MCI-NonConverter: MCI-NC), and NC, from a clinical point of view, it is more practical to build a multi-class classifier.

In neuroimaging studies, while the feature dimension is high in nature, the available sample size is very limited. It has been always an issue for high dimensionality and small sample size in computer-aided AD diagnosis [5,13,22,23]. Thus, dimensionality reduction by means of either subspace learning or feature selection has been one of the core steps in neuroimaging pattern analysis. Methodologically, feature selection methods, *e.g.*, *t*-test and sparse regularized linear regression, select an informative feature subset from the original feature set, while the subspace learning methods, *e.g.*, Fisher's Linear Discriminant Analysis (LDA) [3] and Locality Preserving Projection (LPP) [7], transform the original feature space into a low-dimensional space. As for the interpretability of the results, the feature selection methods are preferable to subspace learning methods, in particular, in neuroimaging studies. However, according to recent studies in machine learning [6,18,19], subspace learning has shown promising performances in various fields.

In this paper, we propose a novel method that efficiently combines the methodologies of feature selection and subspace learning. Specifically, we inject the ideas of two subspace learning methods, *i.e.*, LDA and LPP, into a sparse least square regression framework. The rationale of using both LDA and LPP in our formulation is that LDA considers the global information inherent in the observations with the ratio of within-class-variance and between-class-variance, while LPP reflects the local information by means of graph Laplacian. That is, with the help of global and local information in data, we can select class-discriminative and noise-resistant features that thus help enhance classification performances.

2   Proposed Method

2.1   Multi-class Sparse Discriminative Feature Selection

Let $\mathbf{X} \in \mathbb{R}^{d \times n}$ denote a feature matrix, where d and n are, respectively, the numbers of feature variables and samples, and $\mathbf{Y} \in \mathbb{R}^{c \times n}$ denote a class indicator matrix, *e.g.*, 0-1 encoding, where c is the number of classes. We formulate a multi-class feature selection problem by means of a multi-task learning with a sparse least square regression model as follows:

$$\min_{\mathbf{W}} \frac{1}{2} \|\mathbf{Y} - \mathbf{W}^T \mathbf{X}\|_F^2 + \lambda \|\mathbf{W}\|_{2,1} \tag{1}$$

where $\mathbf{W} \in \mathbb{R}^{d \times c}$ is a regression coefficient matrix and λ is a sparsity control parameter. The $\ell_{2,1}$-norm $\|\mathbf{W}\|_{2,1}$ penalizes the coefficients in the same row of $\mathbf{W}$ together for joint selection or unselection in regressing the response variables in $\mathbf{Y}$. In Eq. (1), the optimal solution assigns a large weight to the important features and zero or a small weight to less important features and this method has been successfully applied for a binary classification [10,12,20]. With respect to the multi-task learning, it has been shown that Eq. (1) utilizes the correlation of different classes [1] by regarding each class as one task. However, in its current form, it cannot guarantee the class-discriminative power of the selected features and the preservation of the neighborhood structure of data points, which are important characteristics for a good classification performance [3,6].

In this section, we propose a novel discriminative feature selection method that considers both the *global* data distribution and the *local* topological relation among data in a sparse least square regression framework. We first utilize a Fisher's LDA that considers the global data distribution based on the ratio between within-class-variance and between-class-variance to find the class-discriminative features. Second, we take the concept of an LPP [7] to preserve the topological relation among data.

Regarding the Fisher's criterion for discriminative feature selection, a straight-forward approach is to penalize the objective function of Eq. (1) with a regularization term defined as follows:

$$R_G = \frac{\mathbf{W}^T \mathbf{\Sigma}_b \mathbf{W}}{\mathbf{W}^T \mathbf{\Sigma}_w \mathbf{W}} \tag{2}$$

where $\mathbf{\Sigma}_w$ and $\mathbf{\Sigma}_b$ denote, respectively, the within-class variance and the between-class variance. However, due to the non-convexity of Eq. (2), it is not trivial to find an optimal solution of the objective function. Fortunately, Ye [15] presented that the multi-class LDA that finds a subspace by maximizing Eq. (2) can be equivalently formulated with a linear regression model by defining the class indicator matrix $\mathbf{Y} = [y_{i,k}]$ in Eq. (1) as follows:

$$y_{i,k} = \begin{cases} \sqrt{\frac{n}{n_k}} - \sqrt{\frac{n_k}{n}}, & \text{if } l(\mathbf{x}_i) = k \\ -\sqrt{\frac{n_k}{n}}, & \text{otherwise} \end{cases} \tag{3}$$

where $l(\mathbf{x}_i)$ denotes a class label of $\mathbf{x}_i$ and n_k is the sample size of the class k. That is, using a class indicator matrix $\mathbf{Y}$ defined as Eq. (3), we can efficiently use the global information, *i.e.*, data distribution in the original space, without changing the formulation. Importantly, we don't transform the original input feature space into a low-dimensional space, in which it is difficult to interpret or investigate the results.

As for the topological relation among data, *i.e.*, local information, we use a graph Laplacian by defining the similarity $s_{i,j}$ between every pair of data points $\mathbf{x}_i$ and $\mathbf{x}_j$ via a heat kernel[1] and define a regularization term as follows:

$$R_L = tr(\mathbf{W}^T \mathbf{X} \mathbf{L} \mathbf{X}^T \mathbf{W}) \tag{4}$$

where $\mathbf{L} = \mathbf{D} - \mathbf{S}$ with a similarity matrix $\mathbf{S} = [s_{i,j}] \in \mathbb{R}^{n \times n}$ and a diagonal matrix $\mathbf{D} = [d_{i,i} = \sum_j s_{i,j}] \in \mathbb{R}^{n \times n}$.

---

[1] $H(\mathbf{x}_i, \mathbf{x}_j) = exp\left[-\frac{\|\mathbf{x}_i - \mathbf{x}_j\|^2}{\sigma}\right]$, where $\sigma \in \mathbb{R}^+$ is a parameter.

Therefore, our final objective function is formulated as follows:

$$\min_{\mathbf{W}} \frac{1}{2}\|\mathbf{Y} - \mathbf{W}^T\mathbf{X}\|_F^2 + \lambda_1 tr(\mathbf{W}^T\mathbf{X}\mathbf{L}\mathbf{X}^T\mathbf{W}) + \lambda_2\|\mathbf{W}\|_{2,1} \qquad (5)$$

where $\mathbf{Y}$ is defined as Eq. (3), and λ_1 and λ_2 are tuning parameters. Here, we should note that Eq. (5) efficiently combines the ideas of subspace learning (LDA and LPP) and feature selection in a unified framework.

Our method can be discriminated from the previous methods in the following senses: (1) Unlike the previous sparse linear regression-based feature selection methods [11,21], the proposed method finds the class-discriminative and noise-resistant regression coefficient matrix thanks to the use of the Fisher's criterion and graph Laplacian. (2) Compared to the subspace learning methods such as Principal Component Analysis (PCA), LDA, and LPP, which all have an interpretational limitation, the proposed method selects features in the original space, and thus it has an advantage of intuitive investigation of the results. (3) Unlike the conventional LDA [3] based on the criterion in Eq. (2), the proposed method uses the Fisher's criterion but still operates in the original feature space, and thus allows for an intuitive interpretation of the selected features. Furthermore, while the conventional LDA finds at most $(c-1)$-dimension features for a c-class classification task, $e.g.$, 2-D space in a three-class classification task, Eq. (5) selects at most d features (in general, $d \gg c$ in the AD study).

2.2   Optimization

Eq. (5) is a convex but non-smooth function. In this work, we solve it by designing a new accelerated proximal gradient method [9,19]. We first conduct the proximal gradient method on Eq. (5) by setting

$$f(\mathbf{W}) = \frac{1}{2}\|\mathbf{Y} - \mathbf{W}^T\mathbf{X}\|_F^2 + \lambda_1 tr(\mathbf{W}^T\mathbf{X}\mathbf{L}\mathbf{X}^T\mathbf{W}) \qquad (6)$$

$$\mathcal{L}(\mathbf{W}) = f(\mathbf{W}) + \lambda_2\|\mathbf{W}\|_{2,1}. \qquad (7)$$

Note that $f(\mathbf{W})$ is convex and differentiable, while $\lambda_2\|\mathbf{W}\|_{2,1}$ is convex but non-smooth [9]. To optimize $\mathbf{W}$ with the proximal gradient method, we iteratively update it by means of the following optimization rule:

$$\mathbf{W}(t+1) = \arg\min_{\mathbf{W}} G_{\eta(t)}(\mathbf{W}, \mathbf{W}(t)), \qquad (8)$$

where $G_{\eta(t)}(\mathbf{W}, \mathbf{W}(t)) = f(\mathbf{W}(t)) + \langle\nabla f(\mathbf{W}(t)), \mathbf{W} - \mathbf{W}(t)\rangle + \frac{\eta(t)}{2}\|\mathbf{W} - \mathbf{W}(t)\|_F^2 + \lambda_2\|\mathbf{W}\|_{2,1}$, $\nabla f(\mathbf{W}(t)) = (\mathbf{X}\mathbf{X}^T + \lambda_1\mathbf{X}\mathbf{L}\mathbf{X}^T)\mathbf{W}(t) - \mathbf{X}\mathbf{Y}^T$, and $\eta(t)$ and $\mathbf{W}(t)$ are, respectively, a tuning parameter and the value of $\mathbf{W}$ obtained at the t-iteration.

By ignoring the terms independent of $\mathbf{W}$ in Eq. (8), we can rewrite it as

$$\mathbf{W}(t+1) = \pi_{\eta(t)}(\mathbf{W}(t)) = \arg\min_{\mathbf{W}} \frac{1}{2}\|\mathbf{W} - \mathbf{U}(t)\|_2^2 + \frac{\lambda_2}{\eta(t)}\|\mathbf{W}\|_{2,1} \qquad (9)$$

where $\mathbf{U}(t) = \mathbf{W}(t) - \frac{1}{\eta(t)} \nabla f(\mathbf{W}(t))$ and $\pi_{\eta(t)}(\mathbf{W}(t))$ is the Euclidean projection of $\mathbf{W}(t)$ onto the convex set $\eta(t)$. Thanks to the separability of $\mathbf{W}(t+1)$ in each row, we can obtain the optimal $\mathbf{W}(t+1)$ by finding a closed form solution of each row [9].

Meanwhile, in order to accelerate the proximal gradient method in Eq. (8), we further introduce an auxiliary variable $\mathbf{V}(t+1)$ as:

$$\mathbf{V}(t+1) = \mathbf{W}(t) + \frac{\alpha(t) - 1}{\alpha(t+1)}(\mathbf{W}(t+1) - \mathbf{W}(t)). \tag{10}$$

where the coefficient $\alpha(t+1)$ is usually set as $\alpha(t+1) = \frac{1+\sqrt{1+4\alpha(t)^2}}{2}$ [9].

3 Experimental Analysis

3.1 Dataset and Feature Extraction

We conducted performance evaluation on a subset (202 subjects: 51 AD, 43 MCI Converter: MCI-C, 56 MCI Non-Converter: MCI-NC, and 52 NC) of the ADNI dataset by comparing the proposed method with the competing methods. We considered two multi-class classification problems: AD vs. MCI (including both MCI-C and MCI-NC) vs. NC and AD vs. MCI-C vs. MCI-NC vs. NC. Regarding the feature extraction, we first sequentially performed spatial distortion, skull-stripping, and cerebellum removal for Magnetic Resonance Imaging (MRI) and Positron Emission Tomography (PET) images. For the MRI images, we further segmented them into three tissue types of gray matter, white matter, and cerebrospinal fluid. By warping a template into a subject's brain image, we parcellated the gray matter into 93 Region-Of-Interests (ROIs). The PET images were spatially aligned to its respective MRI images. Finally, we obtained 93 gray matter tissue volumes from an MRI image and also 93 mean intensities from a PET image. For the modality fusion of MRI and PET (MRI+PET), we concatenated their features into a long vector of 186 features.

3.2 Experimental Setting

We compared our feature selection method with the widely used methods such as Fisher Score (FS for short) [3], LPP [7], LDA [3], and PCA [3]. The FS is categorized as a feature selection method since it selects features in the original feature space based on the score ranking [3]. Meanwhile, LPP, LDA, and PCA are subspace learning methods, which aim, respectively, at preserving the local structures, the maximal variance, and the global structures of the data [3,15]. We also compared the proposed method with the state-of-the-art feature selection methods applied for AD diagnosis: Sparse Joint Classification and Regression (SJCR) [12] and Multi-Modal Multi-Task (M3T) [16]. For these two methods, we followed their papers to apply a 0-1 encoding method for the class indicator matrix.

Table 1. Comparison of classification accuracy ((mean±standard deviation)%) of two classification tasks

Method	AD/MCI/NC			AD/MCI-C/MCI-NC/NC		
	MRI	PET	MRI+PET	MRI	PET	MRI+PET
FS	62.33±1.56	60.11±1.54	62.88±1.31	50.87±1.73	50.44±1.49	51.76±1.58
PCA	63.71±1.30	61.49±1.58	64.61±1.60	51.05±1.64	51.51±1.62	52.20±1.60
LPP	63.21±1.91	61.03±1.22	64.35±1.29	51.72±1.42	51.39±1.58	52.60±1.37
LDA	49.01±1.71	39.02±1.23	51.85±1.66	35.25±1.65	31.82±1.40	36.32±1.64
SJCR	64.02±1.36	61.31±1.73	67.66±1.63	52.13±1.73	51.85±1.68	55.98±1.65
M3T	63.30±1.66	61.32±1.90	67.91±1.91	51.89±1.61	50.91±1.83	54.47±1.67
Proposed	**68.31±1.23**	**65.50±1.50**	**73.35±1.53**	**59.74±1.52**	**56.29±1.53**	**61.06±1.40**

3.3   Classification Results

Table 1 reports the classification accuracy of all the methods for two multi-class classification problems. The experimental results in Table 1 clearly show that the proposed method outperformed all the competing methods in all experiments. For example, in the three-class classification problem, our method improved the classification accuracy by 4.29% (MRI), 4.01% (PET), and 5.44% (MRI+PET), respectively, compared to the best performances among the competing methods. Meanwhile, in the four-class classification problem, the classification improvements were higher than the best performances among the competing methods as much as 7.61% (MRI), 4.44% (PET), and 5.08% (MRI+PET), respectively. Based on these results, we argue that the proposed discriminative and noise-resistant feature selection method helped enhance the classification performances.

Besides, we found that LDA achieved the worst classification performances among all the methods. The main reason was that LDA projected the original high dimensional feature space into only two or three dimensional subspace, respectively. Such low-dimensional space was not enough to correctly classify the neurimaging features. On the other hand, the subspace learning methods, except for LDA, outperformed the feature selection method of FS. This makes it reasonable to integrate subspace learning into the feature selection framework. Moreover, the proposed method clearly outperformed both the conventional feature selection and subspace learning methods thanks to the combination of the two approaches.

3.4   Discussions

We investigated the importance of the brain regions in discriminating among classes based on the frequency of the selected ROIs by the proposed method with MRI+PET. According to our experimental results, we can know that the commonly selected regions in two multi-class classification tasks were uncus right, hippocampal formation right, uncus left, middle temporal gyrus left, hippocampal formation left, amygdala left, middle temporal gyrus right, and amygdala right from MRI, and precuneus right, precuneus left, and angular gyrus left from PET. These regions were also selected by the proposed method with either MRI or PET and almost all the competing methods with MRI+PET. Moreover, these regions have been also shown to be highly related to AD and MCI practical clinical diagnosis [2,8]. In this regard, we can say that these regions can be the potential biomarkers for AD diagnosis.

Meanwhile, the numbers of selected features in three- and four-class classification tasks were, respectively, 50.52 and 34.36 on average. That is, the smaller number of features were used in the classification task of considering the larger number of classes. It is also interesting that the larger number of features from MRI rather than PET was selected in both three- and four-class classification problems. This was also observed in the competing methods. Furthermore, from Table 1, we can see that in general, the MRI-based methods achieved better performance than the PET-based methods. Based on these observations, it is likely that the structural MR image provides more discriminative information in identifying the clinical status related to AD, compared to the functional PET image.

4   Conclusions

In this work, we focused on the issue of discriminative feature selection for multi-class classification in AD diagnosis. Specifically, we proposed a novel feature selection method by integrating subspace learning, which utilized both the global and the local information inherent in the data, into in a sparse least square regression framework. In our experimental results on the ADNI dataset, we validated the efficacy of the proposed method by enhancing the classification accuracies in multi-class classification problems.

Acknowledgements. This study was supported by National Institutes of Health (EB006733, EB008374, EB009634, AG041721, AG042599, and MH100217). Xiaofeng Zhu was partly supported by the National Natural Science Foundation of China under grant 61263035.

References

1. Argyriou, A., Evgeniou, T., Pontil, M.: Convex multi-task feature learning. Machine Learning 73(3), 243–272 (2008)
2. Chételat, G., Eustache, F., Viader, F., Sayette, V.D.L., Pélerin, A., Mézenge, F., Hannequin, D., Dupuy, B., Baron, J.C., Desgranges, B.: FDG-PET measurement is more accurate than neuropsychological assessments to predict global cognitive deterioration in patients with mild cognitive impairment. Neurocase 11(1), 14–25 (2005)
3. Duda, R.O., Hart, P.E., Stork, D.G.: Pattern classification. John Wiley & Sons (2012)
4. Fan, Y., Rao, H., Hurt, H., Giannetta, J., Korczykowski, M., Shera, D., Avants, B.B., Gee, J.C., Wang, J., Shen, D.: Multivariate examination of brain abnormality using both structural and functional MRI. NeuroImage 36(4), 1189–1199 (2007)

5. Franke, K., Ziegler, G., Klöppel, S., Gaser, C.: Estimating the age of healthy subjects from T1-weighted MRI scans using kernel methods: Exploring the influence of various parameters. NeuroImage 50(3), 883–892 (2010)
6. Hastie, T., Tibshirani, R., Friedman, J., Franklin, J.: The elements of statistical learning: data mining, inference and prediction. The Mathematical Intelligencer 27(2), 83–85 (2005)
7. He, X., Cai, D., Niyogi, P.: Laplacian score for feature selection. In: NIPS, pp. 1–8 (2005)
8. Misra, C., Fan, Y., Davatzikos, C.: Baseline and longitudinal patterns of brain atrophy in MCI patients, and their use in prediction of short-term conversion to AD: results from ADNI. NeuroImage 44(4), 1415–1422 (2009)
9. Nesterov, Y.: Introductory lectures on convex optimization: a basic course, vol. 87 (2004)
10. Nie, F., Huang, H., Cai, X., Ding, C.H.Q.: Efficient and robust feature selection via joint $\ell_{2,1}$-norms minimization. In: NIPS, pp. 1813–1821 (2010)
11. Suk, H.-I., Shen, D.: Deep learning-based feature representation for AD/MCI classification. In: Mori, K., Sakuma, I., Sato, Y., Barillot, C., Navab, N. (eds.) MICCAI 2013, Part II. LNCS, vol. 8150, pp. 583–590. Springer, Heidelberg (2013)
12. Wang, H., Nie, F., Huang, H., Risacher, S., Saykin, A.J., Shen, L.: Identifying AD-sensitive and cognition-relevant imaging biomarkers via joint classification and regression. In: Fichtinger, G., Martel, A., Peters, T. (eds.) MICCAI 2011, Part III. LNCS, vol. 6893, pp. 115–123. Springer, Heidelberg (2011)
13. Wang, H., Nie, F., Huang, H., Risacher, S.L., Saykin, A.J., Shen, L., et al.: Identifying disease sensitive and quantitative trait-relevant biomarkers from multidimensional heterogeneous imaging genetics data via sparse multimodal multitask learning. Bioinformatics 28(12), i127–i136 (2012)
14. Wee, C.Y., Yap, P.T., Zhang, D., Denny, K., Browndyke, J.N., Potter, G.G., Welsh-Bohmer, K.A., Wang, L., Shen, D.: Identification of MCI individuals using structural and functional connectivity networks. Neuroimage 59(3), 2045–2056 (2012)
15. Ye, J.: Least squares linear discriminant analysis. In: ICML, pp. 1087–1093 (2007)
16. Zhang, D., Shen, D.: Multi-modal multi-task learning for joint prediction of multiple regression and classification variables in Alzheimer's disease. NeuroImage 59(2), 895–907 (2012)
17. Zhang, D., Wang, Y., Zhou, L., Yuan, H., Shen, D.: Multimodal classification of Alzheimer's disease and mild cognitive impairment. NeuroImage 55(3), 856–867 (2011)
18. Zhu, X., Huang, Z., Shen, H.T., Cheng, J., Xu, C.: Dimensionality reduction by mixed kernel canonical correlation analysis. Pattern Recognition 45(8), 3003–3016 (2012)
19. Zhu, X., Huang, Z., Yang, Y., Shen, H.T., Xu, C., Luo, J.: Self-taught dimensionality reduction on the high-dimensional small-sized data. Pattern Recognition 46(1), 215–229 (2013)
20. Zhu, X., Suk, H.I., Shen, D.: Matrix-similarity based loss function and feature selection for Alzheimer's Disease diagnosis. In: CVPR (2014)
21. Zhu, X., Suk, H.I., Shen, D.: Multi-modality canonical feature selection for Alzheimer's disease diagnosis. In: Golland, P. (ed.) MICCAI 2014, Part II. LNCS, vol. 8674, pp. 162–169. Springer, Heidelberg (2014)
22. Zhu, X., Suk, H.I., Shen, D.: A novel matrix-similarity based loss function for joint regression and classification in AD diagnosis. NeuroImage 14, 1–30 (2014)
23. Zhu, X., Suk, H.-I., Shen, D.: A novel multi-relation regularization method for regression and classification in AD diagnosis. In: Golland, P. (ed.) MICCAI 2014, Part III. LNCS, vol. 8675, pp. 401–408. Springer, Heidelberg (2014)

Context-Aware Anatomical Landmark Detection: Application to Deformable Model Initialization in Prostate CT Images

Yaozong Gao[1,2] and Dinggang Shen[1]

[1] Department of Radiology and BRIC,
University of North Carolina at Chapel Hill, USA
[2] Department of Computer Science,
University of North Carolina at Chapel Hill, USA

Abstract. Anatomical landmark detection plays an important role in medical image analysis, e.g., for landmark-guided image registration, and deformable model initialization. Among various existing methods, regression-based landmark detection method has recently drawn much attention due to its robustness and efficiency. In this method, a regression model is often trained for each landmark to predict the location of this landmark from any image voxel based on local patch appearance, e.g., also the 3D displacement vector from any image voxel to this landmark. During the application stage, the predicted displacement vectors from all image voxels form a displacement field, which is then utilized for final landmark detection with a regression voting process. Accordingly, the quality of predicted displacement field largely determines the accuracy of final landmark detection. However, the displacement fields predicted by previous methods are often spatially inconsistent 1) within each displacement field of same landmark and 2) also across the displacement fields of all different landmarks, thus limiting the final landmark detection accuracy. The main reason is that for each landmark, the 3D displacement of each image voxel is predicted independently, and also for all different landmarks their displacement fields are estimated independently. To address these issues, we propose a two-layer regression model for context-aware landmark detection. Specifically, the first layer is designed to separately provide the initial displacement fields for different landmarks, and the second layer is designed to refine them jointly by using the context features extracted from results of the first layer to impose spatial consistency 1) within the displacement field of each landmark and 2) across the displacement fields of all different landmarks. Experimental results on a CT prostate dataset show that our proposed method significantly outperforms the traditional classification-based and regression-based methods in both landmark detection and deformable model initialization.

1 Introduction

Anatomical landmarks (also landmarks for short) are the distinct points at anatomical structures. The detection of landmarks is important in many medical image analysis tasks, e.g., landmark-guided image registration [1], and deformable

G. Wu et al. (Eds.): MLMI 2014, LNCS 8679, pp. 165–173, 2014.

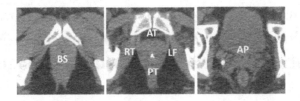

Fig. 1. Example of six prostate landmarks in CT images. BS: base center; RT: right lateral point; LT: left lateral point; AT: anterior point; PT: posterior point; AP: apex center.

model initialization [2]. However, automatic landmark detection is quite challenging due to the variability of anatomical structures across different subjects and also sometimes the indistinct image appearances of landmarks (Fig. 1). Among various methods, learning-based methods have been shown very effective to deal with these challenges. In particular, previous learning-based methods can be roughly categorized into two classes: classification-based [3,4,5,6] and regression-based landmark detection methods [7,8]. In the former class, landmark detection is formulated as a binary classification problem, with voxels near the landmark as positives and the rest as negatives. Then, a strong classifier is typically trained to distinguish landmark voxels from other voxels. For example, Cheng et al. [5] proposed to use classification forest for detecting CBCT dental landmarks. Zhan et al. [6] adopted cascade Adaboost classifiers with Haar wavelet features for MR knee landmark detection. On the other hand, regression-based methods [7,8] learn a regression model (e.g., regression forest) for capturing the non-linear relationship between a voxel's local appearance and its 3D displacement to the target landmark. During the application stage, the learned regression model is used to predict the 3D displacement for each voxel in the testing image, and then obtains a displacement field for the whole testing image[1]. Finally, the landmark location is determined by a voting process using the estimated displacement field. Recent investigation [8] has shown that the regression-based method tends to yield more robust and accurate detection results than the classification-based method in landmark detection. Accordingly, in this paper, we will focus on regression-based landmark detection.

It is clear to see that the accuracy of regression-based landmark detection highly depends on the quality of the predicted displacement field. However, the displacement fields predicted by previous methods [7,8] often suffer from two types of spatial inconsistency, which potentially limit their detection accuracy. **First**, the obtained displacement field of each target landmark is often spatially inconsistent, as the displacement vector from each image voxel to the target landmark is predicted independently. This spatial inconsistency often results in

---

[1] Please note that "displacement field" used in this paper is different from the term often used in the non-rigid image registration. In the latter, each displacement vector indicates the position offset between the two corresponding points in the fixed and moving images, respectively, while the displacement vector in this paper means the position offset from any image point to the target landmark within the same testing image.

non-smooth displacement fields (See the first-layer distance (displacement magnitude) maps in Fig. 2). **Second**, there might also be spatial inconsistency across the obtained displacement fields of all different landmarks since the displacement field for each target landmark is estimated independently. This spatial inconsistency could lead to unreasonable spatial configuration of all detected landmarks. In the literature, researchers often focus on addressing the second spatial inconsistency problem by simply exploiting the inter-landmark spatial relationship in a post-processing step. For example, Zhan et al. [6] proposed a set of linear spatial models to capture the spatial relationship among all different landmarks, and then used it to correct the wrongly detected landmarks. However, due to the lack of appearance information in this post-processing step, these methods can correct only the landmarks that are obviously wrong in their positions. Moreover, the accuracy of those corrected landmarks is often limited due to the use of only the spatial locations of other landmarks for correction. Thus, exploiting the inter-landmark spatial relationship in the post processing step can improve only the robustness of landmark detection, but not the detection accuracy. To improve both robustness and accuracy of landmark detection, it is necessary to incorporate the inter-landmark spatial relationship into the displacement prediction step as proposed in this paper.

Specifically, we propose a two-layer regression model for context-aware landmark detection by imposing the spatial consistency 1) within the displacement field of each landmark, and also 2) across the displacement fields of all different landmarks. In particular, a two-layer regression forest is adopted as a landmark detector for each landmark. Here, the first-layer regression forest is the same as in the traditional regression-based methods, which maps a testing image into a displacement field using only the image appearance features. The displacement fields predicted for all landmarks by the first layer provide the rich context features to assist the refinement of the respective displacement fields in the second layer. That is, since we can roughly know the relative spatial positions of each image voxel to all target landmarks, we can use this valuable information to impose the spatial consistency on the refined displacement fields. Also, by combining high-level context features with low-level appearance features, the second-layer regression forest is able to significantly improve the quality of each predicted displacement field, thus leading to more accurate landmark detection than the traditional regression-based methods (which is also referred in this paper as the one-layer regression model).

2   Methodology

2.1   Regression Forest and Landmark Detection

Regression forest is one type of random forests specialized for non-linear regression tasks. It consists of mutiple independently trained binary decision trees. Each tree is trained with randomness on both features and associated thresholds. The final prediction is the average over the predictions of all individual trees. As an ensemble method, regression forest typically yields robust and accurate predictions.

In the regression-based landmark detection, regression forest is often used to learn the non-linear mapping from a voxel's local appearance to its 3D displacement towards the target landmark. Inspired by the patch-based methods [10], a voxel is often represented by a local patch centered at it. For better characterization of local patch, instead of using only intensities, we also extract Haar-like features from local patch to serve as feature representation for each voxel. The Haar-like features are defined as follows:

$$v(I) = \sum_{i=1}^{Z} p_i \sum_{\|\mathbf{x}-\mathbf{a}_i\|_\infty \leq s_i} I(\mathbf{x}) \tag{1}$$

where $v(I)$ denotes a Haar-like feature, I is a local patch, Z is the number of 3D cubic functions used in this Haar-like feature, and $p_i \in \{-1, 1\}$, $\mathbf{a}_i \in \mathbb{R}^3$ and s_i are the polarity, position and scale of the i-th 3D cubic function, respectively. By changing the values of Z, p_i, $\mathbf{a}_i$ and s_i, we can generate an unlimited number of Haar-like features. During the regression forest training, we randomly sample Z, p_i, $\mathbf{a}_i$ and s_i to generate a feature subset whenever needed. In this work, we limit Z to $\{1, 2\}$, and s_i to $\{3, 5\}$. In order to capture the long-distance context features within the local patch, we do not limit $\mathbf{a}_i$, which can have arbitrary values as long as the 3D cubic function does not move outside the local patch I (of size $30 \times 30 \times 30$).

Regression Voting: Once the appearance-to-displacement mapping is learned by regression forest, we can adopt a regression voting to finally detect the landmark position in the new testing image. The idea of regression voting is simple. For each voxel $\mathbf{x} \in \mathbb{R}^3$ in the testing image, it casts one vote to the discrete position nearest to $\mathbf{x} + \tilde{\mathbf{d}}_\mathbf{x}$, where $\tilde{\mathbf{d}}_\mathbf{x} \in \mathbb{R}^3$ is the predicted displacement vector of voxel $\mathbf{x}$. After voting from all possible image voxels, a voting response map is obtained. Then, the landmark location can be determined as the position that receives the most votes in the voting response map.

Multi-resolution Landmark Detection: To increase both robustness and efficiency of regression-based landmark detection, we can further implement the above algorithm in a multi-resolution way. Specifically, the landmark location detected in the coarser resolution can be used as a good initialization for the next finer resolution. In the finer resolution, regression voting is performed only in a local neighborhood centered at the initialization. In this way, only voxels near the target landmark are involved in the voting, while the far-away voxels are automatically filtered out. This would potentially improve the detection accuracy, as the far-away voxels might not be informative for the detection of the target landmark.

2.2 Context-Aware Landmark Detection

In this section, we first present the training and application of our method. Then, we elaborate how the two types of spatial consistency can be simultaneously enforced in the second-layer regression models by using distance-based context features. Finally, we conclude the contributions of our method compared with previous methods.

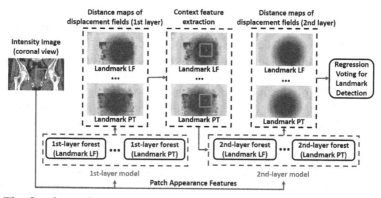

Fig. 2. The flowchart of context-aware landmark detection. Cold and warm color in the color maps indicate the voxels with small and large predicted distances from the target landmark, respectively. Green boxes show the local patches where appearance features and also context features are extracted for the voxel marked as red cross.

Training and Application: In **the training stage**, a two-layer regression forest is trained for each landmark to serve as landmark detector. The first-layer regression forest is trained using only image appearance features (i.e., Haar-like features as defined in Eq. 1), which is the same as in the traditional regression-based landmark detection methods. Then, we can use the trained first-layer forests to estimate an initial displacement field for each landmark, for every training image. By taking L2 norm on the initial displacement field, we can convert the displacement fields into the distance maps. Afterwards, the high-level context features can be jointly extracted from the distance maps of all landmarks and further combined with the previous image appearance features to train the second-layer regression forests. **The application stage** follows the same pipeline as the training stage. To detect a set of target landmarks in a testing image, we will first apply the first-layer regression models to generate an initial distance map for each target landmark. Then, both the initial distance maps of all different target landmarks and the original testing image are taken as input to the second-layer regression forests, which will combine the appearance features extracted from the original testing image with the context features extracted from the initial distance maps of all different target landmarks to refine the respective displacement fields. Once the displacement field for each target landmark is finally obtained, regression voting (Section 2.1) can be adopted to detect the landmark location. Fig. 2 shows the flowchart of our proposed method.

Distance-Based Context Features: The spatial consistency of our context-aware landmark detection comes from two aspects: **1)** spatial consistency within the displacement field of each target landmark, and **2)** spatial consistency across displacement fields of all different target landmarks. Both aspects are simultaneously fulfilled by using the distance-based context features. Different from the traditional context features [9], which are the simple classification responses at the context locations, our context features are Haar-like features (Eq. 1) computed from local patches of distance maps. Specifically, there are two types of context features used in our work, namely **intra-landmark and inter-landmark context features**, respectively. To detect one target landmark, intra-landmark context features refer to the Haar-like features extracted from the initial distance map of the landmark itself. These features are informative in providing the roughly estimated distances of nearby image voxels to the target landmark, and thus can be used for spatially regularizing the displacement field of this landmark. On the other hand, inter-landmark context features refer to the Haar-like features extracted from distance maps of other target landmarks. These features encode the spatial relationship between this landmark and other landmarks, e.g., how far away this landmark is usually from other landmarks. Thus, the use of inter-landmark context features will be effective to impose the spatial consistency across displacement fields of different landmarks. Fig. 2 shows the distance maps of two prostate landmarks before and after imposing two types of spatial consistency as mentioned above. We can clearly observe the improved quality of distance maps by using both types of context features.

Contributions of Our Method: To the best of our knowledge, this is the first paper that utilizes distance-based context features to improve the landmark detection accuracy. The use of distance-based context features not only offers a spatially smooth displacement field for each target landmark, but also enforces the spatial consistency across the predicted displacement fields of all different target landmarks. Compared to previous methods that exploit inter-landmark spatial relationship in a post-processing step, our proposed method can embed the inter-landmark spatial constraint into the displacement prediction step for improving the quality of the predicted displacement fields, and hence the final landmark detection accuracy.

3 Experimental Results

To validate the effectiveness of our context-aware landmark detection, we apply it to detect the six prostate landmarks (Fig. 1) in CT images for deformable model initialization. Specifically, the affine transformation estimated between automatically detected landmarks and their counterparts in the mean shape model will be used for transforming the mean shape model onto the testing image for initialization.

Our dataset consists of 73 pelvic CT images with various image contrasts as shown in Fig. 3. The typical image size is $512 \times 512 \times (60{\sim}80)$ with voxel size $0.938 \times 0.938 \times 3.000\text{mm}^3$. The six landmarks and the whole prostate in each of these 73 images have been manually annotated by an experienced radiation oncologist to serve as ground truth. Four-fold cross validation is used to evaluate our method. In each fold, 54 images are used for training and 19 images are used for testing.

In Table 1, we compared the traditional classification-based ("Cascade") and regression-based ("Regression") landmark detection methods [4,7] with three variants of our methods ("Intra-LM", "Inter-LM", "Both") on the same dataset. All these methods use the same type of appearance features and the same multi-resolution framework for fair comparison. Here, "Intra-LM" imposes only spatial

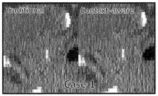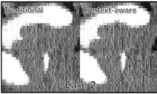

Fig. 3. Qualitative comparison between the traditional regression-based landmark detection with outlier correction ("Traditional") and our proposed method ("Context-aware") on two difference cases (left and right panels). Crosses indicate the positions of landmarks BS, AT, PT and AP after projection onto the central slice of the prostate in the saggital view. **Blue**: ground-truth landmarks. **Red**: detected landmarks by "Traditional". **Green**: detected landmarks by "Context-aware".

consistency within the displacement field of each target landmark by using intra-landmark context features; "Inter-LM" imposes only spatial consistency across the displacement fields of different landmarks by using inter-landmark context features; "Both" is the full version of our method by imposing both types of spatial consistency. On the other hand, to filter out the influence of possibly wrongly detected landmarks (i.e., outliers) on deformable model initialization, we implemented the outlier correction algorithm in [6] to correct the possibly wrongly detected landmarks before deformable model initialization. From Table 1, we can clearly see the accuracy improvments for both landmark detection and deformable model initialization ($p < 0.05$) by imposing spatial consistency either within displacement field of each target landmark or across displacement fields of all different target landmarks. By combining both types of spatial consistency, we can achieve the best performance (as bolded ones in Table 1). In addition, Fig. 3 gives a qualitative comparison between the traditional regression-based landmark detection with outlier correction and our context-aware landmark detection. We can see the importance of utilizing the inter-landmark spatial relationship in the displacement prediction step, instead of a post-processing step.

Table 1. Quantitative comparison between different landmark detection methods on both landmark detection and deformable model initialization. **Cascade**: the traditional classification-based landmark detection; **Regression**: the traditional regression-based landmark detection (also referred as one-layer model); **Intra-LM**: our method with only intra-landmark context features; **Inter-LM**: our method with only inter-landmark context features; **Both**: our method with both types of context features. Error (mm) indicates the landmark detection error. DSC indicates the Dice similarity coefficient between initialized deformable model (e.g., mean shape) and ground-truth. ASD (mm) indicates the average surface distance between the initialized deformable model and ground-truth. * indicates the accuracy without using outlier correction.

		Cascade	Regression	Intra-LM	Inter-LM	Both
Landmark	Error*	6.75 ± 4.81	5.76 ± 2.51	4.98 ± 1.78	4.83 ± 1.93	**4.82 ± 1.89**
Detection	Error	6.70 ± 4.75	5.70 ± 2.59	4.82 ± 1.68	4.73 ± 1.78	**4.67 ± 1.66**
Model	DSC	0.72 ± 0.14	0.78 ± 0.08	0.81 ± 0.07	0.81 ± 0.07	**0.82 ± 0.07**
Initialization	ASD	3.62 ± 1.69	2.82 ± 1.24	2.51 ± 0.83	2.50 ± 1.06	**2.42 ± 0.88**

It is worth noting that, by detecting only six landmarks, our method is able to achieve a fairly good initialization for deformable models (ASD 2.42 ± 0.88mm), which is already better than the inter-user variability of manual delineations of prostate (ASD 3.03 ± 1.15mm [12]). Moreover, it is interesting to see that our landmark-based initialization achieves an accuracy better than several existing prostate segmentation methods (e.g., [11] (ASD 4.19 ± 0.90mm) and [12] (ASD 3.35 ± 1.40mm)), and is comparable to the state-of-the-art prostate segmentation method [13] (ASD 2.37 ± 0.89mm). Although the comparison is not completely fair since different datasets are adopted, it reveals the effectiveness of context-aware landmark detection in deformable model initialization.

The typical runtime of our method to detect a single landmark is 2.35 seconds on an Intel i5 CPU. The detection of six landmarks costs about 14.1 seconds.

4 Conclusion

In this paper, we propose a two-layer regression model for context-aware landmark detection. By imposing the spatial consistency within displacement field of each target landmark, and also across displacement fields of all different target landmarks, our method is able to achieve significant improvement over the traditional classification-based and regression-based landmark detection methods. Experimental results in a CT prostate dataset indicate that our proposed method is very effective for deformable model initialization.

References

1. Johnson, H.J., Christensen, G.E.: Consistent landmark and intensity-based image registration. IEEE TMI 21(5), 450–461 (2002)
2. Zhang, S., Zhan, Y., Dewan, M., et al.: Towards robust and effective shape modeling: Sparse shape composition. Med. Imag. Anal. 16(1), 265–277 (2012)
3. Zheng, Y., Barbu, A., Georgescu, B., Scheuering, M., Comaniciu, D.: Four-Chamber Heart Modeling and Automatic Segmentation for 3-D Cardiac CT Volumes Using Marginal Space Learning and Steerable Features. IEEE TMI 27(11), 1668–1681 (2008)
4. Viola, P., Jones, M.J.: Robust Real-Time Face Detection. IJCV 57(2), 137–154 (2004)
5. Cheng, E., Chen, J., Yang, J., et al.: Automatic Dent-landmark detection in 3-D CBCT dental volumes. In: EMBC 2011, pp. 6204–6207 (2011)
6. Zhan, Y., et al.: Robust Automatic Knee MR Slice Positioning Through Redundant and Hierarchical Anatomy Detection. IEEE TMI 30(12), 2087–2100 (2011)
7. Criminisi, A., Shotton, J., Robertson, D., Konukoglu, E.: Regression Forests for Efficient Anatomy Detection and Localization in CT Studies. In: Menze, B., Langs, G., Tu, Z., Criminisi, A. (eds.) MICCAI 2010. LNCS, vol. 6533, pp. 106–117. Springer, Heidelberg (2011)
8. Cootes, T.F., Ionita, M.C., Lindner, C., Sauer, P.: Robust and Accurate Shape Model Fitting Using Random Forest Regression Voting. In: Fitzgibbon, A., Lazebnik, S., Perona, P., Sato, Y., Schmid, C. (eds.) ECCV 2012, Part VII. LNCS, vol. 7578, pp. 278–291. Springer, Heidelberg (2012)

9. Tu, Z., Bai, X.: Auto-Context and Its Application to High-Level Vision Tasks and 3D Brain Image Segmentation. IEEE PAMI 32(10), 1744–1757 (2010)
10. Coup, P., et al.: Patch-based segmentation using expert priors: Application to hippocampus and ventricle segmentation. NeuroImage 54(2), 940–954 (2010)
11. Rousson, M., Khamene, A., Diallo, M., Celi, J.C., Sauer, F.: Constrained Surface Evolutions for Prostate and Bladder Segmentation in CT Images. In: Liu, Y., Jiang, T.-Z., Zhang, C. (eds.) CVBIA 2005. LNCS, vol. 3765, pp. 251–260. Springer, Heidelberg (2005)
12. Lay, N., Birkbeck, N., Zhang, J., Zhou, S.K.: Rapid Multi-organ Segmentation Using Context Integration and Discriminative Models. In: Gee, J.C., Joshi, S., Pohl, K.M., Wells, W.M., Zöllei, L. (eds.) IPMI 2013. LNCS, vol. 7917, pp. 450–462. Springer, Heidelberg (2013)
13. Lu, C., Zheng, Y., Birkbeck, N., Zhang, J., Kohlberger, T., Tietjen, C., Boettger, T., Duncan, J.S., Zhou, S.K.: Precise Segmentation of Multiple Organs in CT Volumes Using Learning-Based Approach and Information Theory. In: Ayache, N., Delingette, H., Golland, P., Mori, K. (eds.) MICCAI 2012, Part II. LNCS, vol. 7511, pp. 462–469. Springer, Heidelberg (2012)

Optimal MAP Parameters Estimation in STAPLE - Learning from Performance Parameters versus Image Similarity Information

Subrahmanyam Gorthi[1], Alireza Akhondi-Asl[1],
Jean-Philippe Thiran[2], and Simon K. Warfield[1]

[1] Computational Radiology Laboratory, Boston Children's Hospital,
and Harvard Medical School, 300 Longwood Ave. Boston MA 02115, USA
[2] Signal Processing Laboratory (LTS5), École Polytechnique Fédérale de Lausanne
(EPFL), and Department of Radiology, University Hospital Center (CHUV)
and University of Lausanne (UNIL), Lausanne, Switzerland

Abstract. In many medical imaging applications, merging segmentations obtained from multiple reference images (i.e., templates) has become a standard practice for improving the accuracy as well as reliability. Simultaneous Truth And Performance Level Estimation (STAPLE) is a widely used fusion algorithm that simultaneously estimates both performance parameters for each template, and the output segmentation; a more accurate estimation of performance parameters consequently results in more accurate output segmentations. In this paper, we propose a new approach for learning prior knowledge about the performance parameters of each template, and for incorporating it into the Maximum-a-Posteriori (MAP) formulation of the STAPLE, so that more accurate output segmentations can be obtained. More specifically, we propose a new approach to learn, for each structure to be segmented, the relationships between the performance parameters (viz. sensitivity and specificity) and the intensity similarities; we also propose a methodology for transferring this prior knowledge about the performance parameters into the STAPLE algorithm through optimal setting of the MAP parameters. The proposed approach is evaluated for the segmentation of structures in the brain MR images. These experiments have clearly demonstrated the advantages of incorporating such prior knowledge.

Keywords: Medical Imaging, Segmentation, Atlas-based Segmentation, Label Fusion, STAPLE, MAP Formulation, MRI, Brain, Lateral Ventricles.

1 Introduction

It has been shown in many recent works that the automated segmentations obtained based on multiple template images provide more accurate segmentations than the single-template-based methods [1–7]. Multiple-templates-based segmentation can be defined as the alignment of a set of reference images with

G. Wu et al. (Eds.): MLMI 2014, LNCS 8679, pp. 174–181, 2014.

the corresponding segmentations to the target image to be segmented, and followed by the fusion of those aligned segmentations to estimate the reference standard segmentation. Fusion methods can be broadly classified into two categories: (i) voting-based methods [4–7] and (ii) statistically driven methods that simultaneously estimate both the ground-truth and performance-parameters of each template [1–3, 8–10].

Simultaneous Truth and Performance Level Estimation (STAPLE) is a widely used algorithm [1] that belongs to the second category of statistical fusion methods. The Expectation-Maximization (EM) approach used with the classical STAPLE algorithm guarantees convergence to a local optimum solution. However, if we can incorporate appropriate prior knowledge about the performance parameters of the templates into the Maximum-a-Posteriori (MAP) formulation of the STAPLE [9, 10], then it can provide more accurate estimations of both the reference standard and performance parameters.

MAP solution of the STAPLE algorithm is studied previously in a very specific context of missing data [9, 10], where segmentations for the labels of interests are missing in some of the templates; the authors proposed to incorporate this "missing" information into the STAPLE by setting the diagonal elements of the performance matrix close to 1 for the templates that contain the segmentations, and close to 0 for the templates with missing data. As that approach is specifically designed to deal with the fusion problem in the presence of missing data, it cannot distinguish between the performances of the regular templates with no missing data.

In this paper, we introduce a general and powerful framework for learning prior knowledge about the performance parameters of each label in each template, and for using that information to optimally set the MAP parameters of the STAPLE algorithm. More specifically, we propose here a new approach for learning the relationships between the intensity similarities and the performance parameters of each label. This is the first work that deals with learning and incorporating prior knowledge about the performance parameters into a statistical fusion framework, and this approach can be readily incorporated into many of the advanced variants of the STAPLE algorithm, like [2, 3, 8, 10].

The rest of the paper is organized as follows. Section 2 describes our new method. Section 3 presents the evaluation results both on synthetic data, and on real 3D brain images for the segmentation of lateral ventricles. Conclusions are presented in Section 4.

2 Methods

2.1 Framework of the STAPLE Algorithm

Let $D = \{D_1, \ldots, D_i, \ldots, D_N\}$ be a matrix of size $N \times J$, where N and J are respectively the number of voxels and the number of templates. In this matrix, $D_i = [D_{i1}, \ldots, D_{ij}, \ldots, D_{iJ}]'$ and D_{ij} is the label of the template j at voxel i. The goal here is to estimate the reference standard segmentation $T = \{T_1, \ldots, T_i, \ldots, T_N\}$ and the performance parameters $\theta = \{\theta_1, \ldots, \theta_j, \ldots, \theta_J\}$

where θ_j is the matrix of size $S \times S$, $\theta_{js's} = f(D_{ij} = s'|T_i = s)$, and S is the number of segmentation labels. Since both T and θ are unknown, the complete log-likelihood function $Q(\theta|\theta^t) = \sum_i \sum_j \sum_s W_{si}^t \log(\theta_{jD_{ij}s})$ is maximized iteratively using an EM algorithm where W_{si}^t is the posterior probability of the reference standard segmentation T_i for label s. The EM algorithm guarantees convergence to a local optimum. However, incorporating appropriate prior knowledge about the performance parameters of the template images through MAP formulation of the STAPLE could result in more accurate estimation of both the performance parameters and the reference standard. The following subsection presents beta distribution based MAP formulation of the STAPLE.

2.2   Beta Distribution Based MAP Formulation

The MAP formulation of the STAPLE algorithm can be expressed as:

$$Q_{\mathrm{MAP}}(\theta|\theta^t) = Q(\theta|\theta^t) + \gamma \log(p(\theta)). \tag{1}$$

where $p(\theta)$ is the prior probability of the performance parameters and γ is the weighting parameter between the data term and of the MAP prior. As the performance parameters for each template and each label can be considered to be independent of each other [10], $p(\theta)$ can be expressed as a product of the probabilities of each performance parameter denoted by $p(\theta_{js's})$.

Similar to [10], in this paper, we use beta distribution $B_{\alpha,\beta}(x) = \frac{1}{Z}x^{\alpha-1}(1 - x)^{\beta-1}$ for modeling the prior probabilities of each performance parameter. The main advantage of beta distribution is that it facilitates modeling a wide variety of differently shaped characteristics. Using of the beta distribution leads to the following expected value of the complete log-likelihood function:

$$Q_{\mathrm{MAP}}(\theta|\theta^t) = \sum_i \sum_j \sum_s W_{si}^t \log(\theta_{jD_{ij}s})$$
$$+ \gamma \sum_j \sum_{s'} \sum_s [(\alpha_{js's} - 1)\log(\theta_{js's}) + (\beta_{js's} - 1)(\log(1 - \theta_{js's}))]. \tag{2}$$

A detailed description regarding solving the above MAP formulation can be found in [10].

In [9, 10] the authors used the MAP solution for the specific problem of missing data. To this end, they used a set of fixed parameters for all of the templates containing labels, to have priors with probability close to one for diagonal performance parameters, and close to zero for off-diagonal performance parameters. However, in this paper, we are interested in incorporating the prior knowledge about the performance parameters of each label in each template. The following subsection presents our proposed approach for achieving this goal, which is based on learning the relationships between the performance parameters and the image similarity information.

2.3   Learning Performance Parameters vs. Image Similarity Relations

A common underlying assumption for many fusion methods [4–7] is that the accuracy of segmentations obtained from a given template are proportional to it's intensity similarity to the target image to be segmented. In similar lines, we make an assumption here that the performance parameters of a given template are proportional to it's intensity similarity to the target image. We then proceed further by learning the relationships between the performance parameters and the intensity information, by using all templates as our training data.

The training procedure that we propose for learning the prior knowledge is as follows:

1. Select an image from the template database, and treat it as the target image to be segmented.
   Hereafter, we refer to this image as the *pseudo-target*, in order to differentiate it from the actual target image to be segmented. The rest of the images in the database are used as templates for the pseudo-target.
2. Compute the *non-consensus mask* for the pseudo-target image, and compute both the performance parameters over this mask.
   It is easy to notice that instead of deriving the relationships based on the entire image, it is more effective to compute them over the non-consensus mask, which indicates the voxels where at least two of the template images differ in their labeling decisions. Hence, we proposed to compute the performance parameters over the non-consensus mask instead of the entire region.
3. *Observation 1*: As we deal here with the binary labeling problem, the diagonal elements of the performance matrix represent specificity and sensitivity [10], while the off-diagonal elements are (1-specificity) and (1-sensitivity); thus, we only need to learn prior knowledge about sensitivity and specificity.
   Observation 2: Let T' represent the ground truth segmentations for the selected pseudo target. From the definitions of sensitivity ($\Pr(D_{ij} = 1|T' = 1)$) and specificity ($\Pr(D_{ij} = 0|T' = 0)$), we know that they are computed respectively at those voxels where the ground truth labels are 1 and 0.
   Based on these observations, we propose to compute two different masks for intensity similarity calculations; the first mask contains only those voxels in the non-consensus mask for which $T' = 1$, and use this mask for computing the intensity similarity corresponding to sensitivity; similarly, the second mask contains only those voxels in the non-consensus mask for which $T' = 0$, and use this for computing intensity similarity corresponding to specificity.
4. Repeat steps 1 to 3 for each image in the template database using a leave-one-out approach.
5. By the completion of step-4, for a database of J templates, we will have $J(J-1)$ pairs of sensitivity (or specificity) versus similarity values.
   Perform a robust linear regression analysis, and obtain the final parameters representing the overall relation between the sensitivity (or specificity) and the image-similarity.

2.4   MAP Parameters Estimation

We now present how the prior knowledge learned using the approach proposed in Section 2.3 can be incorporated into the MAP formulation of the STAPLE.

The approach that we propose for estimating the performance of each template is as follows: **(1)** Unlike in the learning phase, as we do not know the ground truth segmentation for the target image, we propose to first compute the intensity similarity metric over the entire non-consensus mask (instead of using two different mask as in step 3 of Section 2.3). **(2)** Then, estimate the probable performance parameters for each template using the linear regression parameters computed in the learning phase, and the intensity similarities computed in step-1. **(3)** We further make the assumptions that the mode value of the beta distribution for a given performance parameter occurs at it's estimated value in step-2, and the variance of the beta distribution is equal to the variance of regression fit of the corresponding performance parameter. This implies that for each beta distribution, we know the mode and variance values, and the goal now is to obtain their equivalent α and β values as parameterized in Eq. 2. For this purpose, we use the method that was proposed in [11], and it is as follows.

Let m and σ^2 respectively represent the mode and variance of a beta distribution. Let us define an intermediate variable τ as:

$$\tau = \frac{\sigma^2}{(1-m)^2}. \tag{3}$$

Then, the parameter β of the beta-distribution corresponds to the largest positive real root of the following cubic equation:

$$c_3\beta^3 + c_2\beta^2 + c_1\beta + c_0 = 0, \tag{4}$$

whose coefficients are given by

$$c_0 = -12\tau m^3 + 20\tau m^2 - 11\tau m + 2\tau. \tag{5}$$

$$c_1 = 16\tau m^2 + (2 - 18\tau)m + 5\tau - 1. \tag{6}$$

$$c_2 = -(7\tau + 1)m + 4\tau. \tag{7}$$

$$c_3 = \tau. \tag{8}$$

The other shape parameter α of the fitted beta distribution is given by:

$$\alpha = \frac{(\beta - 2)m + 1}{1 - m}. \tag{9}$$

Thus, the prior knowledge about the performance parameters of each template is incorporated into the MAP formulation of Eq. 2, through α and β parameters of the distribution, computed using Eq. 9 and Eq. 4 respectively.

3   Results

3.1   Experiments on Synthetic Data

We first evaluated the proposed method using synthetic data. For this purpose, we generated 20 template images and their corresponding segmentations using

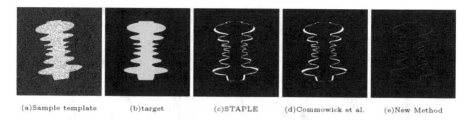

(a)Sample template   (b)target   (c)STAPLE   (d)Commowick et al.   (e)New Method

Fig. 1. Illustration of segmentation results from synthetic data. One of the 20 template images is shown in (a). The target image to be segmented is shown in (b). The misclassified voxels in the output labels from STAPLE [1], MAP-STAPLE of Commowick et al. [10], and our new method are shown in (c), (d) and (e) figures respectively.

the following approach. The target image to be segmented (shown in Fig. 1(b)) is rotated by 0°, 2°, 4°, 6°, 8° (i.e., 5 rotations), with translations of ±1 pixel (i.e., 2 translations), in both x and y directions (i.e., in 2 directions), which resulted in generating 20 templates. We then added white Gaussian noise to the template images with an SNR value of 40dB. One of those 20 templates is shown in Fig. 1(a).

For our new method, we used the local Normalized Cross Correlation (NCC) computed over a radius of 4 (i.e., on a 9×9 regular grid) around each voxel as the intensity-similarity metric. Finally, for setting the weighting parameter γ, we first run the EM-based STAPLE [1], and then set the γ value to the number voxels present in the output label of the STAPLE; by this way, the two terms in the MAP formulation of the STAPLE will have approximately similar weight.

We compared the results from our method with (i)classical EM-based STAPLE [1], and (ii)STAPLE algorithm of Commowick et al. with fixed MAP parameters [10]. The Dice Similarity Coefficient (DSC) values for the results from STAPLE, Commowick et al. and the proposed method are 91.01%, 91.06% and 98.12% respectively. Fig. 1(c), (d), and (e) highlight the differences between the ground truth and the results from each segmentation method, by showing the mis-classified voxels for each method. The number of misclassified voxels from STAPLE, Commowick et al. and our new method are 10931, 10772 and 2251 respectively. Since the method of Commowick et al. with fixed MAP parameters [10] was intended for a different purpose with missing data, we won't be considering it anymore in the later evaluations. In summary, these experiments on the synthetic data clearly illustrated the advantages of our new method.

3.2   Experiments on 3D Brain MR Images

We evaluated the proposed method for the segmentation of left and right lateral ventricles in the 3D brain MR images. These brain MR images are from Open Access Series of Imaging Studies (OASIS), and we got this data as a part of "MICCAI 2012 Grand Challenge and Workshop on Multi-Atlas Labeling[1]." The

---

[1] https://masi.vuse.vanderbilt.edu/workshop2012/index.php/Main_Page

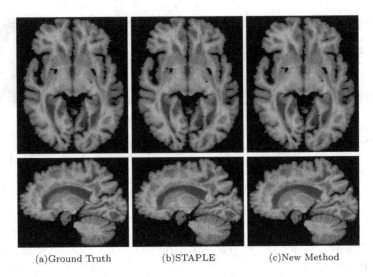

(a)Ground Truth   (b)STAPLE   (c)New Method

Fig. 2. Screen-shots of left and right lateral ventricles segmentation results for one of the target images from the 3D brain MR image database

Table 1. Quantitative evaluation of segmentation results for left and right Lateral Ventricles (LV), obtained from STAPLE and the proposed MAP-based approach. The average size of left and right LV structures are respectively 9424 and 11175 voxels.

| Method | DSC(%) | | Sensitivity(%) | | Avg. mis-class. voxels | |
	Left-LV	Right-LV	Left-LV	Right-LV	Left-LV	Right-LV
STAPLE	84.8 ± 9	87.1 ± 8	91.8 ± 8	92.1 ± 7	2,393	2,715
New Method	88.2 ± 6	89.3 ± 6	92.9 ± 5	93.3 ± 5	1,772	1,945

dataset that we use contained 34 normal brain MR images, and the evaluation is performed on all these images, using a leave-one-out approach. Local NCC is used as the intensity-similarity metric, and it is computed over a neighborhood radius of 4 (i.e., $9 \times 9 \times 9$ regular grid). Finally, we set the weighting parameter γ using the same approach that we have mentioned in the preceding subsection.

Fig. 2 shows the screen-shots of ground-truth segmentations, results from STAPLE, and from our new method, for one of the target images. Table 1 summarizes the quantitative evaluations performed based on - DSC, sensitivity, and the average number of mis-classified voxels. It can be noted from these results that incorporating the prior knowledge using the proposed approach has significantly improved the segmentation results when compared to the original STAPLE. Finally, we also evaluated the statistical significance of the improvements (at 0.05 significance level) using paired t-tests; when compared to STAPLE, the improvements in the DSC value from the proposed method are found to be statistically significant with resulting p values of 5.1×10^{-6} and 2.2×10^{-6} for the left and right lateral ventricles respectively.

4   Conclusions

In this paper, we have a presented a new approach for learning prior knowledge about the performance parameters of each template, and for incorporating it into the MAP-based STAPLE formulation. The advantages of incorporating such prior knowledge are clearly illustrated using both synthetic and 3D brain MR image data. In future work, we will extend this approach to multi-label fusion problem, and also to a local MAP formulation of the STAPLE, as in [10].

Acknowledgments. Subrahmanyam Gorthi is supported by the Swiss National Science Foundation (SNF) under grant P2ELP2_148892.

References

1. Warfield, S., Zou, K., Wells, W.: Simultaneous truth and performance level estimation (STAPLE): an algorithm for the validation of image segmentation. IEEE Transactions on Medical Imaging 23(7), 903–921 (2004)
2. Akhondi-Asl, A., Warfield, S.: Simultaneous truth and performance level estimation through fusion of probabilistic segmentations. IEEE Transactions on Medical Imaging 32(10), 1840–1852 (2013)
3. Asman, A., Landman, B.: Formulating spatially varying performance in the statistical fusion framework. IEEE Transactions on Medical Imaging 31(6), 1326–1336 (2012)
4. Artaechevarria, X., Munoz-Barrutia, A.: Combination strategies in multi-atlas image segmentation: Application to brain MR data. IEEE Transactions on Medical Imaging 28(8), 1266–1277 (2009)
5. Sabuncu, M., Yeo, B., Van Leemput, K., Fischl, B., Golland, P.: A generative model for image segmentation based on label fusion. IEEE Transactions on Medical Imaging 29(99), 1714–1729 (2010)
6. Wang, H., Suh, J., Das, S., Pluta, J., Craige, C., Yushkevich, P.: Multi-atlas segmentation with joint label fusion. IEEE Transactions on Pattern Analysis and Machine Intelligence 35(3), 611–623 (2013)
7. Gorthi, S., Bach Cuadra, M., Tercier, P.A., Allal, A., Thiran, J.P.: Weighted shape-based averaging with neighborhood prior model for multiple atlas fusion-based medical image segmentation. IEEE Signal Processing Letters 20(11), 1034–1037 (2013)
8. Cardoso, M., Leung, K., Modat, M., Barnes, J., Ourselin, S.: Locally ranked STAPLE for template based segmentation propagation. In: Workshop on Multi-Atlas Labeling and Statistical Fusion (2011)
9. Commowick, O., Warfield, S.K.: Incorporating priors on expert performance parameters for segmentation validation and label fusion: A maximum a posteriori STAPLE. In: Jiang, T., Navab, N., Pluim, J.P.W., Viergever, M.A. (eds.) MICCAI 2010, Part III. LNCS, vol. 6363, pp. 25–32. Springer, Heidelberg (2010)
10. Commowick, O., Akhondi-Asl, A., Warfield, S.K.: Estimating a reference standard segmentation with spatially varying performance parameters: Local MAP STAPLE. IEEE Transactions on Medical Imaging 31(8), 1593–1606 (2012)
11. AbouRizk, S.M., Halpin, D.W., Wilson, J.R.: Visual interactive fitting of beta distributions. Journal of Construction Engineering and Management 117(4), 589–605 (1991)

Colon Biopsy Classification
Using Crypt Architecture

Assaf Cohen[1], Ehud Rivlin[2], Ilan Shimshoni[3], and Edmond Sabo[4]

[1] Dept. of Computer Science, Haifa University, Haifa 31905, Israel
[2] Dept. of Computer Science, Technion, Haifa 32000, Israel
[3] Dept. of Information Systems, Haifa University, Haifa 31905, Israel
[4] Dept. of Oncology, Rambam Medical Center and Technion, Haifa 31096, Israel

Abstract. In this paper we introduce a novel method for the detection of diseases in biopsies that contain glandular structures. Most approaches proposed in the literature try to classify the biopsy using the image alone without analyzing its basic elements (such as the nuclei and the glands). The proposed method differs in that it is based on the architecture of the glands in the biopsy and the analysis of each pixel. We demonstrate our novel, three-step method on the task of classifying colon biopsies. First, as described in our previous work, we create a pixel-level classification image, segment the crypts (the glandular structures in the biopsy) using it, and remove false-positive segments. Next, we calculate the crypt architecture using Delaunay triangulation on the crypt centroids and use this architecture to retrieve those crypts that were incorrectly removed in the first step. In the final step, we use the segmented crypts to construct a more accurate architecture and classify each triangle as healthy or cancerous using the classification of the crypts as healthy or cancerous. The method was tested on 54 colon biopsy images: 109 healthy sub-images containing 4944 healthy crypts and 91 cancerous sub-images containing 2236 cancerous crypts. It achieved 92% accuracy in crypt classification and 94% in biopsy region classification.

Keywords: Histology, Colon Crypts, Classification, Architecture.

1 Introduction

Colon cancer is the third most common cancer, with nearly 1.4 million new cases in 2012 worldwide [1]. Early detection of cancer can lead to full recovery. Once a possible cancer is detected, it is diagnosed by a biopsy — pathologist's examination of a tissue sample via a microscope. Due to the implication of this diagnosis for the patient, this process is critical. The pathologist needs to be precise and have the ability to sift through huge amounts of data to detect small anomalies in the biopsy. There is thus a clear need for an automatic tool to draw the pathologist's attention to biopsies with suspicious regions.

Considerable progress has been made in the field of histology image analysis and many surveys on biopsy segmentation and classification have been conducted [2–5]. There are several approaches to this problem. Texture based

G. Wu et al. (Eds.): MLMI 2014, LNCS 8679, pp. 182–189, 2014.

methods [6, 7] classify the biopsy without understanding its structure and basic elements (such as nuclei and crypts). Relying solely on texture can fail due to changes in color between biopsies due to the staining process and fading of colors over time. Architecture based methods [8, 9] classify the biopsy according to an architecture constructed from the nuclei. This type of architecture is too sensitive to errors in nucleus detection and ignores the crypt features. In [10], a method for classification of prostate glands was proposed using structural and contextual information. We believe that classifying the glands alone cannot produce accurate results.

In this paper a novel biopsy classification method is presented. The problem of classifying the biopsy regions as healthy or cancerous is broken into three major steps. Each step relies on the results of the previous steps but uses a higher level of knowledge to overcome any errors that may have occurred. In our previous work, described in Section 2, the image is Classified at the Pixel Level (denoted by PLC). Using the classified pixels, the crypts are then segmented and false positive crypts identified using a classifier that assigns a certainty score to each crypt. In the second step, described in Section 3, the architecture of the crypts is calculated and used to retrieve missing crypts that were removed in the first step. In the third and final step, described in Section 4, a more accurate architecture is constructed using triangulation on the crypt centroids, including the retrieved crypts. Each triangle is classified as healthy or cancerous using geometry, appearance, the classification of the crypts as healthy or cancerous, and features based on the PLC. The main novelty of this method is the architecture created using the segmented crypts. This type of architecture is general and can be used in the detection of diseases in glandular tissue. Section 5 presents the evaluation of the method and results of each step of the proposed classification method on thousands of healthy and cancerous crypts. We conclude in Section 6.

2   Crypt Segmentation

In this study we work with colon tissue images. The colonic biopsy is composed of a stromal intermedium containing glands (called crypts) and immune system cells that surround the crypts (see Figure 1). We model the crypt as an inner area (lumen, goblet cells, and cytoplasm) with an outer layer of nuclei.

In our previous work [11] (included in the supplementary material), we introduced a novel two-step PLC method and a memory based Active Contour algorithm that we used to segment the colon biopsy crypts. The external forces of the active contour are based on the crypt model and the PLC image.

Due to incorrect selection of crypt candidates or incorrect segmentation, false positive crypts are returned. Features describing the shape of the crypt and the distribution of the pixel classes are extracted from each candidate crypt. A RandomForest (RF) [12] classifier trained on these features eliminates the segments that do not satisfy the crypt model and gives a classification certainty score for each crypt. The false-positive rate drops as a result from 63% to 7%, but 15% of the valid crypts are also removed in this phase, whereas prior to this phase, almost all the crypts were retrieved.

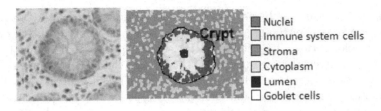

Fig. 1. Healthy colon tissue and crypt structure. A healthy crypt is composed of a lumen and goblet cells in cytoplasm, surrounded by a thin layer of nuclei. The crypt and immune system cells are in the stromal intermedium.

3   Missing Crypt Retrieval Using Crypt Architecture

As described in the previous section, the false-positive crypt elimination step uses only features of a single crypt. These features are local and the errors in eliminating valid crypts can be corrected using a higher level of information – the architecture of the crypts.

The architecture is calculated using Delaunay triangulation where the vertices are the centroids of the crypts. The absence of a crypt results in triangles with a different shape from its valid neighboring triangles and the region between the crypts that define the triangle contains eliminated crypts and pixels of crypt classes (see Figure 2a). In order to identify these triangles, a RandomForest classifier is trained based on the following types of features (see Figure 2b):

- **Triangle geometry.** The average, standard deviation, and median of the side lengths, the standard deviation, median of the angles, largest angle, and the area of the triangle.
- **Crypt inter-area.** The percentage of pixels from each crypt class (nuclei, cytoplasm, goblet cells, lumen) inside the area between the crypts. This percentage is determined from the PLC image.
- **Triangle neighborhood geometry.** The number of neighbors of each vertex, standard deviation and average of the distances of a vertex from its neighbors, and the same for the part of the edge in the crypt inter-area.
- **Probability to contain false negative crypts.** The number of invalid crypts, average certainty of the invalid crypts, and the highest crypt certainty inside the triangle.

The classifier is used to find the triangles suspected of containing false negative crypts (see Figure 2a). The architectural information gives a prior that enables us to lower the threshold for the certainty of a valid crypt. Every eliminated crypt that is in a suspicious triangle and whose certainty is above the new empirically selected threshold is considered valid (see Figure 2c). After this step, the false negative rate drops from 15% to 6.3%. Hence the crypt architecture is more accurate, which is crucial for the partition of the biopsy to cancerous and healthy regions.

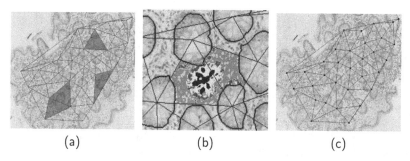

Fig. 2. (a) The architecture of the crypts using Delaunay triangulation on the crypt centroid. In red, the missing crypts. The gray triangles are classified as containing missing crypts. (b) Zoom on a triangle containing a missing crypt. For each triangle, features are extracted on the basis of geometry, content, and similarity to neighboring triangles. (c) The architecture of the crypts after adding those with certainty above the threshold, inside the gray triangles.

4   Biopsy Classification

A biopsy can be healthy or cancerous, but in early stages of cancer development a healthy biopsy might have some cancerous regions (see Figure 6e). In order to accurately segment the biopsy into healthy and cancerous regions, the triangles are classified as healthy or cancerous. This calculated triangle is the smallest unit that has enough information to allow for correct classification. One of the major indications of a cancerous region is that it contains cancerous crypts. In order to use this information in the triangle classification step, we first classify the crypts as healthy or cancerous and then classify the triangles.

4.1   Crypt Classification

In this step, the crypts are classified as cancerous or healthy. A cancerous crypt is larger than a healthy crypt, it does not have a circular shape, its nuclei layer is thicker, and the nuclei pixels are darker. To measure these characteristics, the classifier uses features of the crypt that are extracted from the PLC image:

- **Crypt geometry**. Average radius of the crypt and the distance histogram of the nuclei pixels from the skeleton of the crypt (see Figure 3a).
- **Crypt content**. The percentage of each class of the PLC in the crypt and the thickness of the nucleus layer (see Figure 3b).
- **Crypt appearance**. For each crypt class, the average of the RGB and Lab of the pixels that belong to it (see Figure 3c).

Using the PLC, more accurate features can be extracted: the content and internal structure of the crypt can be measured, as can the thickness of the nucleus layer, and the average of the RGB channels can be calculated for each crypt class (rather than for the entire crypt).

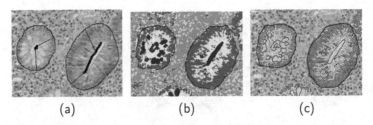

Fig. 3. (a) The radii of the crypt are defined as the distance of the edge pixels from the skeleton. (b) Calculating the percentage of the nucleus, cytoplasm, lumen, and goblet cell pixels. (c) A cancerous crypt has darker nucleus pixels. To measure this characteristic, the average of the RGB pixels is calculated for each of the crypt classes.

The RF classifier gives 92% accuracy. Despite its good performance, there are errors in the classification of the crypts. As can be seen in Figure 4, these errors are sparse. They are dealt with during the triangle classification phase by adding the architecture of the crypts and classification of the neighboring crypts.

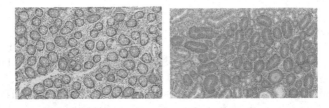

Fig. 4. Results of crypt classification. Left: Healthy biopsy, right: Cancerous biopsy. The green overlay indicates that the crypt is healthy, red indicates that the crypt is cancerous. It can be seen that the classification errors are sparse.

4.2 Biopsy Region Classification

Using the Delaunay triangulation on the crypt centroids, the biopsy is decomposed to small triangular regions that can be used to distinguish cancerous from healthy biopsy regions. A triangle of a cancerous region is larger than that of a healthy region, it differs from neighboring triangles in shape, the crypts that define it are close to each other and different in shape, and the stroma and immune system cell pixels are darker. The classifier uses the following features to measure these characteristics:

- **Triangle geometry and triangle neighborhood geometry.** The same features as in the identification of triangles containing missing crypts, described in Section 3 (see Figure 5a).
- **Crypts' shape similarity.** Variance of the radii of the crypts that define the triangle (see Figure 5a).

- **Crypts' classification.** The classification of the crypts (as described in the previous section) that define the triangle and their classification certainties.
- **Crypt inter-area geometry.** The distance between the edges of the crypts that define the triangle (see Figure 5b).
- **Crypt inter-area content.** The percentage of pixels of each of stroma and immune system cell inside the area between the crypts (see Figure 5b).
- **Crypt inter-area appearance.** The average of RGB and Lab pixels of the stroma and the immune system cells inside the triangle (see Figure 5c).

The RF classifier gives 94% accuracy.

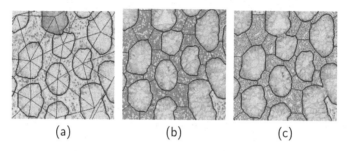

(a)   (b)   (c)

Fig. 5. Triangle Features. (a) Features based on the geometry of the triangles, the similarity of the shape of the crypts that define the triangles, and their classification. (b) Features based on the crypts' intra-area geometry and content. (c) The average of RGB and Lab pixels of the intra-area classes.

5   Results and Discussion

The proposed method is built from three phases. Because each phase relies on the previous phases, in the experiments we evaluate their performance.

Dataset: Since a database with ground truth segmentation of crypts does not yet exist, we collected a database of healthy and cancerous colon biopsies. The biopsies for the database were randomly chosen by E. Sabo MD, a pathologist from the Gyneco-oncology Unit at Rambam Hospital. The database was created by scanning the biopsies under a microscope at x200 magnification. From each scanned biopsy image, sub-images were taken at x4 zoom out. The average size of a sub-image is 800x500 pixels. There were 109 sub-images of healthy colons taken from 33 biopsies and 91 sub-images of cancerous colons taken from 21 biopsies. This database contains 4944 healthy crypts and 2236 cancerous crypts. The ground truth partitioning of the biopsy into cancerous and healthy regions (see Figure 6e) was also confirmed by him.

Missing Crypt Retrieval: The ground truth of the suspicious triangles was created by marking the triangles that contained missing crypts. This step was tested by 5-fold cross-validation on the 200 sub-images and gave 87% accuracy.

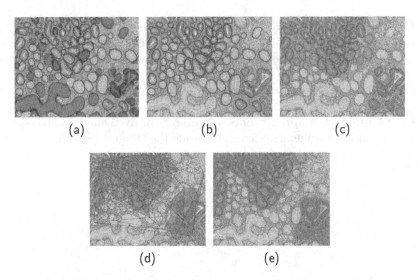

Fig. 6. Example for the steps of the method. (a) Crypt segmentation. The gray overlay indicates that the crypt is classified as false positive. Several valid crypts are misclassified as false positives. (b) Architecture-based retrieval of missing crypts. (c) Crypt classification. (d) Triangle classification. (e) Ground truth image. The red overlay indicates that the region is cancerous.

The following step is retrieving the crypt segments that have certainty above the threshold of being inside the suspicious triangles. This selective crypt retrieval gives significant improvement in the rate of missed crypts, from 15% to 6.3%, with no loss in segmentation accuracy and an increase in the false-positive rate, from 7.2% to 12.4%.

Crypt Classification: The crypt classification was tested using 5-fold cross-validation. The classifier gives 92% accuracy.

Biopsy Region Classification: The classification of triangles was tested using 5-fold cross-validation using balanced datasets. A triangle is considered as cancerous if it intersects with the red overlay in more than 50% of the triangle area. The classifier gives 94% accuracy, when the classification rates of benign and cancerous triangles are similar, 94.6% and 92.8% respectively. Figure 6 displays the steps of this method. For more results see the supplementary material.

To demonstrate the importance of the type of architecture used we compared Delaunay triangulation generated from nuclei which are lower level features (like the ones used by [8]) to triangulation generated from segmented crypts. Using only color statistics for the pixels in the triangle, the classification accuracy was 71% compared to 83%. This demonstrates that relatively high quality classification can be achieved even with naive features when a meaningful triangulation is used. The method for classifying the triangles is also novel by that it uses new features as input for the classification process. When we replaced the simple color statistics with PLC based features that enable us to analyze the color of the pixels and their distribution from each class, the classification accuracy increased from 83% to 91%. Adding the architecture-based features describing the geometry of each triangle and the similarity to its neighborhood, increased the classification rate to our final result of 94%.

6 Conclusions and Future Work

We have presented a novel method to classify colon crypts and biopsies. The contributions of this paper include: (1) an architecture-based method for the identification of crypts misclassified as invalid; (2) new features for crypt classification using the PLC image; (3) biopsy region classification using the segmented crypts and the PLC image.

In contrast to other architectures defined in previous studies, this one is defined on the basis of crypts. Therefore, the proposed method is general and can be used to classify and estimate the severity of other diseases (such as Crohn's and ulcerative colitis), and can be applied to other types of biopsies that contain glandular structures (such as breast, thyroid, and prostate).

References

1. World Health Organization: World cancer statistics,
   http://www.wcrf.org/cancer_statistics/world_cancer_statistics.php
2. Gurcan, M.N., Boucheron, L.E., Can, A., Madabhushi, A., Rajpoot, N.M., Yener, B.: Histopathological image analysis: A review. IEEE Reviews in Biomedical Engineering 2, 147–171 (2009)
3. Demir, C., Yener, B.: Automated cancer diagnosis based on histopathological images: A systematic survey. Rensselaer Polytechnic Institute, Tech. Rep. (2005)
4. Belsare, A., Mushrif, M.: Histopathological image analysis using image processing techniques: An overview. Signal & Image Processing 3(4) (2012)
5. Smochină, C., Herghelegiu, P., Manta, V.: Image processing techniques used in microscopic image segmentation. Technical report, Gheorghe Asachi Technical University of Iaşi (2011)
6. Doyle, S., Feldman, M., Tomaszewski, J., Madabhushi, A.: A boosted bayesian multiresolution classifier for prostate cancer detection from digitized needle biopsies. IEEE Transactions on Biomedical Engineering 59(5), 1205–1218 (2012)
7. Farjam, R., Soltanian-Zadeh, H., Jafari-Khouzani, K., Zoroofi, R.A.: An image analysis approach for automatic malignancy determination of prostate pathological images. Cytometry Part B: Clinical Cytometry 72(4), 227–240 (2007)
8. Doyle, S., Hwang, M., Shah, K., Madabhushi, A., Feldman, M., Tomaszeweski, J.: Automated grading of prostate cancer using architectural and textural image features. In: ISBI, pp. 1284–1287. IEEE (2007)
9. Bilgin, C., Demir, C., Nagi, C., Yener, B.: Cell-graph mining for breast tissue modeling and classification. In: EMBS, pp. 5311–5314. IEEE (2007)
10. Nguyen, K., Sarkar, A., Jain, A.K.: Structure and context in prostatic gland segmentation and classification. In: Ayache, N., Delingette, H., Golland, P., Mori, K. (eds.) MICCAI 2012, Part I. LNCS, vol. 7510, pp. 115–123. Springer, Heidelberg (2012)
11. Cohen, A., Rivlin, E., Shimshoni, I., Sabo, E.: Memory based active contour algorithm using pixel-level classified images for colon crypt segmentation. Submitted to IEEE Transactions on Medical Imaging
12. Breiman, L.: Random forests. Machine Learning 45(1), 5–32 (2001)

Network-Guided Group Feature Selection for Classification of Autism Spectrum Disorder

Veronika Cheplygina[1,3], David M.J. Tax[1], Marco Loog[1,2], and Aasa Feragen[2,3]

[1] Pattern Recognition Laboratory, Delft University of Technology, The Netherlands
[2] The Image Group, University of Copenhagen, Denmark
[3] Machine Learning and Computational Biology Group,
Max Planck Institutes Tübingen, Germany

Abstract. We present an anatomically guided feature selection scheme for prediction of neurological disorders based on brain connectivity networks. Using anatomical information not only gives rise to an interpretable model, but also prevents overfitting, caused by high dimensionality, noise and correlated features. Our method selects meaningful and discriminative groups of connections between anatomical regions, which can be used as input for any supervised classifier, such as logistic regression or a support vector machine. We demonstrate the effectiveness of our method on a dataset of autism spectrum disorder, with an AUC of 0.76, outperforming baseline methods.

1 Introduction

The effect of neurological disorders on structural (and functional) brain connectivity can be studied through magnetic resonance imaging (MRI). Studies often focus on population differences between cases and controls for particular global variables, such as white matter volume [1] or global graph-theoretic properties of brain networks [2,3]. However, the *predictive power* of the selected features is often not tested [3,4], and weak statistical tests which can be inconclusive as to which variables of interest are predictive of the diagnosis [5], leading to poor generalization to unseen data. Classification models are therefore more interesting from a diagnostic perspective [6,7].

Furthermore, *interpretability*, in the sense that prediction should link back to concrete biological markers, is a desirable property. For example, global measures such as small-worldness of networks [3] or histograms of image gradient descriptors [8] may disregard local connectivity changes, and do not provide information about which brain pathways have been altered.

This calls for methods which (i) consider local information and (ii) are predictive. Measuring features on densely sampled regions of interest (ROIs) provides local information, but unfortunately the high dimensionality of the noisy, correlated features can easily lead to overfitting, i.e. predicting perfectly on the training data, but failing to generalize to previously unseen data. It is therefore necessary to reduce the dimensionality, either by clustering ROIs [9], selecting

G. Wu et al. (Eds.): MLMI 2014, LNCS 8679, pp. 190–197, 2014.

features with good predictive performance on the training data [6, 10], and/or using classifiers which penalize complex models [9, 11].

It is important to understand that these techniques do not necessarily lead to good generalization to test data – even feature selection methods can suffer from overtraining due to the large number of potential feature subsets that need to be evaluated using limited training data. Adding constraints to select *groups of features* (i.e. either all or none of the features in a group are selected) helps to reduce the size of this search space. Such an approach is taken in structured sparsity [9, 11], however there the feature selection is implicit and it is not straightforward to control how many feature groups are selected.

In this paper we leverage the advantages of clustering ROIs and group feature selection in order to create a robust predictive model for brain connectivity data. We study features which quantify **ROI-ROI connections**. Clustering ROIs therefore naturally results in groups of connections, which share their start and end clusters. We call the concatenation of all connections within such a feature group a *hyperedge*, see Fig. 1. We cluster the ROIs into data-driven or anatomical clusters, which in both cases may lead to clusters of different sizes. This leads to hyperedges of different dimensionalities. Our goal is to select a set of discriminative hyperedges, i.e. per hyperedge we aim to select all, or none of the features.

By assuming that adjacent ROI-ROI connections are likely to work together in disorders, we further propose to examine *connected* networks of hyperedges. At each step of the feature selection approach, we therefore add a hyperedge that (a) is connected to the already selected hyperedges via one or both of its clusters and (b) leads to the largest improvement in performance on the training set. The performance is evaluated by the nearest mean classifier, which is efficient and insensitive to overfitting.

We contribute an interpretable predictive model for brain connectivity graphs, which selects local discriminative brain connectivity patterns, implicated in neurological disorder. We combat the overfitting problem by grouping ROIs into anatomical or data-driven clusters, and thus grouping ROI-ROI connections into groups of features. We use the cluster assignments to guide the group feature selection process, which, for anatomical clusters, leads to interpretable brain networks. Our method outperforms competing approaches on a dataset of ASD [3, 12].

2   Methods

Each subject's brain graph is represented by a symmetric $m \times m$ matrix which quantifies the brain connectivity between m ROIs in the brain, as illustrated in Fig. 1 (right). Each matrix is a collection of $M = (m^2 + m)/2$ individual connections (including the self-connections on the diagonal). That is, each subject is described by a vector $\mathbf{x}_i \in \mathbb{R}^M$ of M *features*, where each feature is an ROI-ROI fiber count. These m ROIs are associated with G clusters. The clusters organize these M features into $(G^2 + G)/2$ *feature groups* or *hyperedges*. Fig. 1 illustrates the relationship of the ROIs, clusters and the connectivity matrices.

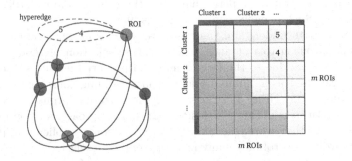

Fig. 1. Illustration of brain network (left) of $m = 6$ ROIs organized into $G = 4$ clusters (by color). Each connection is a feature; all features are summarized in a subject-specific data matrix (right). For each pair of ROI clusters, the set of connections between two clusters, or within a cluster, form a feature group called a *hyperedge*. Due to symmetry, this example has $M = 21$ unique features and 10 hyperedges (outlined in bold) to consider. There are 3 hyperedges with 1 feature, 4 with 2 features, 2 with 3 features, and 1 with 4 features.

For N subjects, this gives an $N \times M$ data matrix $X = (\mathbf{x}_1, \ldots, \mathbf{x}_N)^\mathsf{T}$ and a vector $\mathbf{y} \in \{-1, 1\}^N$ of labels which describe the presence or absence of neurological disorder. Subsets of the features are denoted by X^s, where $s \in S = \{1, \ldots, M\}$. A hyperedge $H_{ij} \subset S$ is the set of indices of all the connections of clusters i and j.

Filter Approach to Feature Selection. We are interested in the feature subset $s^* \subset S$, which maximizes a goodness criterion c on the training data, $s^* = \arg\max_s c(X^s, \mathbf{y})$. Exhaustive evaluation of all choices for s is intractable for large M, while *individual feature selection* does not take feature correlations into account, rendering both approaches unsuitable for brain connectivity. A possible approach is therefore to perform *forward feature selection*: select the best feature, and iteratively grow the feature set with the feature j that leads to the largest improvement in $c(X^{s \cup j}, Y)$.

Network Group Feature Selection. Based on the assumption that discriminative information is contained in networks of anatomical regions, we propose to perform forward selection on *connected feature groups* rather than individual features. This further limits the flexibility of the feature selection methods and therefore helps to reduce overfitting. Furthermore, the selected feature set will be interpretable which is interesting from a diagnostic perspective.

We iteratively grow the feature set by adding the (i,j)-th hyperedge that leads to the largest increase in $c(X^{s \cup H_{ij}}, Y)$, and is adjacent to the already selected hyperedges. For example, in Fig. 1, {blue-green, green-purple} is allowed because the hyperedges are connected at the green cluster, but the feature set {blue-green, purple-orange} is not. A procedure overview is shown in Fig. 2.

Goodness Criterion. The goodness criterion c could be univariate, such as a t-test. However, we need a multivariate c because we want to evaluate groups of hyperedges. We define c as the average cross-validation performance of the nearest mean classifier (NMC) on the training set, $c(X, \mathbf{y}) = \frac{1}{N} \sum_{i=1}^{N} I(f(\mathbf{x}_i) == y_i)$ where $f(\mathbf{x}) = \arg\min_{l \in \{-1,1\}} \|\boldsymbol{\mu}_l - \mathbf{x}\|$ and $\boldsymbol{\mu}_l$ are the class means. This choice has several advantages: NMC is very inflexible and therefore relatively insensitive to overfitting [13], and its performances on different cross-validation folds can be computed very efficiently in matrix form.

The NMC errors are discretized into ranks (equal error = equal rank). To avoid discarding potentially good feature sets when feature sets s and s' have similar errors, we consider all feature sets with rank up to R, therefore reducing the greediness of our method. The added computational effort of this step is compensated by the fact that fewer feature sets need to be evaluated due to the network constraint.

Evaluation Procedure. We perform 10-fold cross-validation, the feature selection is performed only on the training set. The area under the receiver-operating characteristic (AUC) is used for evaluation; random performance is equal to 0.5 and perfect performance is equal to 1.

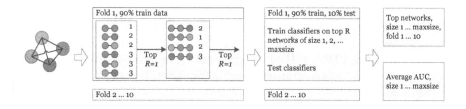

Fig. 2. Overview of procedure. The hyperedges are ranked, then the hyperedges with rank less than or equal to R (here $R = 1$) are selected for the next step. The selected hyperedges are extended to form pairs of hyperedges, which are again ranked. The procedure continues until the desired network size is reached.

3   Experiments and Results

We apply our algorithm to the structural connectivity matrices from the autism spectrum disorder dataset of [3, 12]. Each subject is represented by a 264×264 matrix encoding the number of paths connecting 264 ROIs from a functional atlas [14], where paths are found by deterministic tractography, using the fiber assignment by continuous tracking (FACT) algorithm in Diffusion Toolkit[1]. There are $N = 94$ subjects (51 ASD, 43 TD), matched for factors such as IQ and age. The ROIs are divided into clusters using (a) 88 anatomical regions, based on the coordinates of the 264 ROIs, and (b) 9 data-driven clusters obtained through Louvain modularity on the mean connectivity matrix.

---

[1] http://trackvis.org/dtk

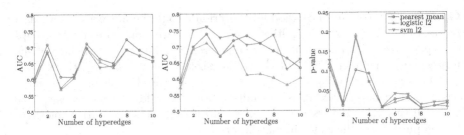

Fig. 3. AUC for an increasing number of hyperedges between data-driven clusters (left), anatomical clusters (middle) and p-values for the anatomical clusters (right). The best result achieved is **AUC of 0.76** for 3 anatomical hyperedges and an SVM.

We evaluate the network group forward selection on both (a) and (b). Fig. 3 shows how the performances change when more hyperedges (best hyperedge, best pair, ...) are added in the two models. As the anatomical clusters achieve superior, less noisy performances and improve interpretability, we use them in further experiments. To test significance of these results, we provide p-values based on a permutation test with 1000 repetitions in Fig. 3 (right).

Comparison. We first compare our method (`fwd-network` with 5 hyperedges and SVM) to filter feature selection with a t-test (`t-test`), minimum redundancy maximum relevance [15] (`mrmr`) from the FEAST toolbox [16] and SVM with recursive feature elimination [17] (`rfe`). We use 300 highest ranked features and an SVM (from PRTools [18]) as a classifier. We also compare to a sparse logistic (`sp-basic`) and group sparse logistic (`sp-group`), both from SLEP toolbox [19], and a tree-structured sparse logistic [9] (`sp-tree`), modified to suit our connectivity data. This method averages correlated groups of connections and enforces that within such correlated groups, all or none of the features are selected. Note that for the sparse methods, it is not possible to control the number of hyperedges explicitly, as in our method. Lastly, we compare to selecting 5 hyperedges without the network constraint (`fwd-group`). The results are shown in Table 1.

Table 1. AUC mean ± std, ×100, of selection of 300 best features (`t-test` to `rfe`), sparse methods (`sp-`) or forward selection (`fwd-`) with 5 hyperedges. 300 features and 5 hyperedges are chosen as default parameters, and NOT to correspond with best performances in Fig. 3.

t-test	mrmr	rfe	sp-basic	sp-group	sp-tree	fwd-network	fwd-group
56.6	52.4	48.9	51.3	47.4	50.1	**73.5**	67.8
± 25.7	± 22.2	± 17.4	± 21.6	± 20.3	± 23.3	**± 16.6**	± 16.2

Interpretation. Table 2 shows the subnetworks frequently selected by our method. In each fold, we record which networks have ranks 1 to 5. Not considered networks are ranked with a 10. By averaging ranks over the folds, we

Table 2. Average ranks (1 = best, 10 = worst) for networks with 1-3 hyperedges. R Putamen (RP), R Superior Parietal Lobule (RSPL), R Parahippocampal Gyrus posterior (RPGp), R Thalamus (RT), L Insular Cortex (LIC), L Planum Temporale (LPT), L Precentral Gyrus (LPG), R Superior Temporal Gyrus posterior (RSTGp), L Inferior Frontal Gyrus pars opercularis (LIGFpo), L Caudate (LC)

Size 1	Rank	Size 2	Rank	Size 3	Rank
RP-RSPL	1.8	LPG-RP-RSPL	2.9	LPG-RP-RSPL-RSTGp	6.2
RPGp-RT	4.5	RP-LIC-LPT	6.7	LC-LPG-RP-RSPL	6.4
LIC-LPT	5.6	RP-RSPL-RSTGp	7.0	LIFGpo-LPG-RP-RSPL	7.6

quantify how frequently a network is selected: if a network is the best in all folds, its average rank is 1, if a network is never selected, its average rank is 10.

4   Discussion and Conclusions

Our method selects groups of connectivity features based on prior anatomical knowledge and outperforms competing approaches which either do not consider groups of features and/or do not select features prior to training a classifier.

Comparison of Classifiers. As expected, methods which select features individually (t-test) perform very poorly because feature interactions are not taken into account. Forward selection methods which add or remove one feature per iteration (mrmr and rfe) perform even worse, because overfitting becomes a problem due to the amount of possible feature subsets that are evaluated. Selecting groups of features in a forward fashion (fwd-) therefore yields superior results, and network selection (fwd-network) outperforms selecting groups without such network constraints (fwd-group).

The sparse classifiers (sp-) perform very poorly. We suspect this is mainly due to the high dimensionality and correlations of the feature space, which lead to overfitting. While structured sparsity aims at selecting few features or feature groups, this cannot be controlled explicitly because a relaxation of the desired l_0 norm is used. Therefore, solutions that are less sparse than desirable could still be chosen. Our method explicitly controls the sparsity by choosing the network size, and therefore removes some potentially harmful solutions. To this end, it would also be interesting to investigate methods from computational biology which explicitly optimize the l_0 norm, such as [20].

In general, we suspect the problems are also caused by the difficulty of the data, because other methods, such as averaging of features for each ROI [7] (AUC ≈ 0.5 on our dataset) or structured sparsity [9], perform well on related problems, but not on this ASD dataset. Perhaps the numbers of fiber tracts do not contain enough discriminative information for this study, because of the differences in the tractography procedure.

Anatomical vs. Data-Driven Clusters. In our method, anatomical ROI clusters outperform data-driven clusters. This may be caused by the dimensionality of the hyperedges, which is higher for the data-driven clusters because the features are divided into less groups, resulting in more features per group. Perhaps more importantly, prior knowledge acts as an intrinsic regularization. We assume that the discriminative information is contained in connected subnetworks of anatomical regions, which reduces the solution search space. The fact that we obtain superior results indicates that the corresponding search space reduction removes solutions (which are not connected subnetworks) that would fit the training data perfectly but not generalize to test data.

Interpretability. Our method selects networks of anatomical regions, and therefore allows interpretation of results from a neurological perspective. The networks selected for this dataset often contain the right putamen. A study of DTI measures in ASD [21], finds significant differences in white matter tracts passing through the putamen (primarily left) to the frontal cortex, which is in part consistent with our results. Other studies of white matter pathways in ASD (reviewed in [22, 23]), find differences in the connections between temporal and occipital lobes and between the cingulate cortex and medial temporal structures. Although we do not find these specific connections, differences in the data acquisition and methodology could also be leading to inconsistencies.

Further Investigation. Age is important in the development of the brain during ASD [4, 22], increasing the variability in brain connectivity inside each class. To this end, we analyzed the correlation of performance, and the similarity of ages in the training and test set. Moderate correlations suggest that it might be advantageous to train age-dependent classifiers. Our initial efforts to do so did not outperform the proposed method, probably because of the even further reduced sample sizes. A remaining question is how to incorporate age in the classification procedure, without splitting the data into smaller subsets.

Conclusions. We propose a network-guided group feature selection method for structural brain connectivity data. The approach reduces overfitting by incorporating prior anatomical knowledge about ROI-ROI connections, and outperforms both methods where group structure is not considered, and data-driven methods. Our method provides interpretable output in the form of connected subnetworks between anatomical regions of the brain, which are discriminative for patients and controls. On a dataset of ASD, we obtain an AUC of 0.76 and select subnetworks which point in the direction of brain areas to be investigated in ASD. Future improvements could include incorporating the subjects' ages into classification.

Acknowledgements. We thank prof. dr. Karsten Borgwardt and dr. Cédric Koolschijn for their valuable advice concerning the paper. Aasa Feragen is supported by The Danish Council for Independent Research — Technology and Production.

References

1. Stigler, K.A., et al.: Structural and functional magnetic resonance imaging of autism spectrum disorders. Brain Research 1380, 146–161 (2011)
2. Bullmore, E., Sporns, O.: Complex brain networks: graph theoretical analysis of structural and functional systems. Nat. Rev. Neurosci. 10(3), 186–198 (2009)
3. Rudie, J., Brown, J., et al.: Altered functional and structural brain network organization in autism. NeuroImage: Clinical (2012)
4. Ghanbari, Y., Smith, A.R., Schultz, R.T., Verma, R.: Connectivity subnetwork learning for pathology and developmental variations. In: Mori, K., Sakuma, I., Sato, Y., Barillot, C., Navab, N. (eds.) MICCAI 2013, Part I. LNCS, vol. 8149, pp. 90–97. Springer, Heidelberg (2013)
5. Rubinov, M., Bullmore, E.: Fledgling pathoconnectomics of psychiatric disorders. Trends in Cognitive Sciences 17(12), 641–647 (2013)
6. Ecker, C., et al.: Investigating the predictive value of whole-brain structural MR scans in autism: a pattern classification approach. Neuroimage 49(1), 44–56 (2010)
7. Ingalhalikar, M., Kanterakis, S., Gur, R., Roberts, T.P.L., Verma, R.: DTI based diagnostic prediction of a disease via pattern classification. In: Jiang, T., Navab, N., Pluim, J.P.W., Viergever, M.A. (eds.) MICCAI 2010, Part I. LNCS, vol. 6361, pp. 558–565. Springer, Heidelberg (2010)
8. Ghiassian, S., et al.: Learning to Classify Psychiatric Disorders based on fMR Images: Autism vs Healthy and ADHD vs Healthy. In: MLINI (2013)
9. Jenatton, R., et al.: Multiscale mining of fMRI data with hierarchical structured sparsity. SIAM J. on Imaging Sciences 5(3), 835–856 (2012)
10. Orrù, G., et al.: Using support vector machine to identify imaging biomarkers of neurological and psychiatric disease: a critical review. Neurosc. Biobeh. Rev. 36(4), 1140–1152 (2012)
11. Bach, F., Jenatton, R., Mairal, J., Obozinski, G.: Structured sparsity through convex optimization. Statistical Science 27(4), 450–468 (2012)
12. Brown, J.A., et al.: The UCLA multimodal connectivity database: a web-based platform for brain connectivity matrix sharing and analysis. Frontiers in Neuroinformatics 6 (2012)
13. Skurichina, M., Duin, R.P.W.: Stabilizing classifiers for very small sample sizes. In: International Conference on Pattern Recognition, vol. 2, pp. 891–896. IEEE (1996)
14. Power, J.D., et al.: Functional network organization of the human brain. Neuron 72(4), 665–678 (2011)
15. Peng, H., Long, F., Ding, C.: Feature selection based on mutual information criteria of max-dependency, max-relevance, and min-redundancy. IEEE TPAMI 27(8), 1226–1238 (2005)
16. Brown, G., et al.: Conditional likelihood maximisation: a unifying framework for information theoretic feature selection. JMLR 13, 27–66 (2012)
17. Guyon, I., Weston, J., Barnhill, S., Vapnik, V.: Gene selection for cancer classification using support vector machines. Machine Learning 46(1-3), 389–422 (2002)
18. Duin, R.P.W., et al.: PRTools, a MATLAB toolbox for pattern recognition (2010), http://www.prtools.org
19. Liu, J., Ji, S., Ye, J.: SLEP: Sparse Learning with Efficient Projections (2009)
20. Azencott, C.A., et al.: Efficient network-guided multi-locus association mapping with graph cuts. Bioinformatics 29(13), i171–i179 (2013)
21. Langen, M., et al.: Fronto-striatal circuitry and inhibitory control in autism: findings from diffusion tensor imaging tractography. Cortex 48(2), 183–193 (2012)
22. Vissers, M.E., et al.: Brain connectivity and high functioning autism: a promising path of research that needs refined models, methodological convergence, and stronger behavioral links. Neurosci. Biobehav. Rev. 36(1), 604–625 (2012)
23. Travers, B.G., et al.: Diffusion tensor imaging in autism spectrum disorder: a review. Autism Research 5(5), 289–313 (2012)

Deformation Field Correction for Spatial Normalization of PET Images Using a Population-Derived Partial Least Squares Model

Murat Bilgel[1,2], Aaron Carass[1],
Susan M. Resnick[2], Dean F. Wong[3], and Jerry L. Prince[1,3]

[1] Image Analysis and Communications Lab., Johns Hopkins University
[2] Lab. of Behavioral Neuroscience, National Institute on Aging, NIH
[3] Dept. of Radiology, Johns Hopkins University School of Medicine,
Baltimore, MD, USA

Abstract. Spatial normalization of positron emission tomography (PET) images is essential for population studies, yet work on anatomically accurate PET-to-PET registration is limited. We present a method for the spatial normalization of PET images that improves their anatomical alignment based on a deformation correction model learned from structural image registration. To generate the model, we first create a population-based PET template with a corresponding structural image template. We register each PET image onto the PET template using deformable registration that consists of an affine step followed by a diffeomorphic mapping. Constraining the affine step to be the same as that obtained from the PET registration, we find the diffeomorphic mapping that will align the structural image with the structural template. We train partial least squares (PLS) regression models within small neighborhoods to relate the PET intensities and deformation fields obtained from the diffeomorphic mapping to the structural image deformation fields. The trained model can then be used to obtain more accurate registration of PET images to the PET template without the use of a structural image. A cross validation based evaluation on 79 subjects shows that our method yields more accurate alignment of the PET images compared to deformable PET-to-PET registration as revealed by 1) a visual examination of the deformed images, 2) a smaller error in the deformation fields, and 3) a greater overlap of the deformed anatomical labels with ground truth segmentations.

Keywords: PET registration, deformation field, partial least squares.

1   Introduction

Deformable medical image registration is essential to aligning a population of images, performing voxelwise association studies, and tracking longitudinal changes. While within-modality spatial normalization of structural medical images has

G. Wu et al. (Eds.): MLMI 2014, LNCS 8679, pp. 198–206, 2014.

been studied extensively, work on anatomically accurate positron emission tomography (PET) spatial normalization remains limited. The anatomical alignment of PET images is a difficult problem since they reflect metabolism and function rather than anatomy, the observed intensities depend on the amount of radiotracer used, and the spatial detail is confounded by radiotracer spillover.

Whenever available, it is preferable to use a structural image (such as a T_1-weighted MRI) co-registered with the subject's PET image for registration purposes and to warp the PET image accordingly. However, it is important to be able to perform PET spatial normalization accurately without guidance from additional images, as structural MR images are not always available due to claustrophobia or MR-incompatible implants. Enabling accurate PET spatial normalization can obviate the need for structural imaging in certain studies, resulting in lower costs, hospitalization time, and patient burden.

Prior work on PET spatial normalization includes modification of the target image intensities using a whole-brain principal component analysis model to match more closely to the moving image intensities [7,9], imposing constraints on the PET deformations via a statistical control point model based on the deformation parameters of PET-to-MR registrations [8], and making use of the 4D data available in dynamic PET studies [3]. While these approaches show improvements over simple 3D PET spatial normalization, they do not take into account the systematic errors present in PET-to-PET registration due to the incorrect inference of anatomical boundaries stemming from spillover effects and the preferential binding of the radiotracer to certain parts within structures.

We present a method for the spatial normalization of PET images based on a deformation correction model learned from structural image registration. The observation motivating our method is: *PET-to-PET registration produces deformations that are systematically biased in certain regions, and these biases can be characterized as a function of location and estimated within small neighborhoods.* The correction operates on the PET-to-PET deformation fields obtained from a deformable registration algorithm and uses partial least squares regression models learned from a population of subjects relating the local PET intensities and deformation fields to the corresponding structural imaging deformation fields. The learned relationship between the deformation fields accounts for the anatomical inaccuracies present in the alignment of PET images, while the use of PET intensity information allows for inter-subject variability in radiotracer binding due to differences in physiology.

2   Method

To construct our model, we need the deformation fields that are to be applied to the PET images and their structural counterparts to bring the images to a common template. Our model is then trained using the resulting deformation fields for the PET and the structural images as well as the warped PET image intensities, yielding a correction that can be applied to PET deformation fields.

2.1   Image Template Generation

To create an anatomically accurate PET template image, we rely on the associated structural images. The structural images S_i ($i = 1, \ldots, N$), are co-registered rigidly with the subject PET images F_i yielding transformation $\boldsymbol{R}_i$, followed by affine registration to a common space with transformation $\boldsymbol{T}_i$.

The affinely coregistered structural images $\hat{S}_i = S_i (\boldsymbol{R}_i \circ \boldsymbol{T}_i)$ are then used to create a structural population template image $\bar{S}$. Let $\boldsymbol{x}$ be in the common space Ω, and $\boldsymbol{\phi}_i$ a diffeomorphism defined on Ω to transform $\hat{S}_i$ into a new coordinate system by $\hat{S}_i \circ \boldsymbol{\phi}_i(\boldsymbol{x}, t)$, with $t \in [0, 1]$ and $\boldsymbol{\phi}_i(\boldsymbol{x}, 0) = \boldsymbol{x}$. The square-integrable and continuous vector field $\boldsymbol{\nu}_i(\boldsymbol{x}, t)$ parameterizes the diffeomorphism such that $\frac{d\phi_i(\boldsymbol{x},t)}{dt} = \boldsymbol{\nu}_i(\boldsymbol{\phi}_i(\boldsymbol{x}, t), t)$ [1]. The population template is

$$\bar{S}, \{\boldsymbol{\phi}_i\} = \underset{\bar{S}, \{\boldsymbol{\phi}_i\}}{\arg \min} \sum_{i=1}^{N} \left(\int_0^1 \|\boldsymbol{\nu}_i(\boldsymbol{x}, t)\|_L^2 \, dt + \int_\Omega -\mathrm{CC} \left(\bar{S}, \hat{S}_i(\boldsymbol{\phi}_i), \boldsymbol{x} \right) d\Omega \right) \quad (1)$$

where L is a Gaussian convolution operator regularizing the velocity field, and $\mathrm{CC}(\bar{S}, \hat{S}_i(\boldsymbol{\phi}_i), \boldsymbol{x})$ is the cross correlation similarity measure with the inner products calculated over a cubic window around $\boldsymbol{x}$ [2].

The affine transformations $\boldsymbol{T}_i$ and diffeomorphisms $\boldsymbol{\phi}_i$ obtained from the structural image template construction are applied to the corresponding PET images in order to bring them into the same template space. The PET template $\bar{F}$ is then defined as the mean of the spatially normalized PET images as

$$\bar{F} = \frac{1}{N} \sum_{i=1}^{N} F_i (\boldsymbol{T}_i \circ \boldsymbol{\phi}_i). \quad (2)$$

2.2   Computing a Training Set

Using a set of subjects for whom both a structural image and a PET image are available, we perform deformable registration to map the PET images onto the PET template. For each subject $i = 1, \ldots, n$ in the training data, the deformable registration consists of an affine transformation $\boldsymbol{T}_i'$ followed by a diffeomorphic mapping $\boldsymbol{\psi}_i(\boldsymbol{x})$ defined on Ω. We denote the PET image registered onto the PET template $\bar{F}$ by $\tilde{F}_i = F_i (\boldsymbol{T}_i' \circ \boldsymbol{\psi}_i)$. Constraining the affine transformation to be the same as that obtained from the PET-to-PET registration, we then perform another registration to find the deformation field $\boldsymbol{\varphi}_i(\boldsymbol{x})$ that must be applied to the structural image such that $S_i (\boldsymbol{R}_i \circ \boldsymbol{T}_i' \circ \boldsymbol{\varphi}_i)$ is in alignment with the structural image template $\bar{S}$.

2.3   Model Training

Our goal is to train a model at each voxel $\boldsymbol{x} \in \Omega$ describing a relationship between the estimated PET deformation field $\boldsymbol{\psi}_i(\boldsymbol{x})$ and the structural image deformation field $\varphi_i(\boldsymbol{x})$ for the training subjects $i = 1, \ldots, n$. To account for the variability in PET intensities across subjects due to differences in function and metabolism, we also include the intensities $\tilde{F}_i(\boldsymbol{x})$ as features in the model.

We denote the row vector whose components are the warped PET intensities at each voxel in the neighborhood $\mathcal{N}(\boldsymbol{x})$ as $\tilde{F}_i(\mathcal{N}(\boldsymbol{x})) \in \mathbb{R}^{|\mathcal{N}|}$, where $|\mathcal{N}|$ is the number of voxels in the neighborhood. Similarly, we denote the row vector whose components are the deformation field components at each voxel in the neighborhood as $\psi_i(\mathcal{N}(\boldsymbol{x})) \in \mathbb{R}^{3|\mathcal{N}|}$. In our setup, we use the input features $\mathbf{X}(\boldsymbol{x}) \in \mathbb{R}^{n \times 4|\mathcal{N}|}$ and the output data $\mathbf{Y}(\boldsymbol{x}) \in \mathbb{R}^{n \times 3}$

$$
\mathbf{X}(\boldsymbol{x}) = \begin{bmatrix} \vdots & \vdots \\ \psi_i(\mathcal{N}(\boldsymbol{x})) & \tilde{F}_i(\mathcal{N}(\boldsymbol{x})) \\ \vdots & \vdots \end{bmatrix} \qquad \mathbf{Y}(\boldsymbol{x}) = \begin{bmatrix} \vdots \\ \varphi_i(\boldsymbol{x}) \\ \vdots \end{bmatrix} \tag{3}
$$

compiled across the n subjects to train a partial least squares regression model for predicting the structural image deformation vector at the center voxel.

Partial least squares (PLS) is a dimensionality reduction technique that seeks to find a small number of latent variables extracted from the input features that best explain the observed data [10]. The number of *latent variables*, or *components*, to be retained in the model is denoted by c. PLS performs linear decomposition of the input features $\mathbf{X} \in \mathbb{R}^{n \times p}$ and observed data $\mathbf{Y} \in \mathbb{R}^{n \times q}$, where n, p, and q are the number of observations, input features, and output features, respectively, to obtain $\mathbf{X} = \mathbf{T}\mathbf{P}^T + \mathbf{V}$ and $\mathbf{Y} = \mathbf{U}\mathbf{Q}^T + \mathbf{W}$, where $\mathbf{T}$ and $\mathbf{U}$ are the $n \times c$ *score matrices* each consisting of orthogonal columns, with *loadings* $\mathbf{P}$ and $\mathbf{Q}$, and *residuals* $\mathbf{V}$ and $\mathbf{W}$. PLS finds the linear decompositions so that the covariance of the extracted score matrices is maximized. The coefficient matrix for the multivariate linear regression of $\mathbf{X}$ on $\mathbf{Y}$ is then given by $\mathbf{B} = \mathbf{X}^T \mathbf{U} (\mathbf{T}^T \mathbf{X}\mathbf{X}^T \mathbf{U})^{-1} \mathbf{T}^T \mathbf{Y}$ [10], which is later used for prediction.

The choice of the number of components c is important: a small value will yield a model that cannot account for the sample variance while a large value will lead to over-fitting. We apply a k-fold cross validation as part of the training to determine the best number of PLS components to retain in our model. The cross validation involves splitting the training subjects into k groups, one of which is used to test the model that is trained on the remaining $k-1$. This training and testing procedure is repeated to obtain predictions on each of the k groups. We find an optimal $\hat{c}$ for each spatial location using the cross validation results:

$$
\hat{c}(\boldsymbol{x}) = \arg \min_c \sum_{i=1}^{n} \|\hat{\varphi}_i(\boldsymbol{x}; c) - \varphi_i(\boldsymbol{x})\|^2. \tag{4}
$$

Here, $\hat{\varphi}_i(\boldsymbol{x}; c)$ is the prediction of the PLS model with c components for test subject i. We use this spatially varying choice $\hat{c}(\boldsymbol{x})$ in the model at each voxel $\boldsymbol{x}$.

3   Results

PET scans were performed on a GE Advance scanner immediately following an intravenous bolus injection of Pittsburgh compound B (PiB), which binds to the beta-amyloid peptide. Dynamic PET data were acquired over 70 minutes, yielding 33 time frames each with $128 \times 128 \times 35$ voxels. Voxel size was $2 \times 2 \times 4.25$ mm^3. Each time frame was cropped to $118 \times 118 \times 33$ images. The images corresponding to the first 20 minutes were averaged to create a static PET image for each subject. Early time frames were chosen as they are mostly reflective of cerebral blood flow and show clearer anatomic boundary less vulnerable to modification by beta-amyloid. For structural images, we used MPRAGE scans performed on a Philips Achieva 3T scanner with the following acquisition parameters: TR = 6.8 ms, TE = 3.2 ms, $\alpha = 8°$ flip angle, 256×256 matrix, 170 sagittal slices, 1×1 mm^2 in-plane pixel size, 1.2 mm slice thickness. Three subjects had their MPRAGE scan 4 years after the PET, and one subject 2 years after the PET. The remaining subjects had both scans during the same visit.

The inhomogeneity corrected [11] MPRAGE images for each subject were rigidly aligned onto the corresponding static PET and skull-stripped [4]. The intensities of the PET images were normalized by the mean intensity within the volume, and thresholded at 80% to remove background noise. The MPRAGE and PET population templates were constructed using the ANTs package using 79 subjects (http://picsl.upenn.edu/software/ants/). The diffeomorphic registration of each subject onto the population template was performed using SyN [1], with the same parameters for MPRAGE and PET. The model was validated using 10-fold cross validation on 79 subjects. Input features for PLS were obtained over $3 \times 3 \times 3$ neighborhoods, and within each training set, an additional $k = 10$-fold cross validation was used to pick the number of components to keep in the model.

We compared our method against PET-to-PET template registration and an implementation of [7] that involved first creating a PET template using corresponding MRIs as in our approach, constructing a whole-brain PCA model from the spatially normalized PET images, affinely registering the subject's PET onto the template, modifying the template using the PCA model to resemble more closely to the subject, and finally performing deformable registration using the modified template. Sample PET and MPRAGE images warped by deformation fields obtained from the different methods are presented in Fig. 1. Ventricle size is overestimated in both PET-to-PET registration and the method described in [7], whereas our method achieves better registration as revealed by the difference images. The putamen, a structure that exhibits higher activity in the PET image and thus causes spillover, is also better aligned by our method.

A comparison of the root mean square (RMS) error of the deformation fields is presented in Fig. 2. The deformation field φ obtained from the registration of MPRAGE onto the MPRAGE template is used as ground truth in the RMS error calculation. Our method achieves the lowest overall RMS error.

To assess the accuracy of anatomical alignment, the FreeSurfer [5] segmentations of the original MPRAGE images were brought into the template space

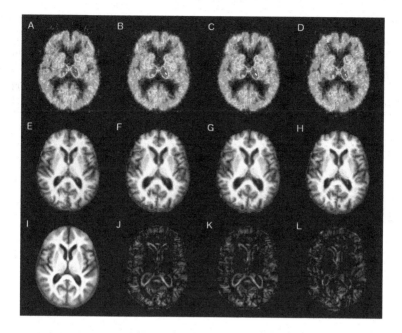

Fig. 1. Visual comparison of deformed images for a sample subject. First row: PET deformed using (A) the deformation φ from MPRAGE-to-MPRAGE template registration, (B) the deformation ψ from PET-to-PET template registration, (C) the deformation given by [7] (D) the deformation $\hat{\varphi}$ predicted using our PLS model. Second row: MPRAGE deformed using (E) φ, (F) ψ, (G) the deformation given by [7] and (H) $\hat{\varphi}$. Third row: (I) MPRAGE template, (J) difference of E and F, (K) difference of E and G (L) difference of E and H.

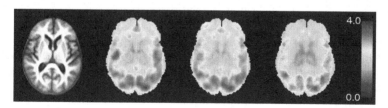

Fig. 2. Root mean square (RMS) error (in mm) of the PET deformation fields, calculated across 79 subjects. Left to right: MPRAGE template, RMS error of ψ, RMS error of the deformation given by [7], and RMS error of $\hat{\varphi}$ predicted using our PLS model.

by applying the mappings from the previously performed registrations. Using the FreeSurfer labels deformed according to φ as ground truth, we calculated the Dice coefficients [6] for the deformed labels. Table 1 shows the summary statistics for Dice coefficients for gray matter, white matter, and ventricular corticospinal fluid (CSF). Dice coefficients for our method are statistically different ($p < 0.01$ for all three tissue types) from both compared methods. Fig. 3 shows the Dice coefficient box plots for cortical regions. While the method proposed by

Table 1. Dice coefficients (mean ± st. dev., $N = 79$) for major brain tissue types

	PET-to-PET	PCA method by [7]	Our method
Gray matter	0.64 ± 0.02	0.64 ± 0.03	0.65 ± 0.02
White matter	0.76 ± 0.02	0.76 ± 0.02	0.78 ± 0.02
Ventricular CSF	0.77 ± 0.05	0.78 ± 0.04	0.80 ± 0.04

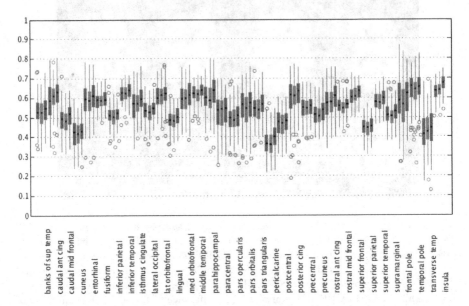

Fig. 3. Box plots of Dice coefficients for cortical labels across 79 subjects calculated using the deformations obtained from PET-to-PET registration (blue), the method proposed by [7] (green), and our method (red).

[7] yields mixed results, our method consistently achieves higher Dice coefficients than either of the methods compared against. Dice coefficients for our method are statistically different ($p < 0.05$) from both compared methods for all regions except for cuneus, paracentral lobule, precentral gyrus and temporal pole.

4   Discussion and Conclusion

In our dataset, PET-to-PET registration consistently yielded larger ventricles compared to MPRAGE-to-MPRAGE registration. We also observed smaller brains and larger subcortical gray structures in PET-to-PET registered volumes, but these effects were subtle (Fig. 1).

We presented a deformation correction method to improve the anatomical alignment of PET images. Cross validation results show that our deformation correction method reduces the deformation field error and improves the anatomical alignment of PET images as evidenced by the higher Dice coefficients calculated using the deformed segmentations. Our method can compensate for errors in PET-to-PET registration by learning locally from the structural image registrations. While we used SyN for registration purposes, the method can be applied to any deformable PET-to-PET registration method.

Our method is particularly suited for spatial normalization of PET images in datasets where only a subset of the subjects have structural images. Subjects with both PET and structural images can be used to train the model, and those with PET images only can then be registered onto the PET template, taking into account the deformation correction provided by the model. If the dataset contains no concurrent PET and structural images, our deformation correction can still be applied given a PET template and an associated deformation field correction model that has already been constructed using a separate dataset.

The proposed approach could be applied to improve the deformable registration of other types of medical images with low resolution, poor contrast, geometric distortions, or inadequate anatomical content by using a model trained on corresponding medical images that are largely free of such effects.

Acknowledgment. This research was supported in part by the Intramural Research Program of the NIH.

References

1. Avants, B.B., Epstein, C.L., Grossman, M., Gee, J.C.: Symmetric diffeomorphic image registration with cross-correlation: evaluating automated labeling of elderly and neurodegenerative brain. Medical Image Analysis 12(1), 26–41 (2008)
2. Avants, B.B., Yushkevich, P., Pluta, J., Minkoff, D., Korczykowski, M., Detre, J., Gee, J.C.: The optimal template effect in hippocampus studies of diseased populations. NeuroImage 49(3), 2457–2466 (2010)
3. Bieth, M., Reader, A.J., Siddiqi, K.: Atlas construction for dynamic (4D) PET using diffeomorphic transformations. In: Mori, K., Sakuma, I., Sato, Y., Barillot, C., Navab, N. (eds.) MICCAI 2013, Part II. LNCS, vol. 8150, pp. 35–42. Springer, Heidelberg (2013)
4. Carass, A., Cuzzocreo, J., Wheeler, M.B., Bazin, P.L., Resnick, S.M., Prince, J.L.: Simple paradigm for extra-cerebral tissue removal: algorithm and analysis. NeuroImage 56(4), 1982–1992 (2011)
5. Desikan, R.S., Ségonne, F., Fischl, B., Quinn, B.T., Dickerson, B.C., Blacker, D., Buckner, R.L., Dale, A.M., Maguire, R.P., Hyman, B.T., Albert, M.S., Killiany, R.J.: An automated labeling system for subdividing the human cerebral cortex on MRI scans into gyral based regions of interest. NeuroImage 31(3), 968–980 (2006)
6. Dice, L.R.: Measures of the amount of ecologic association between species. Ecology 26(3), 297–302 (1945)
7. Fripp, J., Bourgeat, P., Acosta, O., Jones, G., Villemagne, V., Ourselin, S., Rowe, C., Salvado, O.: Generative atlases and atlas selection for C11-PIB PET-PET registration of elderly, mild cognitive impaired and Alzheimer disease patients. In: ISBI 2008, pp. 1155–1158 (2008)
8. Fripp, J., et al.: MR-less high dimensional spatial normalization of ^{11}C PiB PET images on a population of elderly, mild cognitive impaired and alzheimer disease patients. In: Metaxas, D., Axel, L., Fichtinger, G., Székely, G. (eds.) MICCAI 2008, Part I. LNCS, vol. 5241, pp. 442–449. Springer, Heidelberg (2008)

9. Lundqvist, R., Lilja, J., Thomas, B.A., Lötjönen, J., Villemagne, V.L., Rowe, C.C., Thurfjell, L.: Implementation and validation of an adaptive template registration method for 18F-flutemetamol imaging data. Journal of Nuclear Medicine 54(8), 1472–1478 (2013)
10. Rosipal, R., Krämer, N.: Overview and recent advances in partial least squares. In: Saunders, C., Grobelnik, M., Gunn, S., Shawe-Taylor, J. (eds.) SLSFS 2005. LNCS, vol. 3940, pp. 34–51. Springer, Heidelberg (2006)
11. Sled, J.G., Zijdenbos, A.P., Evans, A.C.: A nonparametric method for automatic correction of intensity nonuniformity in MRI data. TMI 17(1), 87–97 (1998)

Novel Multi-Atlas Segmentation by Matrix Completion

Gerard Sanroma, Guorong Wu, Kim Thung, Yanrong Guo, and Dinggang Shen

Department of Radiology and BRIC, University of North Carolina at Chapel Hill

Abstract. The goal of multi-atlas segmentation is to estimate the anatomical labels on each target image point by combining the labels from a set of registered atlas images via label fusion. Typically, label fusion can be formulated either as a reconstruction or as a classification problem. Reconstruction-based methods compute the target labels as a weighted average of the atlas labels. Such weights are derived from the representation of the target image patches as a linear combination of the atlas image patches. However, the related issue is that the optimal weights in the image domain are not necessarily corresponding to those in the label domain. Classification-based methods can avoid this issue by directly learning the relationship between image and label domains. However, the learned relationships, describing the common characteristics of all the training atlas patches, might not be representative for a particular target image patch, and thus undermine the labeling results. In order to overcome the limitations of both types of methods, we innovatively formulate the patch-based label fusion problem as a matrix completion problem. By doing so, we can jointly utilize (1) the relationships between atlas and target image patches (thus taking the advantage of the reconstruction-based methods), and (2) the relationships between image and label domains (taking the advantage of the classification-based methods). In this way, our generalized paradigm can improve the label fusion accuracy in segmenting the challenging structures, e.g., hippocampus, compared to the state-of-the-art methods.

1 Introduction

Multi-atlas segmentation (MAS) is commonly used for automated labeling of anatomical structures from the target images. It consists of two steps, namely, image registration and label fusion. In the registration step, either linear or non-linear registration is used to spatially normalize all atlas images to the target. In the label fusion step, the latent labels in the target image are determined by utilizing image appearance and fusing the label information from each registered atlas.

Typically, label fusion can be solved either as a reconstruction or a classification problem. Reconstruction-based methods compute the target labels as a weighted average of the atlas labels. The weights are often derived from the reconstruction coefficients used to represent the target image patch from a set of atlas image patches [1]. However, the optimal weights used for patch reconstruction in the image domain might not be optimal for fusing labels in the label domain. On the other hand, classification-based methods have no such issue since they determine the target labels based on a learned mapping function from the image appearance domain to the label

G. Wu et al. (Eds.): MLMI 2014, LNCS 8679, pp. 207–214, 2014.

domain. Such mapping is learned from the observed atlas image patches and ground-truth (manual) labels [2]. However, the relationships learned using the whole training set might not be representative enough for a new specific target patch under consideration. Fortunately, this issue can be alleviated by utilizing the correlation between the target image patch and each atlas image patch, which is the essential idea in reconstruction-based methods.

It is apparent that the reconstruction-based and classification-based methods can help each other to overcome their respective limitations. This is exactly the goal of this paper, i.e., improving the label fusion accuracy by integrating the advantages of both types of methods. To achieve this goal, we formulate label fusion as a matrix completion problem, where the latent target labels are the missing entries in a four-quadrant matrix. Specifically, we first stack each atlas image patch and its respective (ground-truth) label into a column vector. We do similarly for the target image patches, but leaving the label entries blank. Then, we build a matrix by arranging these column vectors in a column-wise manner, where the four parts in the matrix are the atlas image patches, atlas labels, target image patches, and latent target labels (to be estimated), respectively. According to the assumptions made by the reconstruction- and classification-based methods, the four-quadrant matrix is highly correlated in both column-wise and row-wise manners, and thus it has low rank. In this way, the problem of estimating the missing entries (i.e., the latent target labels) in the matrix can be solved with the rank minimization technique, as commonly used by matrix completion [3]. It is worth noting that we can now leverage both column-wise correlations (i.e., representing a target image patch by all atlas image patches) and row-wise correlations (i.e., mapping the image appearance domain to the label domain) to predict more reasonable values for the target patches (i.e., values for those missing entries).

Furthermore, we also propose two additional strategies to make our new label fusion method more robust: **(1)** instead of estimating only the labels for the center of target patches, we estimate labels for the whole target patch in a set of target patches simultaneously. In this way, we provide additional useful sources of correlation among the observed data to be leveraged by the matrix completion technique; and **(2)** instead of treating each atlas label equally, we assign a confidence for each atlas label based on its distance to the corresponding boundary of the manually-labeled structure, since labels far from the boundary are more reliable of conveying the correct label information. We have comprehensively evaluated the labeling accuracy of our method on both ADNI and LONI datasets obtaining much better results than the state-of-the-art patch-based label fusion methods.

2   Method

Given a target image I_T and a set of atlas images I_i along with their respective label maps B_i, $i = 1 \dots M$, which have been registered to the target image, the conventional label fusion approaches estimate the target label f at each voxel $u \in \Omega$ of target image I_T in a patch-wise manner. Denote t as a (column) vector of intensities in the target image patch (centered at voxel u), and $A = \left[A_1^1, \dots, A_j^i, \dots, A_n^M \right]_{i=1\dots M, j=1\dots n}$ as a dictionary of n candidate atlas image patches with centers in a local search neighborhood of voxel u. Note that, each column vector A_j^i contains the j-th image patch from the i-th atlas image I_i. Corresponding to A, $l = \left[l_1^1, \dots, l_j^i, \dots, l_n^M\right]_{i=1\dots M, j=1\dots n}^{\mathsf{T}}$ is a (column) vector of labels at the patch centers, with each element $l_j^i \in \{-1, 1\}$ indicating absence or presence of certain label at the center of the respective atlas image patch A_j^i.

As mentioned, label fusion can be regarded as a reconstruction or classification problem. In the reconstruction case, each target label f is approximated as a linear combination of the atlas labels [1], i.e., $f = w^{\mathsf{T}} l$, where w is a weighing vector to combine the atlas labels. Weights in w can be computed as the reconstruction coefficients of the target patch t by the atlas patches A, i.e., $\begin{bmatrix} t \\ 1 \end{bmatrix} \approx \begin{bmatrix} A \\ 1^{\mathsf{T}} \end{bmatrix} w$. Note that we add the trailing 1 in the target and atlas patches to enforce the weighting vector w will add up to one. On the other hand, in the classification case, given the target image patch t, its central label is determined only based on the mapping function learned from the atlas image patches and ground-truth labels [2], i.e., $f = w^{\mathsf{T}} \begin{bmatrix} t \\ 1 \end{bmatrix}$, where the trailing 1 allows to include the bias term of the linear mapping in the last entry of w. The linear mapping function w can be learned by minimizing the discrepancies between the predicted labels and ground-truth labels in the training stage, i.e., $l^{\mathsf{T}} \approx w^{\mathsf{T}} \begin{bmatrix} A \\ 1^{\mathsf{T}} \end{bmatrix}$.

Instead of predicting only the label at the center of each target patch, we also estimate the labels for the entire target image patch. Following the same order as in A, we can arrange the label vector L_j^i of each atlas patch A_j^i into the atlas label matrix $L = \left[L_1^1, \dots, L_j^i, \dots, L_n^M\right]_{i=1,\dots,M, j=1,\dots,n}$. Moreover, instead of labeling each target patch independently, we go one step further to simultaneously label a large group of target image points with similar anatomical characteristics. To achieve it, we first group the target image into several partitions based on the image intensities. Then, we label the target image in a group-by-group manner. For each group, we use $T = [T_1, \dots, T_m]$ and $F = [F_1, \dots, F_m]$ to denote m intensity vectors and their respective missing label vectors of all target image points in the group.

Construction of the Four-Quadrant Matrix. Fig. 1 illustrates the construction of the four-quadrant matrix $Z^0 = \begin{bmatrix} \begin{bmatrix} A \\ 1^{\mathsf{T}} \end{bmatrix} & \begin{bmatrix} T \\ 1^{\mathsf{T}} \end{bmatrix} \\ L & F \end{bmatrix}$. This matrix consists of four parts (from top to bottom, left to right): the atlas image patch matrix A, the atlas label matrix L, the target image patch matrix T, and the target label matrix F (for the sake of simplicity, we consider the trailing ones along with the intensity vectors as a whole). Our goal is to complete the missing values in the target label matrix F by using matrix completion (MC) techniques. In this way, label fusion can be formulated as the recovery of the missing entries in F by imposing the low-rank constraint upon Z^0.

Advantages of Label fusion by Matrix Completion. As mentioned earlier, the reconstruction-based methods assume that each target-patch column can be represented by a linear combination of atlas-patch columns, while classification-based methods assume that each label-patch row can be represented by a linear combination of image-patch rows. In order to leverage the significant row-wise and column-wise correlations, label fusion can be regarded as finding the entries in F that make the four-quadrant matrix Z^0 the lowest rank possible. As a result, matrix F is the result of a blend of row-wise and column-wise combinations. Since the column-wise correlations describe the relationships between atlas and target image patches as in the reconstruction-based methods and also the row-wise correlations encode the mapping between image and label domains as in the classification-based methods, our MC-based label fusion approach inherits the advantages of both reconstruction- and classification-based methods.

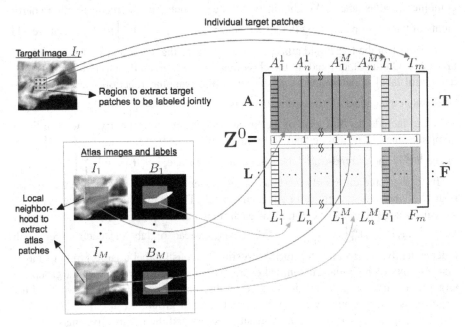

Fig. 1. Construction of the four-quadrant matrix

Label Fusion by Matrix Completion. As mentioned above, label fusion by MC consists in finding the missing entries in F so that the rank of Z^0 is minimized. To improve the robustness to noise in the observed data, we also allow for small deviations in the entries corresponding to the observed data that further help reducing the rank. Therefore, the objective of label fusion by MC is to find the new four-quadrant matrix Z which satisfies (1) the rank of Z is low; and (2) the residual between the observed data in Z and Z^0 is small. Due to the different natures of the data contained in matrix Z^0 (i.e., image data and label data) it is more convenient to use different cost functions for evaluating the residuals regarding each one of the types. To that end, we define Θ_I and Θ_L as the sets of matrix indices pointing to the entries in Z^0 (i.e., pairs of row and column coordinates) corresponding to the observed image data and the observed label data, respectively. Accordingly, $Z^0_{a,b}$, $(a,b) \in \Theta_I$ corresponds to the image-intensity value at position (a,b) in matrix Z^0 (i.e., in either the red or blue quadrants of Fig. 1), and $Z^0_{a,b}$, $(a,b) \in \Theta_L$ corresponds to a label-value at position (a, b) in matrix Z^0 (i.e., in the yellow quadrant of Fig. 1). As shown by [3], the above objectives can be stated by a convex optimization problem as:

$$\underset{Z}{\text{minimize}} \quad \mu \|Z\|_* + \frac{1}{|\Theta_1|} \Sigma_{(a,b) \in \Theta_I} c_I(Z_{a,b}, Z_{a,b}^0) + \frac{\lambda}{|\Theta_2|} \Sigma_{(a,b) \in \Theta_L} c_L(Z_{a,b}, Z_{a,b}^0) \quad (1)$$

where $\|\cdot\|_*$ denotes the nuclear norm, which is responsible for the minimization of the rank of matrix Z, and $c_I(\cdot)$ and $c_L(\cdot)$ are the loss functions regarding the image reconstruction errors (across the indices in Θ_I) and label reconstruction errors (across the indices in Θ_L), respectively, which are responsible for the minimization of the discrepancies between the observed entries of Z and Z^0. Equation (1)(1) represents a trade-off between leveraging the row- and column-wise correlations to reproduce the data in the matrix, and minimizing the residual error between the reproduced and the original matrix (balanced by scalars μ and λ, respectively).

Similarly as in [3], we use the squared loss to penalize the image reconstruction errors, i.e., $c_I(Z_{a,b}, Z_{a,b}^0) = (Z_{a,b} - Z_{a,b}^0)^2 / 2$, $(a, b) \in \Theta_I$ since it is suitable for the continuous values in the intensity images, and logistic loss to penalize the label prediction errors, i.e., $c_L(Z_{a,b}, Z_{a,b}^0) = \log(1 + \exp(-Z_{a,b}^0 Z_{a,b}))$, $(a, b) \in \Theta_L$ since it is suitable for the binary values in the label maps.

Confidence Measurements for the Atlas Labels. Logistic loss assumes binary atlas labels $B_i(v) \in \{-1, 1\}$ $v \in \Omega$ in the label images B_i for each atlas. Since different points act different roles in label fusion, we further propose to measure the importance of each atlas label by assigning high confidence degrees to labels distant to the structure boundary. Thus, we replace the binary label maps B_i by the signed distance maps (SDM) D_i when building the new four-quadrant matrix Z^0, where $D_i(v)$, $v \in \Omega$ contains the signed distance of voxel v in the i-th atlas to the boundary of the structure. Given the new four-quadrant matrix Z^0 (with the atlas label matrix L containing signed distances from D_i instead of binary labels from B_i), we compute the probability that a signed distance, $Z_{a,b}^0$, $(a, b) \in \Theta_L$, corresponds to a voxel inside a structure, by using the sigmoid function, as proposed in [4]:

$$P(Z_{a,b}^0) = \frac{1}{1 + \exp(-\alpha Z_{a,b}^0)} \quad , (a, b) \in \Theta_L \quad (2)$$

Therefore, voxels deep inside/outside the structure will be considered with high confidence to belong/not belong to the structure (i.e., $P \to 1$ / $P \to 0$) and voxels within a neighborhood of the boundary will be considered with less confidence to belong/not belong to the structure (i.e., $P \in (0,1)$). The size of this neighborhood is determined by the scalar α. Fig. 2 shows an example of this representation.

Given the observed signed distance, $Z_{a,b}^0$, $(a, b) \in \Theta_L$, and the estimated one by MC, $Z_{a,b}$, $(a, b) \in \Theta_L$, we define the new loss $c_L(Z_{a,b}, Z_{a,b}^0)$ as the negative of the probability of both agreeing in their relative position w.r.t. the boundary of the structure, as follows:

$$c_L(Z_{a,b}, Z_{a,b}^0) = -\left(P(Z_{a,b})P(Z_{a,b}^0) + \left(1 - P(Z_{a,b})\right)\left(1 - P(Z_{a,b}^0)\right)\right) \quad (3)$$

The difference between logistic loss and the proposed loss function is that, with logistic loss, errors are penalized equally across all voxels, whereas with equation (3), errors at pixels deep inside/outside the structure are penalized higher.

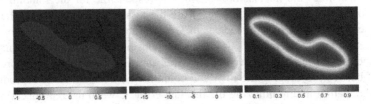

Fig. 2. The confidence map of a 2D synthetic hippocampus. From left to right: binary labels as in B_i, signed distance map as in D_i and confidence map as computed by eq. (2).

MC Optimization. The optimization of equation (1) can be solved by an iterative algorithm that alternates between a gradient step and a shrinkage step. In the gradient step, the matrix is updated so as to decrease the residual error, and in the shrinkage step, the rank of the matrix is reduced. Since it is a convex optimization problem, convergence to the global optimum is guaranteed [3].

Determine the Target Labels after Matrix Completion. As result of MC, we get a low rank matrix Z containing continuous target labels in F. Discretization is straightforwardly applied to each target label by using the sign function (in the case of using both binary labels and SDMs). Since we predict the target label for the entire target patch, we end up with multiple estimations from the neighboring points for each target image point. We use the majority voting rule to determine the final label for each target image point.

3   Experiments

We evaluate the performance of the proposed method in the segmentation of the left and right hippocampi in the ADNI[1] and LONI LPBA40[2] datasets. The ADNI dataset is provided by the Alzheimer's Disease Neuroimaging Initiative and the size of each image is $256 \times 256 \times 256$. The LONI LPBA40 dataset is provided by the Laboratory of Neuro-Imaging at UCLA and contains 40 brain images of size $220 \times 220 \times 184$. Manual annotations of the left and right hippocampi for all the subjects are available in both datasets. These manual annotations are used as the labels for the atlases and as gold standard to evaluate the segmentation performance in the target images.

In order to evaluate the performance of the proposed method we compare the following methods: (i) non-local weighted voting label fusion (**NLWV**) [5] (i) Linear

---

[1] http://www.adni-info.org/
[2] http://www.loni.usc.edu/atlases/Atlas_Detail.php?atlas_id=12

reconstruction with sparsity constraints (**Rec**), which falls into the reconstruction-based methods with ℓ_1 regularization; (ii) logistic regression with group sparsity (**Class**), which is one of the classification-based methods with $\ell_{1,2}$ regularization on the weighting vector; (iii) matrix completion with SDMs (**MCFull**), which is the full version of our proposed method. We tested the label fusion performance of the different methods under two different registration scenarios: (1) linear (affine) registration by FLIRT [6], and (2) non-linear registration by diffeomorphic demons [7]. After registration, we selected the best 15 atlases to label each target image according to the normalized mutual information criterion.

We include results for both point-wise estimation (i.e., only central label) and multi-point estimation (i.e., entire label patch). In the multi-point case, we use the same patch size ($5 \times 5 \times 5$) for image patch and label patch. The local search neighborhoods are set to $5 \times 5 \times 5$ for linear registration and $3 \times 3 \times 3$ for non-linear registration, respectively, in order to adapt to their different accuracies. We use $\alpha = 1$ for measuring the confidence value as in equation (2). We have experimentally set the trade-off parameters for the MC optimization to $\mu = 10^{-4}$ and $\lambda = 0.05$, respectively.

Tables 1 and 2 show the Dice ratios obtained by the compared methods in segmenting of both hippocampi in the ADNI dataset using linear and non-linear registration, respectively. Tables 3 and 4 show results obtained in the LONI dataset, similarly using linear/non-linear registration. There are four columns in Tables 1-4, with each column showing the Dice ratio of the left/right hippocampi with multipoint/point-wise estimation.

Table 1. Dice Ratio in the **ADNI** database using **linear** registration

	Right, multipoint	Left, multipoint	Right, point-wise	Left, point-wise
NLWV	78.00	76.42	75.67	73.63
Rec	78.93	78.19	74.87	74.17
Class	79.01	77.34	76.67	74.82
MCFull	**80.02**	**78.47**	**77.34**	**75.83**

Table 2. Dice Ratio in the **ADNI** database using **non-linear** registration

	Right, multipoint	Left, multipoint	Right, point-wise	Left, point-wise
NLWV	81.68	80.21	81.06	79.59
Rec	81.96	80.89	79.63	78.40
Class	82.21	80.69	81.16	79.69
MCFull	**82.88**	**81.54**	**81.95**	**80.59**

Table 3. Dice Ratio in the **LONI** database using **linear** registration

	Right, multipoint	Left, multipoint	Right, point-wise	Left, point-wise
NLWV	79.84	80.86	78.33	79.39
Rec	80.74	81.45	78.48	78.92
Class	80.68	81.42	79.06	79.90
MCFull	**81.21**	**81.91**	**79.39**	**79.93**

Table 4. Dice Ratio in the **LONI** database using **non-linear** registration

	Right, multipoint	Left, multipoint	Right, point-wise	Left, point-wise
NLWV	80.92	80.70	80.23	80.09
Rec	81.29	81.25	79.72	79.56
Class	81.38	81.26	80.32	80.10
MCFull	**81.83**	**81.66**	**80.79**	**80.60**

In order to get further insights, we also report results of matrix completion using binary labels instead of SDMs (**MCBin**) in the multipoint estimation case. In the ADNI dataset, MCBin achieved average Dice ratios of 79.28 and 82.06 with linear and non-linear registration, respectively. In the LONI dataset, MCBin achieved average Dice ratios of 81.41 and 81.73 with linear and non-linear registration, respectively. As we can see the use of the SDMs improves $\sim 0.2\%$ in the non-linear registration case. Regarding the comparison with the rest of the methods, in the ADNI dataset our proposed method achieved improvements w.r.t. the 2nd best performing method of $> 1\%$ and $\sim 0.7\%$ with linear and non-linear registration, respectively. In the LONI dataset, our method achieved improvements of $\sim 0.5\%$ with both linear and non-linear registration.

4   Conclusions

In this paper, we have presented a novel label fusion method that inherits the benefits of the reconstruction and classification-based approaches by posing the label fusion problem as a matrix completion problem. By doing so, we fully utilize not only the correlation between atlas and target image patches but also the relationship between image patches and ground-truth labels. Promising labeling results have been achieved in ADNI and LONI datasets.

References

1. Zhang, D., Guo, Q., Wu, G., Shen, D.: Sparse Patch-Based Label Fusion for Multi-Atlas Segmentation. In: Yap, P.-T., Liu, T., Shen, D., Westin, C.-F., Shen, L. (eds.) MBIA 2012. LNCS, vol. 7509, pp. 94–102. Springer, Heidelberg (2012)
2. Hao, Y., et al.: Local Label Learning (LLL) for subcortical structure segmentation. Human Brain Mapping, n/a–n/a (2013)
3. Goldberg, A.B., et al.: Transduction with Matrix Completion: Three Birds with One Stone. In: NIPS (2010)
4. Pohl, K.M., Fisher, J., Shenton, M.E., McCarley, R.W., Grimson, W.E.L., Kikinis, R., Wells, W.M.: Logarithm Odds Maps for Shape Representation. In: Larsen, R., Nielsen, M., Sporring, J. (eds.) MICCAI 2006. LNCS, vol. 4191, pp. 955–963. Springer, Heidelberg (2006)
5. Coupe, P., et al.: Patch-based segmentation using expert priors: Application to hippocampus and ventricle segmentation. NeuroImage 54(2), 940–954 (2011)
6. Jenkinson, M., et al.: Improved Optimization for the Robust and Accurate Linear Registration and Motion Correction of Brain Images. NeuroImage 17(2) (2002)
7. Vercauteren, T., et al.: Diffeomorphic demons: efficient non-parametric image registration. NeuroImage 45 (2009)

Structured Random Forests for Myocardium Delineation in 3D Echocardiography

João S. Domingos[1], Richard V. Stebbing[1], Paul Leeson[2], and J. Alison Noble[1]

[1] Department of Engineering Science, University of Oxford, U.K.
[2] Department of Cardiovascular Medicine, John Radcliffe Hospital, Oxford, U.K.

Abstract. Delineation of myocardium borders from 3D echocardiography is a critical step for the diagnosis of heart disease. Following the approach of myocardium segmentation as a contour finding task, recent work has shown effective methods to interpret endocardial edge information in the left ventricle. Nevertheless, these methods are still prone to preserve irrelevant edge responses and would struggle to overcome chief ventricle anatomical challenges. In this paper we adapt Structured Random Forests, borrowed from computer vision, for fast and robust myocardium edge detection. This method is evaluated on a dataset composed of short-axis slices from 25 End-Diastolic echocardiography volumes. Results show that the proposed ensemble model outperforms standard intensity-based and local phase-based edge detectors, while removing or significantly suppressing irrelevant edges triggered by ultrasound image artefacts and blood pool anatomical structures.

1   Introduction

In this paper we propose a fast and effective method to perform myocardial boundary detection in short-axis slices of 3D Echocardiography (3DE) volumes by integrating structural information of pixel neighbourhoods in classification random forests. These novel Structured Random Forests (SRFs) were introduced in [1] for fast edge detection in computer vision and were adapted here to demonstrate their value in the task of enhancing myocardial boundary. While a truly 3D analysis would be more consistent, slice-by-slice analysis does not lead to notably misaligned contours from observation. Any error has to be traded with the computational cost of a 3D implementation.

Delineation of myocardium borders is a critical step for accurate left ventricle (LV) segmentation and cardiac function quantification. Although LV border delineation has been a widely researched topic, it remains a challenging task mainly due to the anatomical presence of papillary muscles and trabeculae. In addition, there are 3DE image limitations such as speckle, low signal-to-noise ratio, low contrast images and stitching artefacts. In this context, development of computer aided ventricle delineation and segmentation frameworks aimed at improving volumetric analysis in 3DE is of particularly relevance.

Following the approach of myocardium segmentation as a contour finding task, it has previously been shown that intensity-invariant phase-based methods

G. Wu et al. (Eds.): MLMI 2014, LNCS 8679, pp. 215–222, 2014.
© Springer International Publishing Switzerland 2014

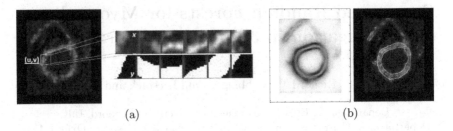

(a)   (b)

Fig. 1. [a] Training data examples as used in our proposed SRFs. While standard random forests associate only the centre label at position (u,v) to an image patch **x**, we incorporate the topology of the local label neighbourhood (**y**) and hence learn relevant labelling transitions between myocardium and blood pool. A rich set of structured labels are then used by the ensemble model to select splits in the decision trees. [b] LV myocardial edge probability map (*left*) from the slice in [a], obtained from our SRFs, and its non-maximal suppression version (*right*).

offer a good alternative to underperforming intensity gradient-based ones in ultrasound images. In [2] a 3D edge detection method was proposed based on a local-phase Feature Asymmetry (FA) measure using the monogenic signal. Motivated by the principle that only the edges that contribute to the myocardium boundary are relevant for segmentation, a 3D Boundary Fragment Model-based method is proposed in [3] to perform anatomical heart boundary delineation. Nevertheless, when accurate myocardium delineation is required, these methods still preserve irrelevant edges. The proposed SRFs use the topological information in local image patches (Figure 1[a]) to selectively suppress spurious edge responses and learn only relevant local image neighbourhoods that encode the myocardial boundaries in a structured learning-based approach [4].

2   Methods

2.1   Structured Random Forests

Following a data-driven learning approach, we could firstly propose semantic myocardial boundary detection as a simple binary classification problem. The idea being that a given input image patch can be classified as a positive patch if its centre pixel contains an edge and negative otherwise. Nevertheless, this binary approach ignores valuable local structural information about edges. A multiclass classification approach could then be proposed by simply clustering label (Ground Truth, GT) patches into patch classes. Upon reaching a leaf node, a standard Random Forest (RF) classifier [5] could then directly predict, from a distribution over the labels, the most likely patch class correspondent to the input patch image. With the proposed SRFs, we directly predict local structure of a given image patch, at the cost of a high dimensional output space. As such, standard RFs need to be extended to arbitrary structured output spaces $\mathcal{Y}$.

In RFs the information stored at a leaf node can be arbitrary [1]: binary, multiclass or structured labels. Moreover, inference in SRFs is actually identical to inference in standard RFs, the only difference being is what information is stored at the leaf nodes and how it is used. For multiclass classification, the standard information gain criterion may also not be well defined over structured labels, $y \in \mathcal{Y}$, that encode the local image annotations of image patches $x \in \chi$. As a result of this, in [1] the authors propose a straightforward two-step mapping approach (defined below): firstly $\mathcal{Y} \to \mathcal{Z}$ and then $\mathcal{Z} \to \mathcal{C}$.

Intermediate Mapping and Information Gain Criterion. Given that our required information gain criterion depends on the similarity over $\mathcal{Y}$, we assume that for many structured output spaces, including for structured learning of myocardium edge detection, we can define a mapping Π of $\mathcal{Y}$ to an *intermediate* space $\mathcal{Z}$, $\Pi : \mathcal{Y} \to \mathcal{Z}$, in which the Euclidean distance in $\mathcal{Z}$ can be measured.

Considering that an approximate measure of information gain is sufficient to train an effective random forest classifier, our goal is to map a set of structured labels $y \in \mathcal{Y}$ into a discrete set of labels $c \in \mathcal{C}$, where $\mathcal{C} = \{1, ..., k\}$, in a way that labels with similar $\mathcal{Y}$ are assigned to the same discrete label c. Given that these discrete labels can be binary ($k = 2$) or multiclass ($k > 2$), we can use standard information gain measures such as Shannon entropy or Gini impurity [5]. The discretization step ($\mathcal{Z} \to \mathcal{C}$) yielding the discrete label set $\mathcal{C}$ given $\mathcal{Z}$ is computed independently when training each node and depends on the distribution of labels at each node. To do this, z is quantized based on the top $log_2(k)$ PCA dimensions, effectively assigning z a discrete label c according to the orthant into which z falls [1].

Because $\mathcal{Z}$ can be of high dimension and computationally expensive to deal with, and since an approximate distance measure is sufficient, we perform dimensionality reduction by sampling m dimensions of $\mathcal{Z}$ which yields a reduced mapping $\Pi_\phi : \mathcal{Y} \to \mathcal{Z}$ parametrised by ϕ. While training, we randomly generate and apply a unique mapping Π_ϕ to training labels y at each node. By sampling $\mathcal{Z}$, we not only make Π_ϕ faster to compute than Π, but also improve diversity of trees by injecting additional randomness into the learning process [1].

Ensemble Model. The structured ensemble model merges a set of n labels $y_1...y_n \in \mathcal{Y}$ into a single prediction both for training, upon association of labels with nodes, and testing i.e. merging of multiple predictions. After sampling a selected m dimensional mapping Π_ϕ and computing $z_i = \Pi_\phi(y_i)$ for each i, we finally select the label y_k whose z_k is the medoid i.e. the medoid z_k that minimizes $\sum_{ij}(z_{kj} - z_{ij})^2$. Because we only need an approximate distance measure to estimate the dissimilarity of y, by reducing $\mathcal{Z}$ dimensionality, the medoid only needs to be computed for small n, which means that an approximate distance metric is sufficient to select an effective element y_k. Notice that the ensemble model is incapable of synthesising new labels without added information about $\mathcal{Y}$. Hence, every prediction $y \in \mathcal{Y}$ must have been observed during training.

2.2 3D Echocardiogram Database

25 End-Diastolic (ED) 3D echocardiograms (224x208x208 voxels) of healthy volunteers (ranging from 19 to 26 years old) were recorded using a Philips iE33 xMATRIX System (X3-1 and X5-1 probes). LV myocardial boundary references (segmentation masks or GT shown in Figure 1[a]) were manually drawn for these. All the Structured Edge Detector (SED) models learned in this paper underwent 3-fold cross validation (CV) (divided as 8,8,9 randomly selected datasets). For example, these were trained on say 16 volumes on every 5th short-axis slice of each volume and tested on the remaining 9 volumes, hence there was no correlation between training and testing volumes and slices.

2.3 Myocardium Boundary Detection

Given an input short-axis slice from an ED echocardiography volume, the proposed SED task is to label each pixel with a binary variable indicating whether it belongs to an edge or not. This is done by predicting a structured 24×24 segmentation patch from a larger 48×48 image patch (fixed for all experiments). This patch size was empirically determined to give best edge delineations, and is a result of the need to look at more global information, i.e. contribution of more neighbourhood pixel votes, in order to effectively avoid local irrelevant edge responses.

Regarding the input feature pool, each image patch was augmented with multiple channels of information yielding a feature vector $x \in \mathbb{Z}^{48 \times 48 \times K}$ where K is the number of channels. Two types of features were used: pixel lookups $x(i, j, k)$ and pairwise differences $x(i_1, j_1, k) - x(i_2, j_2, k)$. A similar set of gradient channels used in [6] were implemented in this work. We computed the normalised gradient magnitude at 2 scales (original and half resolution) and each of these channels is then split into 4 channels based on orientation. The channels were blurred and then downsampled by a factor of 2. The resulting K consists of 11 channels (1 grayscale, 2 magnitude and 8 orientation channels). Pairwise difference features were obtained by sampling a blurred and downsampled (7×7) version of the previous candidate pairs, and computing their differences.

Upon training our SRF, and because the Euclidean distance over binary edge maps yields a weak distance measure, we define our mapping Π by sampling a pair of locations $j_1 \neq j_2$, where $1 \leq j \leq 256$ denote the jth pixel of segmentation mask $y(j)$ (Figure 1[a]), and check if $y(j_1) = y(j_2)$. This defines $z = \Pi(y)$ as a large binary vector encoding $[y(j_1) = y(j_2)]$ for every distinct pair of indices $j_1 \neq j_2$. Hence, a subset of $m = 256$ dimensions of the high dimensional $\mathcal{Z}$, and $k = 2$, were found to effectively capture the similarity of segmentation masks.

Given that we can store edge maps (any arbitrary information) at the leaf nodes, we finally averaged these to compute a soft edge response. The resulting ensemble model is computationally efficient because it uses structured labels, capturing information for an entire image neighbourhood, thus reducing the number of decision trees T that need to be evaluated per pixel. The structured output was computed on the image with a stride of 2 pixels. Since both the inputs and outputs of each tree overlapped, we trained T=8 trees and evaluated an alternating set of 4 trees at each adjacent location.

Motivated by [7], we finally performed classical multiscale of our SED by averaging the result of three probability edge maps at the original, half (robust but poor localisation), and double resolution (detail-preserving detection but sensitive to endocardial boundary artefacts) version of a given input image. Prior to evaluation, we performed standard non-maximal suppression on the resulting edge maps to obtain thinned edges.

Finally, a SRF ensemble model, *SED1*, was trained on LV myocardial boundary references, and hand-optimized with the parameters previously discussed and a maximum depth of $D = 64$. In addition, a second model, *SED2*, was trained on the same volumes but on LV endocardial boundaries only. After 3-fold CV of results from both SEDs, we evaluated them qualitatively by comparing endocardial edge strength and enhancement against the best (hand-optimized) standard 2D and 3D local phase-based FA measure [2] (parameters: centre frequency: 0.25mm, and 2 octaves) and intensity-based Canny edge detector (magnitude of a Gaussian derivative operator) [8]. In the latter we used the "CannyEdgeDetectionImageFilter" from ITK (parameters: variance: 0.25, lower threshold: 0, upper threshold 1.0, maximum error: 0.0125). For the quantitative evaluation of *SED2*, we computed the Hausdorff distance between the detected endocardium boundaries (non-maximally suppressed) and their correspondent GT. The same was performed for the other two standard edge detectors. To compare these, we used a *masking procedure* in which we mask (GT contour filled and dilated) the (2D and 3D) FA and Canny edge responses to include all responses inside the GT and to explicitly exclude epicardium or other edge responses exterior to the myocardium that could have made the Hausdorff distances bogus.

3   Experimental Results and Discussion

Qualitative Evaluation. Examples of unseen test cases with visible papillary muscles and trabeculation in the blood pool were selected for comparison between the proposed SED ensemble models and the best (thresholded) 3D FA measure. As depicted in Figure 2[a], the proposed *SED1* significantly outperformed the best standard FA and Canny methods in the sense that where responses fade in the local phase-based measure (known to respond well to ultrasound images since they are intensity invariant), *SED1* yielded myocardium edges with high probability. Non-maximal suppression computation of these allowed to better delineate the myocardium. In our method, the stronger edge responses were derived from the topological knowledge gathered by the SRF from each edge pixel neighbourhood ($24 \times 24 = 576$ pixel votes), and therefore contribute to the completeness of the LV and RV blood pools. In addition, it is illustrated how our *SED1* was able to significantly suppress or, in most cases, completely remove any spurious or irrelevant edge responses that result from image artefacts or the presence of papillary muscles and trabeculations in the LV and RV blood pool. In the typical case where accurate myocardium delineation

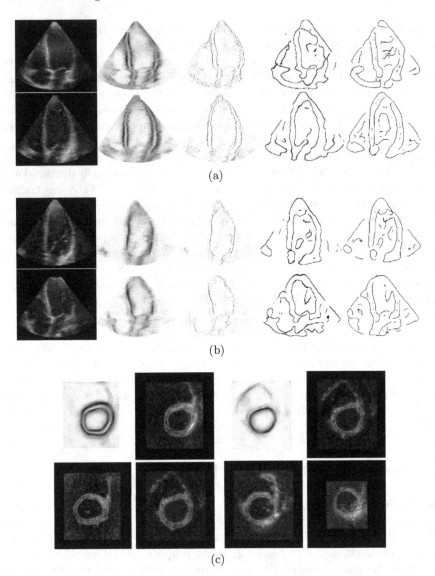

Fig. 2. [a] From *left* to *right*: unseen testing examples with GT (red); LV myocardial edge probability maps from *SED1*; non-maximal suppressed versions of the previous; 3D FA-based edge maps; 3D Canny edge maps. [b] From *left* to *right*: unseen testing examples; LV endocardial edge probability maps from *SED2*; non-maximal suppressed versions of the previous; 3D FA-based edge maps; 3D Canny edge maps. [c] Unseen testing examples of LV myocardial (endocardium and epicardium) boundary detection from *SED1* and single endocardial boundary detection from *SED2* on short-axis slices. Where shown, GT (red) boundaries are superimposed on the detected ones (green) by the proposed SEDs.

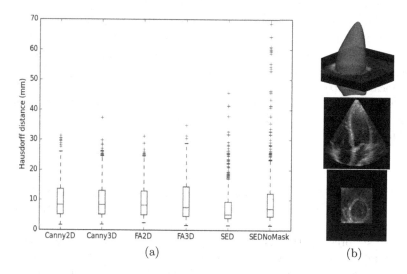

(a)   (b)

Fig. 3. [a] Comparison of the Hausdorff distance distribution between the detected myocardial boundaries (*SED2*) and the GT for different edge detectors. [b] Fitting a biquadratic B-spline surface [3] to the detected epicardial boundaries of an LV blood pool test example. This demonstrates that our *SED2* allows for fast and robust heart segmentation and volumetric quantification.

is required, both the FA and Canny methods preserve irrelevant edges which can be seen inside the blood pool of both ventricles in Figure 2[a,b].

Unsurprisingly, when we fitted a deformable anatomical model to the LV blood pool, depicted in Figure 3[b], we found that convergence of surfaces to detected endocardial boundaries was complete for our *SED2*, while in both FA and Canny methods, irrelevant edge responses will prevent deformable models from growing and converging to boundaries. A more extensive analysis of this method for LV volumetric quantification can be found in [9].

In Figure 2[c], our SEDs demonstrated the ambiguity existent in the segmented masks (GT) since in some cases it is arguable that our method performed a better endocardial boundary detection than the GT, which could be due to the blurring and thus smoothing process occuring at the feature extraction level.

Quantitative Evaluation. Because the *masking procedure* preserves all the responses interior to the endocardium, the Hausdorff distance measures whether or not the different methods detect erroneous edges in the blood pool, which is the primary driver for our method. As depicted in Figure 3[a], our *SED2* method ([4.1 5.3 9.5] mm) outperformed the standard FA (2D:[5.1 8.3 12.9] mm; 3D:[4.7 7.6 14.4] mm) and Canny (2D:[5.3 8.5 13.7] mm; 3D:[5.3 8.5 13.1] mm) methods at every percentile (25th, 50th and 75th). More interestingly, even when not masked to exclude epicardium or other edge responses exterior to the myocardium, the proposed *SED2* ([4.7 7.1 12.2] mm) was still able to outperform the standard methods. Note that ultrasound images have been shown to respond well to local phase-based methods, such as the 3D FA measure, and still our unmasked SED did slightly better when it comes to endocardial boundary detection and enhancement. The higher number of outliers in the *SEDNoMask* was related to some detected RV endocardial boundaries in short-axis slices where RV endocardial structure resembled the LV one.

Finally, at runtime, a 224x208x208 image volume took only 6.7s to generate the myocardial edge probability and orientation volumes on a single core of an Intel Mobile 4930MX (or 4.2s on 8 cores).

4   Conclusion

A novel structured learning approach borrowed from computer vision is shown to perform fast and robust myocardial edge detection. Qualitative and quantitative results demonstrate that our method outperforms standard edge detectors, effectively suppressing the prediction of irrelevant endocardial edge responses, and allowing deformable models and contour-based approaches to more stably converge to the detected myocardial boundaries, enabling computation of more accurate LV clinical indices. Future work will evaluate how accurate the proposed ensemble model is in performing wall thickness measurements.

Acknowledgments. This work was supported by the RCUK CDT in Healthcare Innovation, EPSRC grant EP/G030693/1, and Rhodes Trust.

References

1. Dollár, P., Zitnick, C.L.: Structured forests for fast edge detection. In: ICCV (2013)
2. Rajpoot, K., Grau, V., Noble, J.: Local-phase based 3D boundary detection using monogenic signal and its application to real-time 3-D echocardiography images. In: IEEE International Symposium on Biomedical Imaging: From Nano to Macro, ISBI 2009, pp. 783–786. IEEE (2009)
3. Stebbing, R.V., Noble, J.A.: Delineating anatomical boundaries using the boundary fragment model. Medical Image Analysis 17(8), 1123–1136 (2013)
4. Nowozin, S., Lampert, C.H.: Structured learning and prediction in computer vision, vol. 6. Now Publishers Inc. (2011)
5. Criminisi, A., Shotton, J., Konukoglu, E.: Decision forests: A unified framework for classification, regression, density estimation, manifold learning and semi-supervised learning. Foundations and Trends® in Computer Graphics and Vision 7(2-3), 81–227 (2012)
6. Lim, J.J., Zitnick, C.L., Dollár, P.: Sketch tokens: A learned mid-level representation for contour and object detection. In: 2013 IEEE Conference on Computer Vision and Pattern Recognition (CVPR), pp. 3158–3165. IEEE (2013)
7. Ren, X.: Multi-scale improves boundary detection in natural images. In: Forsyth, D., Torr, P., Zisserman, A. (eds.) ECCV 2008, Part III. LNCS, vol. 5304, pp. 533–545. Springer, Heidelberg (2008)
8. Canny, J.: A computational approach to edge detection. IEEE Transactions on Pattern Analysis and Machine Intelligence (6), 679–698 (1986)
9. Domingos, J., Stebbing, R., Noble, J.: Endocardial segmentation using structured random forests in 3D echocardiography. In: MICCAI Challenge on Endocardial Three-dimensional Ultrasound Segmentation (2014)

Improved Reproducibility of Neuroanatomical Definitions through Diffeomorphometry and Complexity Reduction

Daniel Tward[1], Jorge Jovicich[2], Andrea Soricelli[3], Giovanni Frisoni[4], Alain Trouvé[5], Laurent Younes[1], and Michael Miller[1]

[1] Center for Imaging Science, Johns Hopkins University, Baltimore MD USA
[2] Center for Mind/Brain Sciences, University of Trento, Italy
[3] University of Napeles Parthenope and IRCSS Fondazione SDN, Naples Italy
[4] Geneva University Hospitals and University of Geneva, Geneva, Switzerland
IRCCS Fatebenefratelli, Brescia, Italy
[5] CMLA, ENS Cachan - CNRS (UMR 8536), F-94235 Cachan Cedex

Abstract. We present an algorithm for passing from dense noisy neuroanatomical segmentations, directly to a complexity-reduced representation with respect to a deformed smooth template surface, bypassing the need for triangulation of any target data. We demonstrate the utility of this algorithm toward improving reproducibility of hippocampal definitions, using a dataset containing 4 MR images per subject, two within the same visit on each of two dates, with dense segmentations provided by unedited longitudinal Freesurfer analysis. We quantify reproducibility of intra-visit and inter-visit variability through L2 distances and Hausdorff distances between pairs of segmentations, and show that our method results in a statistically significant improvement by a factor of 1.63 to more than 3-fold.

Keywords: Complexity reduction, reproducibility, diffeomorphometry, LDDMM, neuroanatomy, neuroimaging.

1 Introduction

Medical imaging data is necessarily high dimensional. Reduction of its inherent complexity is essential for machine learning applications—overcoming the curse of dimensionality in model estimation, multiple comparison corrections in statistical hypothesis testing, and building and communicating intuition with medical practitioners comprise a few compelling reasons.

When studying anatomical structures, one observes that imaging modalities only provide information about shape through their gradients and discontinuities. In neuroimaging this corresponds to boundaries between grey matter, white matter, and cerebrospinal fluid, the remainder of the images being relatively homogeneous in intensity. This leads to a natural reduction in complexity by representing subcortical structures by triangulated surfaces defined on their boundaries, rather than through dense imagery defined everywhere in space.

G. Wu et al. (Eds.): MLMI 2014, LNCS 8679, pp. 223–230, 2014.

However, dense voxelized imaging data, including the unedited anatomical segmentations generated by longitudinal Freesurfer analysis [1] used here, is widely available. Making use of such data is important, despite its quality often being low for shape analysis. An example of a typical voxelized hippocampus segmentation is shown in Fig. 1. Note the lack of smoothness, the appendages, the isolated components, and the concavities which are not reflective of real anatomy and can be considered noise.

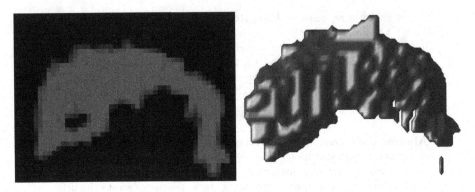

Fig. 1. A typical example of a voxel based segmentation of left hippocampus shown as a slice (left) and an isosurface rendering (right)

In this work we present a method for passing from structural definitions in terms of dense voxelized data in the presence of such noise, directly to a representation defined with respect to a deformed smooth template surface. This approach is novel as compared to other surface based analyses in that it bypasses the need for triangulation of segmentations, and allows working with the voxelized data directly. This complexity reduction solves the problem of ambiguity in defining deformations within the homogeneous interiors of the subcortical structures. We demonstrate its application to improvement in reproducibility of hippocampal definitions for repeated scans—both within a single visit and between repeated visits—the hippocampus being a clinically important structure for the detection of Alzheimer's disease onset [2]. Quantifying and improving reproducibility is an important challenge facing the shape analysis community [3].

2   Anatomical Shape Model

We work within the large deformation diffeomorphic metric mapping framework [4] referred to as diffeomorphometry, characterizing shapes by the action of a group of diffeomorphisms on a template. Machine learning applications within this framework have been explored for building classifiers from medical imaging data based an anatomical structure. Examples include identifying patients with Alzheimer's disease [5], or healthy patients who are likely to develop Alzheimer's disease in the future [6,7]. Here we consider a template consisting of a smooth surface $\mathcal{M} \subset \mathbb{R}^3$, representing the left hippocampus, estimated as the average of the population [8] (to remove bias associated with a single subject template), along with a corresponding dense segmentation image, a function I_0 from a subset Ω of $\mathbb{R}^3$ to $[0, 1]$. The segmentation image may not be strictly binary due to interpolation. The surface is represented by the coordinate chart $f_0 : U \subset \mathbb{R}^2 \to \mathcal{M}$, with $u \mapsto f_0(u)$.

We describe target anatomy by acting on the template with diffeomorphisms φ_1 generated by smooth time varying velocity fields v_t, with $\varphi_0 = Id$ and the dynamics

$$\dot{\varphi}_t = v_t(\varphi_t). \tag{1}$$

The reduction in complexity arises by modelling the dense velocity field as indexed to the surface $\mathcal{M}$ through a kernel K (here a Gaussian with standard deviation chosen heuristically to be 4mm) and a function $p_t(u)$ which we call the momentum

$$v_t(x) = \int_U K(x, f_t(u))p_t(u)du. \tag{2}$$

As described in [9], we consider only flows corresponding to geodesics in the diffeomorphism group, allowing us to describe the shape of target anatomy through the value of p_0. This describes our forward model—given a value for p_0, we can generate φ_t and a realization of anatomy, with $I_t - I_0 \circ \varphi_t^{-1}$, $f_t = \varphi_t(f_0)$, and p_t satisfying the geodesic equation $\dot{p}_t = -Dv_t^*(f_t)p_t$.

3   Complexity Reduction Algorithm

The problem of interest will be to estimate the reduced representation p_0, given the atlas data f_0 and I_0, and a dense anatomical segmentation of a target subject J (like I_0, J is a function from $\Omega \to [0, 1]$). We assume that J has been rigidly registered to I_0, which is accomplished by calculating the rigid body transform minimizing the sum of square error between I_0 and J. If J represents a right hippocampus, it is reflected to the left side before rigid alignment. We solve this problem using a variational approach to minimize the cost function

$$E = \frac{1}{2}\|p_0\|_{V^*}^2 + \frac{1}{2\sigma_I^2}\|I_1 - J\|_{L^2}^2 \tag{3}$$

where $\|p_0\|_{V^*}^2 = \iint_{U \times U} p_0^*(u)K(f_0(u), f_0(u'))p_0(u')dudu'$ is a norm enforcing smoothness of the velocity field. The parameter σ_I^2, which expresses the trade-off between accuracy and smoothness, is chosen heuristically to be 0.5. We enforce the system dynamics—the images evolving under the optical flow equation $\dot{I}_t = -DI_t v_t$, the manifold moving with the velocity field as $\dot{f}_t = v_t(f_t)$, and the momentum satisfying the geodesic equation—through time varying Lagrange multipliers (also called co-state variables) $\lambda_{ft}, \lambda_{pt}, \lambda_{It}$ in the augmented cost

$$C = \frac{1}{2}\|p_0\|_{V^*}^2 + \frac{1}{2\sigma_I^2}\|I_1 - J\|_{L^2}^2 + \int_0^1 \int_\Omega \lambda_{It}^*(x)[-DI_t(x)v_t(x) - \dot{I}_t(x)]dx$$

$$+ \int_U \lambda_{ft}^*(u)[v_t(f_t(u)) - \dot{f}_t(u)] + \lambda_{pt}^*(u)[-Dv_t^*(f_t(u))p_t(u) - \dot{p}_t(u)]dudt \quad (4)$$

We extremize the cost function with respect to each variable, giving co-state dynamics and boundary conditions, and use an adjoint method as in [10,11] to calculate the gradient of the cost with respect to p_0. We optimize with gradient descent.

4 Experiment

We expect this reduction in complexity to be a powerful tool in overcoming sensitivity to noise that voxelized data is vulnerable too. We evaluate the performance of our algorithm in terms of accuracy, and reproducibility in the definition of the hippocampus across repeated scans.

We use a subset of five subjects from the data described in [13]. The mean subject age is 59 ± 3.5 years, with 2 females and 3 males. Subjects were scanned with a 3T Siemens Biograph mMR, and a 12 channel body RF coil. A 256^3 mm volume at 1 mm isotropic resolution was acquired with a 3D sagittal MPRAGE sequence (TR/TI=2300/900 ms, flip angle 9 degrees, no fat suppression, full k-space, no averages). Subjects returned for a retest scan after 19 ± 15 days, and each visit included two acquisitions. For each of these four scans, subcortical structures were segmented using longitudinal Freesurfer analysis [1]. In this study we consider only the left and right hippocampus, giving 40 target segmentation images total.

We verify the accuracy of our method by examining volume bias, as well as sum of square error. We quantify reproducibility by measuring the square of the L_2 distance (i.e. volume of disagreement in mm^3 or sum of square error) and Hausdorff distance (i.e. maximum distance between segmentations in mm). The intra-visit variability is calculated as the average of two distances (distance between repeats on visit 1, and distance between repeats on visit 2), whereas the inter-visit variability is calculated as the average of four distances (distance between repeat i on visit 1 and repeat j on visit 2, for $i, j \in \{1, 2\}$).

The statistical significance of results is determined using the non-parametric signed rank test for paired data.

5 Results

Three typical results of our complexity reduction algorithm are shown in Fig. 2. One can see the segmentations overlap well with the target, capturing their shape. At the same time they inherit the smoothness of our template and effectively filter out the noise.

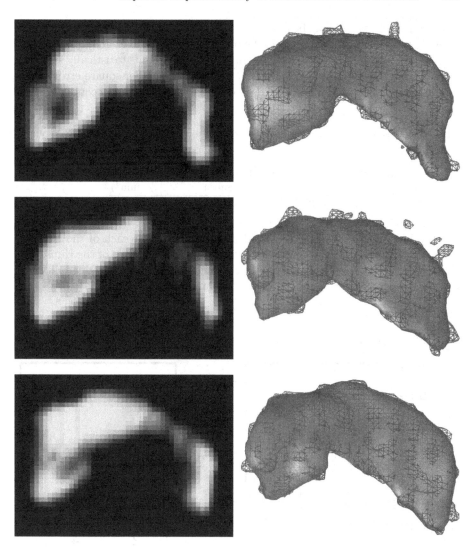

Fig. 2. Three typical results of our complexity reduction algorithm are shown (rows). At left a slice through the deformed template I_1 is shown in green, summed in RGB space with the target J in red. Where they overlap their color appears yellow. At right is the deformed template surface f_1 shown in green, overlaying a red mesh isosurface rendering of the target J.

The accuracy of our segmentations is quantified in terms of mean absolute volume bias ($\text{vol}[I_1] - \text{vol}[J]$), mean relative volume bias ($(\text{vol}[I_1] - \text{vol}[J])/(0.5(\text{vol}[I_1] + \text{vol}[J]))$), and mean sum of square error ($\|I_1 - J\|_{L_2}^2$), and is summarized in Table 1. This accuracy should be compared with the intra-visit square error, $276 \pm 64\text{mm}^3$, a measure of the intrinsic variability of our Freesurfer segmentations. The volume bias $-34 \pm 16\text{mm}^3$ is quite small compared to this intrinsic variability, and may be partly explained by avoiding contouring the noisy appendages as visible for example in the top two rows of Fig. 2. The square error, $243 \pm 17 \, \text{mm}^3$, is comparable to this intrinsic variability (but statistically smaller, $p = 0.0423$ in a non-parametric ranksum test). Much smaller square error could be interpreted as over fitting noise, so we consider this accuracy acceptable.

Table 1. Accuracy of our segmentations, as quantified through volume bias and square error

Relative Volume Bias (%)	Absolute Volume Bias (mm^3)	Square error (mm^3)
-0.81 ± 0.38	-34 ± 16	243 ± 17

Reproducibility is quantified in L_2 distance squared, for each of the five patients, left then right, in Fig. 3. It is quantified similarly in terms of the Hausdorff distance in Fig. 4. Note that our method provides improved reproducibility for both measures, for every patient, left and right.

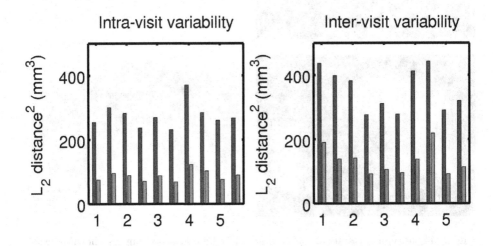

Fig. 3. The square of L2 distance between segmentations is shown for each of the five patients, left then right, with target segmentations in red and our results in green.

The means of these results, along with p-values demonstrating statistical significance, are shown in Table 2. Note that our results show an improvement of a factor of two or more in each case, except inter-visit Hausdorff distance where the improvement is by a factor of 1.63.

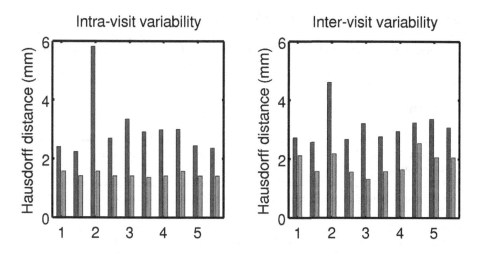

Fig. 4. The Hausdorff distance between segmentations is shown for each of the five patients, left then right, with target segmentations in red and our results in green

Table 2. Mean intra- and inter-visit variability is shown in terms of the squared L_2 distance, and the Hausdorff distance. The p-values are calculated from a paired nonparametric signed rank test.

Method	L_2 distance^2 (mm^3)	p-value	Hausdorff distance (mm)	p-value
Freesurfer intra-visit	275.7	4.8e-05	3.0	4.7e-05
Surface based intra-visit	87.5		1.5	
Freesurfer inter-visit	354.6	9.8e-04	3.1	9.8e-04
Surface based inter-visit	132.4		1.9	

6 Conclusions

We have presented an algorithm to directly reduce the complexity of voxel based neuroanatomical segmentations, by interpreting them as a deformation defined with respect to a template triangulated surface. We bypass the need for triangulating target segmentations, and work with the widely available dense data directly. We have shown that this method is able to smooth out noise while still capturing overall shape effectively, and maintain accuracy with minimal volume bias. Furthermore, we have shown how this method can be used to improve reproducibility of anatomical definitions for scans acquired within a single visit and between visits, a challenge for high dimensional data and shape analysis. We expect this complexity reduction to have important implications for machine learning applications based on anatomical shape.

Acknowledgements. The research leading to these results has received funding from the European Community's Seventh Framework Programme (FP7/2007-2013) for the Innovative Medicine Initiative under Grant Agreement No 115009. This work was supported by NIH grant P41 EB015909.

References

1. Reuter, M., Schmansky, N.J., Rosas, H.D., Fischl, B.: Within-Subject Template Estimation for Unbiased Longitudinal Image Analysis. Neuroimage 61(4), 1402–1418 (2012)
2. Csernansky, J.G., et al.: Preclinical detection of Alzheimer's disease: hippocampal shape and volume predict dementia onset in the elderly. NeuroImage 25(3), 783–792 (2005)
3. Gau, Y., Riklin-Raviv, T., Bouix, S.: Shape Analysis, A Field in Need of Careful Validation. Hum. Brain Mapp. (in press, 2014), doi:10.1002/hbm.22525
4. Beg, M.F., Miller, M.I., Trouvé, A., Younes, L.: Computing Large Deformation Metric Mappings via Geodesic Flows of Diffeomorphisms. Int. J. Comput. Vision 61(2), 139–157 (2005)
5. Wang, L., et al.: Large Deformation Diffeomorphism and Momentum Based Hippocampal Shape Discrimination in Dementia of the Alzheimer type. IEEE Trans. Med. Imaging 26(4), 462–470 (2007)
6. Singh, N., Wang, A.Y., Sankaranarayanan, P., Fletcher, P.T., Joshi, S.: Genetic, Structural and Functional Imaging Biomarkers for Early Detection of Conversion from MCI to AD. In: Ayache, N., Delingette, H., Golland, P., Mori, K. (eds.) MICCAI 2012, Part I. LNCS, vol. 7510, pp. 132–140. Springer, Heidelberg (2012)
7. Tang, X., et al.: Detecting, quantifying, and predicting. Hum. Brain Mapp. (2014), doi: 10.1002/hbm.22431
8. Ma, J., Miller, M.I., Younes, L.: A bayesian generative model for surface template estimation. Int. J. Biomedical Imaging 2010, ID 974957, 14 pages (2010)
9. Miller, M.I., Trouvé, A.: Geodesic Shooting for Computational Anatomy. Journal of Mathematical imaging and Vision 24(2), 209–228 (2006)
10. Vailard, F.-X., Risser, L., Rueckert, D., Cotter, C.J.: Diffeomorphic 3D Image Registration via Geodesic Shooting Using an Efficient Adjoint Calculation. Int. J. Comput. Vision 97(2), 229–241 (2011)
11. Durrleman, S., Allassonnière, S., Joshi, S.: Sparse adaptive parameterization of variability in image ensembles. Int. J. Comput. Vision 101(1), 161–183 (2013)
12. Staniforth, A., Côté, J.: Semi-Lagrangian integration schemes for atmospheric models—a review. Mon. Wea. Rev. 119(9), 2206–2223 (1991)
13. Jovicich, J., et al.: Brain morphometry reproducibility in multi-center 3 T MRI studies: A comparison of cross-sectional and longitudinal segmentations. Neuroimage 83, 472–484 (2013)

Topological Descriptors of Histology Images

Nikhil Singh, Heather D. Couture, J.S. Marron,
Charles Perou, and Marc Niethammer

The University of North Carolina, Chapel Hill, USA

Abstract. The purpose of this study is to investigate architectural characteristics of cell arrangements in breast cancer histology images. We propose the use of topological data analysis to summarize the geometric information inherent in tumor cell arrangements. Our goal is to use this information as signatures that encode robust summaries of cell arrangements in tumor tissue as captured through histology images. In particular, using ideas from algebraic topology we construct topological descriptors based on cell nucleus segmentations such as persistency charts and Betti sequences. We assess their performance on the task of discriminating the breast cancer subtypes Basal, Luminal A, Luminal B and HER2. We demonstrate that the topological features contain useful complementary information to image-appearance based features that can improve discriminatory performance of classifiers.

1 Introduction

Clinical diagnosis of cancer is performed by assessing properties of biopsied tissue. For breast cancer, architectural criteria based on the organization and arrangement of cells, form critical cues for a pathologist to assess and grade tissue samples. Methods to automatically and objectively analyze architectural characteristics of human tissue from histology images are therefore needed to aid pathologists and to computationally *quantify* tissue architecture.

A variety of geometric approaches to pattern or shape recognition have been investigated over the last 15 years. Of these, topological data analysis (TDA) enables the investigation of structural characteristics of high-dimensional data [1,3,4]. The strength of TDA lies in its two core ideas: (a) representing objects based on their topology making it invariant to small changes in shapes and hence robust to noise, and (b) considering *a range* of coarse to fine scales of topological changes, thereby, summarizing large *and* small scale objects.

This paper explores to which extent TDA can characterize cell organization and tissue in breast cancer histology images. We study how to analyze nuclear arrangements through TDA to distinguish genetically derived breast cancer subtypes. These subtypes can be used to guide personalized treatments. We propose topological methods for feature extraction and present a method to combine topological summaries with other imaging features thereby demonstrating that topological features can add information over local image-based descriptors. We first review the necessary background of computational topology for TDA in § 2.1

G. Wu et al. (Eds.): MLMI 2014, LNCS 8679, pp. 231–239, 2014.

and present its application to the analysis of breast cancer histology images in § 2.2. In § 3, we discuss and evaluate the extracted topological summaries.

2 Methodology

2.1 Background on Topological Data Analysis and Homology Groups

Topological data analysis uses concepts from algebraic topology [10,3] and provides methods to characterize geometric information in the data. The classical way is to represent the data in the form of combinatorial objects called simplicial complexes to form a topological space. TDA then studies connectivity information and characterizes loops, voids and higher dimensional surfaces within the space [4]. To analyze tissue architecture the simplicial complex is built, for example, based on the center points of segmented cell nuclei, which define a point-cloud. See the section on the Vietoris-Rips filtration on point clouds below. We review the necessary concepts in topological data analysis in what follows.

Simplicial Complexes and Filtration. A simplicial complex consists of a collection of simplices, such as vertices, edges, triangles or d-dimensional simplices, which is closed under inclusion. More precisely, a simplicial complex is a collection, K of d-dimensional simplices, τ, such that if $\tau \in K$, all its faces, $\sigma \subset \tau$, are also in K. A subcollection L of simplices from K which itself is a simplicial complex, forms a subcomplex of K, denoted as $L \hookrightarrow K$. A nested sequence of simplicial subcomplexes that ascends from an empty set all the way up to K is called a *filtration* of K. An N-step filtration is therefore denoted by the sequence,

$$\emptyset = \mathscr{F}_0 K \hookrightarrow \mathscr{F}_1 K \hookrightarrow \mathscr{F}_2 K \hookrightarrow \ldots \hookrightarrow \mathscr{F}_{N-1} K \hookrightarrow \mathscr{F}_N K = K.$$

Topological Summaries Using Homology Groups. The representation of data by a simplicial complex, K, allows for its characterization through homology groups, which we denote as $H_d(K)$. $H_d(K)$ is the collection of d-dimensional holes. Homology groups consist of groups of d-dimensional homology generators, e.g., 1D connected components for $d = 0$, 2D loops for $d = 1$, 3D cavities for $d = 2$, and so on. The rank of $H_d(K)$ is called the d-th *Betti number*. We now discuss a simple example of a filtration of a 2D simplicial complex formed by point cloud data entities, which will form the basis of our analysis of tissue data.

Example of Vietoris-Rips Filtration on Point Cloud Simplicial Complex. Consider a set of points, $C \subset R^d$ (Fig. 1, left) and define the largest possible simplicial complex, K_C, consisting of all subsets of C. We construct a subcomplex by using a threshold on the pairwise distances between any two points. We define a simplicial subcomplex as a function of filtration scale, s. The subcomplex $\mathscr{F}_s K_c$ consists of a subcollection of points with pairwise distance between them less than s. It is helpful to think of this subcollection of points obtained when the balls of radius, s, centered at each point intersect (Fig. 1,

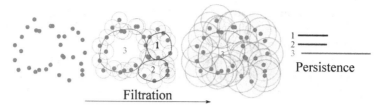

Fig. 1. Vietoris-Rips filtration of a point cloud. Two steps of filtration that depict topological features forming and disappearing (left). Three loops as H_1 formed during filtration persist for different length of filtration (right).

center). Increasing the ball radii results in a chain of subcomplexes defining a filtration of K_c. For a given s, the 0-dimensional homology group consists of the set of independent components. The 1-dimensional group consists of the loops. The rank of $H_0(K_c)$ is the count of connected components and the rank of $H_1(K_c)$ is the count of loops (Fig. 1, right). These topological objects can be summarized in terms of their persistence during the filtration steps. This results in a signature representation of topology of the data in the form of persistent diagrams or bar charts [2].

2.2   Cell Architecture, Nuclei Arrangement and Topology

Clinical diagnosis of breast cancer is usually performed by analyzing H&E-stained histology images. The arrangement of cells and other structures are some of the cues guiding a pathologist to characterize tissue and assess prognosis. Hence, TDA as described in Sec. 2.1 seems a natural choice to quantify such arrangements. In previous work, TDA has been applied to microarray data. Nicolau et al. [12] propose cluster analysis of persistence charts derived from the simplicial complex of microarray data to identify breast cancer subtypes. However, the topological characterizations of nuclear arrangements in tumor

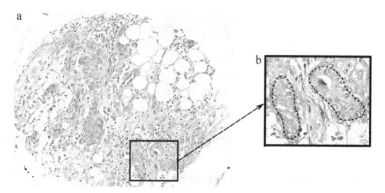

Fig. 2. Example of a histology image for a tumor of subtype, Basal. The highlighted loops formed due to the arrangement of nuclei are an example of architectural feature.

tissue has not yet been investigated. Fig. 2 suggests that such an approach could capture architectural characteristics, using an example H&E stained histology image. The patterns in the organization of cells is evident simply by observing the nuclei in a region (Fig. 2, b). Distinct topological object characterizations such as nuclear connectivity and loops based on the Vietoris-Rips filtration of nuclei centers look promising as summaries of the arrangement of nuclei in tissue.

3   Experiments

We present our topological analysis of nuclei arrangements using a dataset of breast cancer microarray tissue samples, imaged at the University of British Columbia from a Washington University cohort of patients [13]. The dataset consists of 111 subjects with two images each. Subtypes of Basal, Luminal A, Luminal B, and HER2 have been assigned to each sample by molecular means. The ensemble has 38 Basal, 35 Luminal A, 18 Luminal B and 17 HER2 cases and our goal is to assess whether these subtypes differ in terms of their topological characteristics. We combine the features extracted from two images to construct a single patient level representation.

Constructing Topological Summaries of Homology Images. As discussed in § 2.1, we define the simplicial complex by representing the collection of nuclei as point clouds such that the center of mass of each nucleus denotes a vertex. We perform the Vietoris-Rips filtration of this complex by growing balls centered at each vertex. The initial start radius of a ball is proportional to the mass of its nucleus. Since each nucleus has a different size, such an initialization ensures that at the first step, the balls approximately encircle the respective nuclei. We successively increase the radii of all balls with equal rates and stepsizes. Beginning at the start scale, where the number of connected components is equal to the number of nuclei, this filtration computes the generators of zero (H_0: connected components) and one dimensional (H_1: loops) homology groups. We use the Perseus software [11,9] to perform the filtration on the Rips complex.

We summarize the resulting topological objects into a sequence of Betti numbers, e.g., Fig. 3 a and b. We convert the Betti numbers into densities, by dividing them by the area of the tissue in the image making the representation invariant to tissue size. Fig. 3 b suggests that loops exhibit the most dynamics with changing filtration scale. Thus, in another representation, we consider the bar chart representation, called the persistence diagram, based on birth and death of loops during filtration (Fig. 3 c and d). Small bars can be considered as noise artifacts in imaging and segmentation. For robustness, we consider the top few persistent bars (lengthwise), arranged in the order of their birth, as features.

3.1   Evaluating Topological Features

We perform leave-one-out cross-validation experiments to demonstrate the discriminatory capabilities of the topological features to classify tissue images into subtypes. We use distance weighted discrimination (DWD) [8] as a classifier.

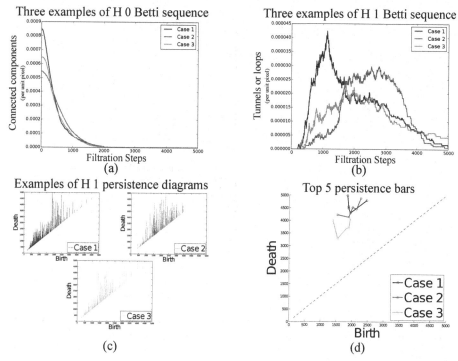

Fig. 3. Different topological summaries for nuclei arrangements in histology images demonstrated for three different examples. (a) and (b) display the Betti densities for H_0 and H_1 homology as a function of filtration steps, while (c) shows the corresponding persistence diagrams, and (d) shows how those are summarized into just the 5 longest bars, in birth order (connecting line segments represent the order of arrangement).

For each pair of subtypes, we evaluated the prediction accuracy using the two classifiers on Betti densities, top 5 and top 75 persistent bars. The best results were obtained for the Basal vs Luminal A classification using Betti density features and for Luminal B vs HER2 classification using the top 5 persistent bars. For Basal vs Luminal A, we achieved a classification accuracy of 69.86%, an improvement of 17.80% over the baseline accuracy of predicting the subtype based on the proportion of the samples of the largest class. For Luminal B vs HER 2 subtype classification, the topological features improved the prediction accuracy by 17.14% over the baseline, giving an overall accuracy of 68.57%.

3.2   Joint Analysis of Topological and Other Imaging Features

Besides topological connectivity and nuclei arrangements, a histology image has other potentially complementary information about tumor tissue. We augment the topological features with those extracted from local image intensities: we construct another set of features learned directly from image patches. A dictionary is learned by modeling 9×9 pixel image patches as sparse linear combinations of

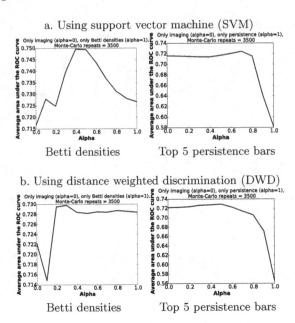

Fig. 4. Repeated 5-fold cross validation for Basal vs Luminal A: combining TDA with patch-based image features suggests improvement in performance for certain cases

dictionary elements [7]. Each patch of an image is encoded with this dictionary. The frequency of usage of each dictionary element is summarized with a 128 bin histogram resulting in a 128-dimensional feature vector for each image.

We define the combined feature space as a product space of topological features, represented as a matrix T, and the patch based image feature space, represented as a matrix I. In these matrices, let rows represent samples and columns represent features. We construct a convex combination of columnwise concatenated features, to form the augmented feature matrix, $C = (\alpha T \ (1 - \alpha)I)$, where α controls the feature weight; α is a relative weight when both feature matrices are normalized to have unit variance. This is achieved by mean centering and dividing the two matrices by the sum of their eigenvalues. Another possibility is to use a multi-kernel approach to combine complementary features [5].

To investigate whether topological features and the image based-features provide complementary information relevant to cancer subtypes, we assess the receiver operator characteristics (ROC) of the classifiers over the entire range of $\alpha \in [0, 1]$. Note that ROC analysis is not applicable to leave-one-out crossvalidation since we get test prediction only on a single test sample for each trained model. Hence, we perform Monte-Carlo (MC) repetitions of 5-fold crossvalidation using both SVM and DWD classifiers for 3500 repetitions. We choose the average area under the ROC curve (AUC) as the metric of performance. AUC is a more stable performance measure than accuracy as it considers the whole range of thresholds for a classifier [6]. For each MC iteration, we compute the false positive (FPR) and true positive (TPR) rates for every crossvalidation run

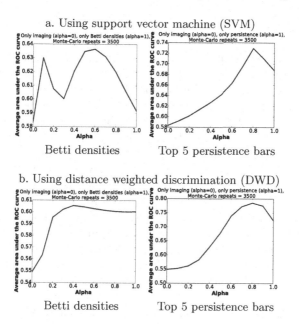

a. Using support vector machine (SVM)

Betti densities   Top 5 persistence bars

b. Using distance weighted discrimination (DWD)

Betti densities   Top 5 persistence bars

Fig. 5. Repeated 5-fold cross validation for Luminal B vs. HER2: combining TDA with patch-based image features suggests improvement in performance for certain cases

for the test data, resulting in an average FPR and TPR to give a mean AUC. We test this for the classification tasks that resulted in the best performance with the leave-one-out classification using only the topology features in § 3.1, i.e., Basal vs Luminal A and Luminal B vs HER2. The trends in AUC as a function of α suggest that, for some cases, the topological Betti features perform better when compared to the patch based image-appearance features for both the classification tasks using either of the classifiers. (Fig. 4 and Fig. 5). In terms of AUC, the Betti features perform better than the persistence summaries, for discriminating Basal from Luminal A. However, the persistence summaries outperform the Betti features, in average AUC metric, for Luminal B vs HER2 discrimination. Another observation is that the AUC peaks in the middle for some of the plots suggesting that a combination of the two features may provide useful information. The results on average accuracy metric as a function of α did not match for all cases with those obtained for the AUC metric. For the top 5 persistence summaries for Luminal B vs HER2 with DWD, both the average AUC and the accuracy analyses suggest that topological features massively outperform the image-appearance features. In particular, using top 5 persistence summaries with DWD improve the AUC by 43% and the accuracy by 22% over imaging features and their combination further adds 13% and 8% improvements, respectively. Additional results are in the supplementary material at http://www.cs.unc.edu/ nsingh/publications/nsingh2014topology_breast_cancer_supplementary.pdf.

4   Discussion

We proposed the use of topological methods to summarize architectural features of cancerous tissue. We constructed geometric features that quantitatively capture arrangements of nuclei as seen in histology images. We explored multiple topological features derived from the homology groups resulting from filtrations of simplicial complexes defined using nuclei locations. Our experiments suggest that, for most cases, topological features perform as good as the patch based features on the task of discriminating cancer subtypes. We also demonstrate that for certain combinations, the topological features provide complementary information, which in turn improves the performance of classifiers. Our future work will include exploring more informative features from the persistence diagram and will repeat the analysis on bigger datasets. A possibility could be to use persistent bars from the chart but maintain their order of filtration. This would result in a sparse feature vector of size equal to the number of filtration steps.

We believe that the topological study of histology image data provides complementary information to image-appearance about tissue properties. It holds promise to improve our understanding of cytological and architectural differences in tissues. In the context of cancer a topological characterization of tumor tissue could potentially aid clinicians in cancer diagnosis and treatment planning.

Acknowledgements. Data collection used in this article was funded by the Strategic Partnering to Evaluate Cancer Signatures (SPECS) group. This research is supported by grants, NSF EECS-1148870, NSF EECS-0925875, and NIH P41-EB002025.

References

1. Carlsson, G.: Topology and data. Bulletin of the American Mathematical Society 46(2), 255–308 (2009)
2. Cohen-Steiner, D., Edelsbrunner, H., Harer, J.: Stability of persistence diagrams. Discrete Comput. Geom. 37(1), 103–120 (2007)
3. Edelsbrunner, H., Harer, J.: Computational topology: an introduction. American Mathematical Soc. (2010)
4. Edelsbrunner, H., Letscher, D., Zomorodian, A.: Topological persistence and simplification. Discrete Comput. Geom. 28(4), 511–533 (2002)
5. Gönen, M., Alpaydın, E.: Multiple kernel learning algorithms. The Journal of Machine Learning Research 12, 2211–2268 (2011)
6. Ling, C.X., Huang, J., Zhang, H.: Auc: a statistically consistent and more discriminating measure than accuracy. In: IJCAI, vol. 3, pp. 519–524 (2003)
7. Mairal, J., Bach, F., Ponce, J., Sapiro, G.: Online learning for matrix factorization and sparse coding. The Journal of Machine Learning Research 11, 19–60 (2010)
8. Marron, J., Todd, M.J., Ahn, J.: Distance-weighted discrimination. Journal of the American Statistical Association 102(480), 1267–1271 (2007)
9. Mischaikow, K., Nanda, V.: Morse theory for filtrations and efficient computation of persistent homology. Discrete Comput. Geom. 50(2), 330–353 (2013)

10. Munkres, J.R.: Elements of algebraic topology, vol. 2. Addison-Wesley, Reading (1984)
11. Nanda, V.: Perseus: The Persistent Homology Software, http://www.sas.upenn.edu/~vnanda/perseus (accessed April 30, 2014)
12. Nicolau, M., Levine, A.J., Carlsson, G.: Topology based data analysis identifies a subgroup of breast cancers with a unique mutational profile and excellent survival. Proceedings of the National Academy of Sciences 108(17), 7265–7270 (2011)
13. Parker, J.S., Mullins, M., Cheang, M.C., Leung, S., Voduc, D., Vickery, T., Davies, S., Fauron, C., He, X., et al.: Supervised risk predictor of breast cancer based on intrinsic subtypes. Journal of Clinical Oncology 27(8), 1160–1167 (2009)

Robust Deep Learning for Improved Classification of AD/MCI Patients

Feng Li[1], Loc Tran[1], Kim-Han Thung[2],
Shuiwang Ji[3], Dinggang Shen[2], and Jiang Li[1]

[1] Department of ECE, Old Dominion University, Norfolk, VA
[2] Department of Radiology, University of North Carolina at Chapel Hill, NC
[3] Department of Computer Science, Old Dominion University, Norfolk, VA

Abstract. Accurate classification of Alzheimer's Disease (AD) and its prodromal stage, Mild Cognitive Impairment (MCI), plays a critical role in preventing progression of memory impairment and improving quality of life for AD patients. Among many research tasks, it is of particular interest to identify noninvasive imaging biomarkers for AD diagnosis. In this paper, we present a robust deep learning system to identify different progression stages of AD patients based on MRI and PET scans. We utilized the dropout technique to improve classical deep learning by preventing its weight co-adaptation, which is a typical cause of overfitting in deep learning. In addition, we incorporated stability selection, an adaptive learning factor and a multi-task learning strategy into the deep learning framework. We applied the proposed method to the ADNI data set and conducted experiments for AD and MCI conversion diagnosis. Experimental results showed that the dropout technique is very effective in AD diagnosis, improving the classification accuracies by 6.2% on average as compared to classical deep learning methods.

1 Introduction

Alzheimer's disease is the sixth-leading cause of death in the United States [1]. AD patients usually undergo progressive stages of cognitive and memory function impairment, including prodromal, MCI and AD. For each of these stages, significant amount of research has been conducted aiming to understanding the underlying pathological mechanisms. In addition, imaging biomarkers have been identified using different imaging modalities such as magnetic resonance imaging (MRI) [2], positron emission tomography (PET) [3], and functional MRI (fMRI) [4]. Imaging biomarkers are a set of indicators computed from image modalities and can be used for early detection of AD disease. It has been shown that fusing these different modalities may lead to more effective imaging biomarkers [5].

Deep learning is a new breakthrough in machine learning. The first successful deep learning framework, auto-encoder, was developed in 2006 [6]. It was subsequently used in other application fields and achieved state-of-the-art performance in speech recognition, image classification and computer vision [7]. Deep learning itself also evolves after 2006. For instance, the multimodal deep learning framework boosted speech classification by learning a shared representation between

G. Wu et al. (Eds.): MLMI 2014, LNCS 8679, pp. 240–247, 2014.

video and audio modalities [8]. A dropout technique further improved zip code recognition, document classification and image recognition [9].

In this paper, we developed a robust deep learning framework for AD diagnosis by fusing complementary information from MRI and PET scans. These 3D scans were preprocessed and features were extracted. We first applied the principle component analysis (PCA) to obtain PCs as new features. We then utilized the stability selection technique [10] together with the least absolute shrinkage and selection operator (Lasso) method [11] to select the most effective features for the diagnosis. The selected features were subsequently processed by the deep learning structure. Model weights in the deep structure were first initialized by unsupervised training and then fine-tuned by AD patient labels. During the fine-tune phase, the dropout technique was employed to improve the model's generalization capability. Finally, the learned feature representation was used for AD/MCI classification by a support vector machine (SVM).

In addition to the discrete patient labels (AD, MCI or Healthy), there are two additional clinical scores, namely Minimum Mental State Examination (MMSE) and Alzheimer's Disease Assessment Scale-Cognitive subscale (ADAS-Cog) associated with each patient. We configured the deep learning structure as a multi-task learning (MTL) framework, and treated the learning of class label, MMSE and ADAS-Cog as related tasks for improved main task (class label) prediction. We evaluated the proposed method on the ADNI data set and compared it with a similar deep learning system, where the auto-encoder was used as a feature learning method for AD diagnosis [5].

2   Materials and Methods

The proposed system consists multiple components including PCA, stability selection, unsupervised feature learning, multi-task deep learning and SVM training as shown in Fig. 1. We will detail each of these components in the following subsections.

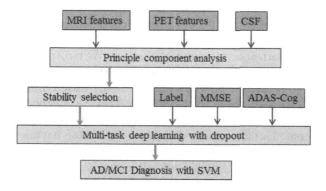

Fig. 1. Diagram of the proposed multi-task deep learning framework

2.1 Data Preprocessing

We utilized the public ADNI data set [1] to validate our proposed deep learning framework. The data set consists of MRI, PET, and CSF data from 51 AD patients, 99 MCI patients (43 MCI patients who converted to AD (MCI.C), and 56 MCI patients who did not progress to AD in 18 months (MCI.NC)) as long as 52 healthy normal controls. In addition to the crisp diagnostic result (AD or MCI), this data set contains two additional clinical scores, MMSE and ADAS-Cog for each patient. A typical procedure of image processing was applied to the 3D MRI and PET volume [2,12,13] including anterior commissure-posterior commissure correction, skull-stripping, cerebellum removal and spatially normalization. Finally, we extracted 93 features from MRI and PET volume, respectively, and three CSF biomarkers, $A\beta_{42}, t-$tau, and p-tau were computed, resulting in 189 features for each subject.

2.2 Principle Component Analysis and Stability Selection

We first applied PCA to the 189 features and used the resulting PCs as new features. PCs are linear combinations of all original individual features that may preserve more information for the subsequent diagnosis. However, not all PCs are effective for the diagnosis. We applied Lasso [11] to reduce the dimensionality of the new feature vector. Lasso tries to minimize the following cost function for feature selection:

$$\min_{\mathbf{w}} ||\mathbf{y} - \mathbf{wx}||_2^2 + \lambda ||\mathbf{w}||_1 \qquad (1)$$

where $y \subset \{1, -1\}$ is the desired class label, $\mathbf{x}$ is the feature vector and $\mathbf{w}$ is the weight vector in the linear model. Because of the L_1 norm constraint on the weight magnitude, the solution minimizing the above cost function is usually sparse, meaning that if a feature in the feature vector $\mathbf{x}$ is not correlated with the target variable, $\mathbf{y}$, the feature will have a zero weight such that being excluded, and features having none zero weights will be selected.

It is well known that the solution of L_1 norm based optimizations are sensitive to the choice of λ. A recent breakthrough [10] sheds a light on selecting the right amount of regularization for stability selection. We incorporate the stability selection concept into the AD patient diagnosis in this paper. In particular, we repeated the Lasso procedure 50 times and each time with a different value for the parameter λ (We used the SLEP toolbox for Lasso [2]). A probability for each feature was computed by counting the frequency of the feature being selected in the 50 experiments. The final selected features were those having probabilities above a threshold t. It has been shown experimentally and theoretically that the stabilized selection results vary little for sensible choices in a range of the cut-off value for t [10].

---

[1] Available at http://www.loni.ucla.edu/ADNI
[2] Available at http://www.public.asu.edu/ jye02/Software/SLEP/index.htm

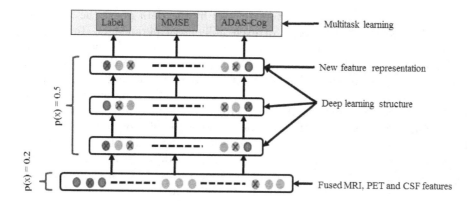

Fig. 2. Multi-task deep learning with dropout. "x" denotes a dropped unit.

2.3   Multi-task Deep Learning

In contrast to the traditionary three-layer neural network (shallow structure), deep learning is based on a deep architecture consisting of many layers of hidden neurons for modelling. A shallow architecture would involve a lot of duplications of effort to express things and such a fat architecture has been shown to suffer from the problem of over-fitting, which leads to a poor generalization capability. Instead, deep architecture could more gracefully reuse previous computations and discover complicated relations of the input [14].

To train the deep architecture, the standard Backpropagation (BP) algorithm did not work well with randomly initialized weights because the error feedback becomes progressively noisier as it goes back to lower levels, making the low level weight updates less effective. In 2006, a breakthrough in deep learning has made the deep architecture training possible [6] by utilizing the restricted Boltzmann machine to initialize multiple hidden layers one layer at a time in an unsupervised manner. With unsupervised learning, deep learning is trying to understand the data first, i.e., to obtain a task specific representation for the data so that a better classification can be achieved. It has experimentally proven that the unsupervised learning step in deep learning plays a critical role in the success of the training in deep learning [7].

In multi-task learning, related tasks are learnt simultaneously by extracting and utilizing appropriate shared information across tasks. It is worth noting that neural network can simultaneously model multiple outputs making deep learning a natural multi-task learning framework [6]. The proposed multi-task deep learning framework is shown in Fig. 2, where we treated class label, MMSE and ADAS-Cog as three different tasks but modeling them simultaneously. We also utilized the dropout technique to improve the training.

2.4   Dropout with Adaptive Adaption

Deep learning achieved excellent results in many applications where training data size is large. For small sized data sets such as the one in this paper, it is still possible for a deep structure to over-fit the data given the fact that it usually has tens of thousands or even millions of parameters. To improve the generalization capability of a model, the dropout technique tries to prevent weight co-adaptation by randomly dropping out some units in the model during training [9]. We incorporated the dropout technique in the multi-task learning context to improve AD diagnosis as shown in Fig. 2. In the training process, each hidden unit in the model was dropped with a probability of 0.5 when a batch of training cases were present. Previous experiments [9] showed that it is also beneficial if we apply the "dropout" process to the input layer but with a lower probability (0.2 in this paper). In the testing procedure, all hidden units and inputs were used to compute model outputs for a testing case with appropriate compensations, i.e., weights between inputs and the first hidden layer were scaled by 0.8 and all other weights were halved.

During the multi-task fine-tune step, the stochastic gradient descent method with a fixed learning factor is usually utilized as [6],

$$w(j,i) = w(j,i) + \triangle w(j,i) = w(j,i) - \alpha \frac{\partial E}{\partial w(j,i)}, \qquad (2)$$

where $w(j,i)$ is the weight connecting the ith node and jth node in two consecutive layers. $\frac{\partial E}{\partial w(j,i)}$ is the gradient of the cost function E and α is a learning factor. Sometimes, the weights update may contain a momentum term [9]. We proposed to use an adaptive learning factor to speed up the adaptation. The motivation of the adaptive learning is that the learning factor should be large at location where gradient is small and vice verse. Based on the motivation, an adaptive learning factor α can be determined as $\alpha = \frac{\beta E}{\sum_i \sum_j [\frac{\partial E}{\partial w(j,i)}]^2}$, which decreases E by $\beta\%$.

There are usually two ways to increase the generalization capability of a learned model, adding regularization (L_1 or L_2 norm) on weights or using committee machine. However, solving the regularization problem is usually challenging especially in the deep learning context. In addition, the committee machine technique requires averaging many separately trained models to compute a prediction for a testing case, which is time consuming for deep learning. The dropout procedure does the both (constraint and committee machine) simultaneously in a very efficient way. 1) Each sub-model in training is a sampled model from all possible ones and all sub-models share weights. The weight sharing property is equivalent to the L_1 or L_2 norm constraint on weights, and 2) The testing procedure is an approximation of averaging all trained sub-models for a testing case but it does not separately store them because they share weights. This is an extremely efficient and a smart implementation of a committee machine [9].

3   Results and Discussion

3.1   Experimental Setup

We consider three classification tasks including AD patients vs Healthy Control subjects (AD vs HC), MCI patients vs HC (MCI vs HC) and MCI-converted vs

MCI-non converted (MCI.C vs MCI.NC). For each task, we utilised a ten-fold cross-validation (CV) scheme to evaluate the proposed method. In the ten-fold CV, we randomly divided the data set into 10 parts and for one run, we separated one part for testing and applied the proposed framework to the remaining data to train a classification model. This procedure was repeated 10 times so that each part was tested once. Finally, testing accuracies were computed. To obtain a more realizable estimate of the performance, we repeated the ten-fold CV ten times for each task with different random data partitions and computed average accuracy as the performance metric. To compare different classification models, we kept the same data partitions in the ten-fold CV and utilized the paired-t test to evaluate if there is a significant performance difference.

We did preliminary experiments to determine the structure of the deep learning model. For all the three classification tasks, it was found that a three hidden layers with hidden units of 100-50-20 worked the best among the candidate structures considered, then all tasks used the same structure. For the SVM classifier, we tried different kernels and a linear kernel was chosen. We also did a grid search for the "soft margin" parameter in the linear kernel SVM model but it did not improve the classification accuracies. Therefore, in all experiments, we utilized a three hidden-layer model with a structure of 100-50-20 for feature learning and a linear SVM with default soft margin as classifier.

There are four components in the proposed framework including PCA, stability selection, dropout and multi-task learning. Inspired by "sensitivity analysis" and "impact assessment", we identified the impact of each component by evaluating classification performances without the component being included in the framework.

3.2   Performance Evaluation

Table 1 shows the overall performances of the proposed method and the impact of each component in the framework. The proposed method performed the best in diagnosing AD and MCI patients with accuracies of 91.4% and 77.4%, respectively, and it is significantly better than the baseline method that obtained accuracies of 86.4% and 72.1% for the diagnosis. The baseline method consists of all components in the proposed method except deep learning. In the MCI conversion diagnosis (MCI.C vs MCI.NC), the PCA component slightly degraded the proposed method (from 58.1% to 57.4%) but it is still significantly better than the baseline method (57.4% vs 50.6%).

Among those components, it is obvious that "dropout" has the most significant impact on the performances. Without "dropout", deep learning did not improve the baseline method (69.2% vs 69.7% in terms of average acc.). The least important component is "PCA", the average acc. slightly dropped from 75.4% to 74.7% without the PCA component. Without "stability selection" and "multi-task learning", the average accuracy dropped from 75.4% to 73.8% and 74.2%, respectively.

We conducted a paired-t test between results by the proposed method and those from classical deep learning ("-Dropout"). Table 2 lists the improvements

Table 1. Performance comparison (in%) of the competing methods. The proposed method consists of four components. "-PCA" stands for "the proposed method without the PCA component" and "SS" stands for stability selection, "Baseline" denotes the framework without the deep learning component.

Tasks	Proposed	-PCA	-Dropout	-SS	-MultTask	Baseline
AD vs HC	**91.4**(1.8)	89.6(1.3)	84.2(3.0)	89.4(1.6)	90.3(1.7)	86.4(2.0)
MCI vs HC	**77.4**(1.7)	76.4(1.5)	73.1(3.1)	74.3(1.6)	75.6(1.7)	72.1(3.0)
MCI.C vs MCI.NC	57.4(3.6)	**58.1**(1.8)	50.2(3.3)	57.7(1.8)	56.7(3.0)	50.6(4.7)
Average	**75.4**	74.7	69.2	73.8	74.2	69.7

Table 2. Paired-t test between results of the proposed method vs deep learning without dropout. The methods of "SAEF" and "LLF+SAEF" were proposed by Suk [5]. "SAEF" stands for Stacked Auto-Encoder Features and "LLF" denotes Low Level Features.

Tasks	Proposed	-Dropout	Improvement	p-value	SAEF	LLF+SAEF
AD vs HC	**91.4**(1.8)	84.2(3.0)	7.2	$< 10^{-3}$	83.2(2.7)	85.3(3.2)
MCI vs HC	**77.4**(1.7)	73.1(3.1)	4.3	0.0034	70.1(2.8)	76.9(2.3)
MCI.C vs MCI.NC	57.4(3.6)	50.2(3.3)	7.2	$<10^{-3}$	58.4(4.1)	**60.3**(2.3)
Average	**75.4**	69.2	6.2	N/A	70.6	74.2

and p-values. The average improvement is 6.2% and the improvements for all the three classification tasks are significant. The work by Suk [5] on the same data set is also shown in Table 2, where "SAEF" corresponds to the method using features learned by a deep auto-encoder and "LLF+SAEF" represents the method that combines original features with the SAEF features for AD diagnosis.

The proposed method (75.4%) outperformed the SAEF method (with an average accuracy of 70.6%). By combining SAEF with LLF (LLF+SAEF), the average accuracy was increased to 74.2% [5]. The SAEF method is a similar deep learning method in which feature representations for MRI, PET and CSF were learned separately and combined by a linear SVM classifier. It is worth to note that the proposed method used the learned representation only. In [5], utilizing the multi-kernel SVM (MK-SVM) to combine SAEF features from MRI, PET and CSF boosted the performances to 95.9%, 85.0% and 75.8% for the three tasks, respectively. Since the dropout technique improved upon the basic deep learning significantly in this paper, we are currently investigating if the MK-SVM can further boost the performance of the proposed system.

4 Conclusion

Our proposed method achieved 91.4%, 77.4% and 57.4% accuracies for AD, MCI and MCI conversion diagnosis, respectively. The framework consists of multiple components including PCA, stability selection, dropout and multi-task deep learning. We showed that dropout is the most effective one. This is not surprising because the size of ADNI data is relatively small compared to that of the deep structure utilized in this paper. Classical deep learning cannot help but with the dropout technique, the average accuracy was improved by 6.2% on average. We are incorporating MK-SVM [5] into our method for improved AD diagnosis.

References

1. Alzheimer's Association: 2012 Alzheimer's disease facts and figures. Alzheimer's & Dementia 8(2), 131–168 (2012)
2. Davatzikos, C., Bhatt, P., Shaw, L.M., Batmanghelich, K.N., Trojanowski, J.Q.: Prediction of MCI to AD conversion, via MRI, CSF biomarkers, and pattern classification. Neurobiology of Aging 27, 2322.e19–2322.e27 (2011)
3. Nordberg, A., Rinne, J.O., Kadir, A., Langstrom, B.: The use of PET in Alzheimer disease. Nature Reviews Neurology 6(2), 78–87 (2010)
4. Greicius, M.D., Srivastava, G., Reiss, A.L., Menon, V.: Default-mode network activity distinguishes Alzheimer's disease from healthy aging: Evidence from functional MRI. Proceedings of the National Academy of Sciences of the United States of America 101(13), 4637–4642 (2004)
5. Suk, H.-I., Shen, D.: Deep learning-based feature representation for AD/MCI classification. In: Mori, K., Sakuma, I., Sato, Y., Barillot, C., Navab, N. (eds.) MICCAI 2013, Part II. LNCS, vol. 8150, pp. 583–590. Springer, Heidelberg (2013)
6. Hinton, G.E., Grivastava, Osindero, S., Teh, Y.W.: A fast learning algorithm for deep belief nets. Neural Computation 18(7), 1527–1554 (2006)
7. Bengio, Y., Courville, A., Vincent, P.: Representation learning: A review and new perspectives. PAMI 35(8), 1798–1828 (2013)
8. Ngiam, J., Khosla, A., Kim, M., Nam, J., Lee, H., Ng, A.: Multimodal deep learning. In: ICML, pp. 689–696 (2011)
9. Hinton, G.E., Srivastave, N., Krizhevsky, A., Sutskever, I., Salakhutdinov, R.R.: Improving neural networks by preventing co-adaptation of feature detectors. arXiv:1207.0580 (2012)
10. Meinshausen, N., Buhlmann, P.: Stability selection. J. R. Statist. Soc. B, 417–473 (2010)
11. Tibshirani, R.: Regression shrinkage and selection via the Lasso. Journal of the Royal Statistical Society, Series B 58(1), 267–288 (1996)
12. Kabani, N., MacDonald, D., Holmes, C., Evans, A.: A 3D atlas of the human brain. NeuroImage 7(4), S717 (1998)
13. Hinrichs, C., Singh, V., Xu, G., Johnson, S.C.: Predictive markers for AD in a multi-modality framework: An analysis of MCI progression in the ADNI population. NeuroImage 55(2), 574–589 (2011)
14. Erhan, D., Bengio, Y., Courville, A., Manzagol, P.A., Vincent, P., Bengio, S.: Why does unsupervised pre-training help deep learning? Journal of Machine Learning Research 11, 625–660 (2010)
15. Caruana, R.: Multitask learning: A knowledge-based source of inductive bias. Machine Learning 28, 41–75 (1997)

Subject Specific Sparse Dictionary Learning for Atlas Based Brain MRI Segmentation

Snehashis Roy[1,*], Aaron Carass[2], Jerry L. Prince[2], and Dzung L. Pham[1]

[1] Center for Neuroscience and Regenerative Medicine, Henry Jackson Foundation
[2] Department of Electrical and Computer Engineering, Johns Hopkins University

Abstract. Quantitative measurements from segmentations of soft tissues from magnetic resonance images (MRI) of human brains provide important biomarkers for normal aging, as well as disease progression. In this paper, we propose a patch-based tissue classification method from MR images using sparse dictionary learning from an atlas. Unlike most atlas-based classification methods, deformable registration from the atlas to the subject is not required. An "atlas" consists of an MR image, its tissue probabilities, and the hard segmentation. The "subject" consists of the MR image and the corresponding affine registered atlas probabilities (or priors). A subject specific patch dictionary is created by learning relevant patches from the atlas. Then the subject patches are modeled as sparse combinations of learned atlas patches. The same sparse combination is applied to the segmentation patches of the atlas to generate tissue memberships of the subject. The novel combination of prior probabilities in the example patches enables us to distinguish tissues having similar intensities but having different spatial location. We show that our method outperforms two state-of-the-art whole brain tissue segmentation methods. We experimented on 12 subjects having manual tissue delineations, obtaining mean Dice coefficients of 0.91 and 0.87 for cortical gray matter and cerebral white matter, respectively. In addition, experiments on subjects with ventriculomegaly shows significantly better segmentation using our approach than the competing methods.

Keywords: Image synthesis, intensity normalization, hallucination, patches.

1 Introduction

Magnetic resonance imaging (MRI) is a widely used noninvasive modality to image the human brain. Postprocessing of MR images, such as tissue segmentation, provides quantitative biomarkers for understanding many aspects of normal aging, as well as progression and prognosis of diseases like Alzheimers' disease and multiple sclerosis. Finite mixture models of the image intensity distributions is the basis of many image segmentation algorithms, where the intensity

* Support for this work included funding from the Department of Defense in the Center for Neuroscience and Regenerative Medicine and by the grants NIH/NINDS R01NS070906, NIH/NIBIB R21EB012765.

G. Wu et al. (Eds.): MLMI 2014, LNCS 8679, pp. 248–255, 2014.

histogram is fitted with a number of distributions, e.g. Gaussians, [1]. Other algorithms model the tissue intensities using fuzzy C-means (FCM) [2], partial volume models [3] etc. Prior information on the spatial locations of the tissue are usually incorporated using statistical atlases [4,2], which captures their spatial variability. Since there is no tissue-dependent global MR image intensity scale (unlike computed tomography), the intensity range and distribution varies significantly across scanners and imaging protocols. Thus it is sometimes unclear if a particular model is optimal for MR images with different acquisition protocols. Instead of trying to fit image intensities into pre-defined models, we rely on similar looking examples from expert segmented images.

In this paper, we propose an example based brain segmentation method, combining statistical atlas priors into sparse dictionary learning. The *atlas* comprises an MR image, corresponding stastistical priors, and the hard segmentation into tissue labels, e.g, cerebral gray matter(GM), cerebral white matter (WM), ventricles, cerebro-spinal fluid (CSF) etc. An image patch from the subject MR along with the corresponding patches from the affine registered statistical priors in the subject space, comprise of an image feature. A sparse patch dictionary is learnt using the atlas and subject image features. For every subject patch, its sparse weight is found from the learnt dictionary. Corresponding atlas hard segmentation labels are weighted by the same weights to generate the tissue membership of the subject patch.

In a previous example based binary segmentation method [5], prior information about spatial location of a tissue is obtained from a deformable registration of the atlas to the subject image. A binary dictionary-based labeling method was proposed for hippocampal segmetation in [6]. Our method is similar in concept to this approach, but we perform whole brain segmentation using a single dictionary encompassing multiple tissue classes using statistical priors without the need for deformable registration between subject and atlas.

Since the previous example based methods [5,6] are only applicable to binary segmentation, we compare our method with two state-of-the-art publicly available whole brain multi-class segmentation methods, Freesurfer [3] and TOADS [2], and show that segmentation accuracy significantly improves with our example based method. We also experimented on 10 subjects with ventriculomegaly and show that when the anatomy between atlas and subject is significantly different (e.g., enlarged ventricles), our method is more robust.

2   Method

We define an *atlas* as a $(n+1)$-tuple of images, $\{a_1, \ldots, a_{n+1}\}$, where a_1 denotes the T_1-w MR scan, a_{n+1} denotes the hard segmentation, and a_2–a_n denotes $(n-1)$ statistical priors. At each voxel, a 3D patch can be defined on every atlas image and are rasterized as a $d \times 1$ vector $\mathbf{a}_k(i)$, where $i = 1, \ldots, M$, is an index over the voxels of the atlas. A subject MR image is denoted by s_1. Atlas a_1 is affine registered to s_1, and the priors a_2–a_n are transformed to the subject space by the same affine transformation. The transformed priors are denoted by $\{s_2, \ldots, s_n\}$. The subject patches are denoted by $\mathbf{s}_k(j)$, $j = 1, \ldots, N$. The idea is to use these images $\{a_1, \ldots, a_{n+1}, s_1, \ldots, s_n\}$ to generate a segmentation $\hat{s}_{n+1}$. The priors can be weighted, i.e., $s_k \leftarrow w \times s_k$, where w is a scalar multiplying the prior images.

An atlas patch dictionary is defined as $A_1 \in \mathbb{R}^{nd \times M}$, where the ith column of A_1, $\mathbf{f}(i)$, consists of the ordered concatenation of atlas patches $(\mathbf{a}_k(i))$, i.e., $\mathbf{f}(i) = [\mathbf{a}_1(i)^T \ldots \mathbf{a}_n(i)^T]^T$. Thus the $nd \times 1$ vectors $\mathbf{f}(i)$ becomes the atlas feature vectors. Similarly, the subject feature vectors are denoted by $\mathbf{b}(j) = [\mathbf{s}_1(i)^T \ldots \mathbf{s}_n(i)^T]^T$, $\mathbf{b}(j) \in \mathbb{R}^{nd}$. We also refer to the $nd \times 1$ feature vector as a "patch". A patch encodes the intensity information of a voxel and its neighborhood, as well as its spatial information via the use of statistical atlases. The atlas segmentation image is also decomposed into patches $\mathbf{a}_{n+1}(i)$, which forms the columns of the segmentation dictionary A_2.

2.1 Sparse Dictionary Learning

If the atlas and the subjects have similar tissue contrasts, we can assume that for every subject patch $\mathbf{s}_1(j)$, a small number of similar looking patches can always be found from the set of atlas patches $(\mathbf{a}_1(i))$ [7,8]. We extend this assumption for the $nd \times 1$ feature vectors $\mathbf{b}(j)$ as well, enforcing the condition that every subject feature can be matched to a few atlas feature vectors, having not only similar intensities but similar spatial locations as well. This idea of sparse matching can be written as

$$\mathbf{b}(j) \approx A_1 \mathbf{x}(j), \text{for some } \mathbf{x}(j) \in \mathbb{R}^M, ||\mathbf{x}(j)||_0 \ll M, \forall j. \qquad (1)$$

Previous methods [6,5] try to enforce the similarity in spatial locations by searching for the similar patches in a small window around the jth voxel. We obviate the need for such windowed searching by adding statistical priors in the features. The non-negativity constraints in the weight $\mathbf{x}(j)$ enforces the similarity in *texture* between the subject patch and the chosen atlas patches.

The combinatorics of the ℓ_0 problem in Eqn. 1 makes it infeasible to solve directly, but it can be transformed into an ℓ_1 minimization problem,

$$\hat{\mathbf{x}}(j) = \arg\min_{\mathbf{x} \geq \mathbf{0}} \left\{ ||\mathbf{b}(j) - A_1 \mathbf{x}(j)||_2^2 + \lambda ||\mathbf{x}(j)||_1 \right\}, \text{subject to } ||\mathbf{f}(i)||_2^2 = 1 \quad (2)$$

However, $\mathbf{x}(j)$ is a $M \times 1$ vector, where M is the number of atlas patches, typically $M \sim 10^7$. Thus solving such a large optimization for every subject patch is computationally intensive. We use sparse dictionary learning to generate a dictionary of smaller length $D_1 \in \mathbb{R}^{nd \times L}$, from A_1, which can be used instead of A_1 in Eqn. 2 to solve for $\mathbf{x}(j)$. We have chosen $L = 5000$ empirically.

The advantage of learning a dictionary is twofold. First, although the dictionary elements are not orthogonal, all the subject patches $(\mathbf{b}(j))$ can be sparsely represented using the dictionary elements. Second, the computational burden of Eqn. 2 for every subject patch is reduced. The sparse dictionary is learnt using training examples from the subject such that all subject patches can be optimally represented via the dictionary [9]. The dictionary learning approach is an alternating minimization to solve the following problem,

$$\{\hat{\mathbf{x}}(j), \hat{D}_1\} = \arg\min_{\mathbf{x} \geq \mathbf{0}, D_1} \sum_{j=1}^{N} \left\{ ||\mathbf{b}(j) - D_1 \mathbf{x}(j)||_2^2 + \lambda ||\mathbf{x}(j)||_1 \right\}, \text{s.t } ||\mathbf{f}(i)||_2^2 = 1. \ (3)$$

INITIAL DICTIONARY   FINAL DICTIONARY

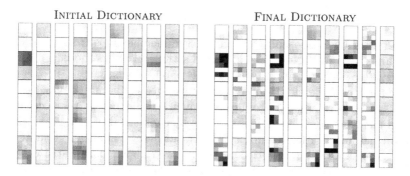

Fig. 1. The left image shows middle sections of 100 randomly chosen $3 \times 3 \times 3$ patches from $D_1^{(0)}$, while on the right are the same atlas patches learnt from the subject after five iterations of Eqn. 5

$\mathbf{f}(i), i = 1 \ldots, M$ are the columns of D_1. Eqn. 3 can be solved in two alternating steps. First, keeping D_1 fixed, we solve for $\mathbf{x}(j)$ for each j, as in Eqn. 2. Then keeping $\mathbf{x}(j)$ fixed, we solve

$$\hat{D}_1 = \arg\min_{D_1} \sum_{j=1}^{N} ||\mathbf{b}(j) - D_1\mathbf{x}(j)||_2^2. \tag{4}$$

A gradient descent approach leads to the following update equation,

$$D_1^{(t+1)} = D_1^{(t)} + \eta \sum_{j=1}^{N} (\mathbf{b}(j) - D_1^{(t)}\mathbf{x}(j))\mathbf{x}(j)^T, \tag{5}$$

where η is the step-size and t denotes iteration numbers. We note that η should be chosen carefully so that $D_1^{(t)} > 0$ always, since the columns of D_1 contains MR intensities and statistical priors. $D_1^{(0)}$ is generated using L randomly chosen columns of A_1. The segmentation dictionary D_2 is generated using corresponding columns of A_2.

Once the dictionary is learnt after the convergence of Eqn. 5, Eqn. 2 is solved for every subject patch $\mathbf{b}(j)$ using $\hat{D}_1$ instead of A_1, to find the sparse representation $\mathbf{x}(j)$. Every atlas patch in the learnt dictionary D_1 has a corresponding segmentation patch in D_2. Thus the columns of D_2 contain segmentation labels $\{2, \ldots, k\}$. It can be shown that $||\mathbf{x}(j)||_1$ follows a Laplace distribution with mean 1. Empirically, the variance is found to be very small (~ 0.005). Thus we weigh the segmentation labels according to their weights in $\mathbf{x}(j)$ to generate tissue memberships,

$$\mathbf{p}_k = (\mathbb{1}_{D_2}(k))\frac{\mathbf{x}(j)}{||\mathbf{x}(j)||_1}, k = 2, \ldots, n, \tag{6}$$

where $\mathbb{1}_{D_2}(k)$ denotes the indicator matrix having the same size as D_2, whose elements are 1 if the corresponding element in D_2 is k, 0 otherwise. $k = 2, \ldots, n$ denotes $(n - 1)$ tissue labels. We only take the central voxel of $\mathbf{p}_k$ to generate the full membership image p_k.

2.2   Updating Statistical Priors in the Segmentation

We have described a method to obtain tissue memberships from a set of MR images and statistical priors. Usually, fixed statistical priors should be non-zero and fuzzy, leaving a possibility that a CSF patch can be matched to a ventricle patch, which have similar intensity as well as similar prior. On the other hand, less fuzzy priors will introduce too much dependence on the accurate initial alignment between the atlas and the subject. Instead of using a fixed prior based on the initial atlas-to-subject registration, we dynamically update it by iterating the same patch selection method stated above. The statistical priors ($\{s_2, \ldots, s_n\}$) at each iteration is replaced by a Gaussian blurred version of the obtained memberships p_k [10]. The blurring relaxes the localization of the tissues in the memberships by increasing the capture range in the priors. The algorithm can be written as,

1. At $t = 0$, start with $\{a_1, \ldots, a_{n+1}, s_1, s_2^{(0)} \ldots, s_n^{(0)}\}$, where $s_k^{(0)}$ are the registered atlas priors, $k = 2, \ldots, n$.
2. Generate dictionaries $\hat{D}_1$ and D_2 from Eqn. 5 using $\{a_1, \ldots, a_{n+1}, s_1, s_2^{(0)} \ldots, s_n^{(0)}\}$. The subject patches are denoted by $\mathbf{b}^{(0)}(j)$.
3. At $t \leftarrow t + 1$, for each subject patch $\mathbf{b}^{(t)}(j)$, generate the sparse coefficient $\mathbf{x}^{(t)}(j)$ using $\hat{D}_1$ from Eqn. 2.
4. Generate memberships $\{p_2^{(t)}, \ldots, p_n^{(t)}\}$ using $\mathbf{x}^{(t)}(j)$s from Eqn. 6
5. Generate new statistical priors $s_k^{(t)} \leftarrow G_\sigma \star p_k^{(t)}, k = 2, \ldots, n.$ $\sigma = 3$mm is chosen empirically.
6. Generate $\mathbf{b}^{(t+1)}(j)$ using the new $\{s_1, s_2^{(t)}, \ldots, s_n^{(t)}\}$
7. Stop if $\frac{1}{N}\sum_{j=1}^{N} \|\mathbf{x}^{(t)}(j) - \mathbf{x}^{(t-1)}(j)\| < \epsilon$, else go to step 3.

3   Results

The run-time is approximately $\frac{1}{2}$hours on 2.7GHz 12-core AMD processors for $181 \times 217 \times 181$ sized 1mm^3 images. SparseLab is used to solve Eqn. 2. We used $3 \times 3 \times 3$ patches in all our experiments, and empirically chose the atlas weight w as 0.10. λ for Eqn. 2 and η for Eqn. 5 are chosen as 0.01 and 0.001, respectively. All images are skull-stripped [11] and corrected for any intensity inhomogeneity [12]. All MR images are intensity normalized so that their modes of WM intensities are unity [13]. WM intensity modes are found by fitting a smooth kernel density estimator to the histograms.

An example of the learnt dictionary is shown in Fig. 1, where $D_1^{(0)}$ is compared with $D_1^{(5)}$. Clearly, after learning from the subject patches, there are more edges in $D_1^{(5)}$ patches, compared to the "flat"-looking patches in $D_1^{(0)}$, indicating $D_1^{(5)}$ can represent any unknown subject patch better than $D_1^{(0)}$. Fig. 2 shows the effect of iteratively updating the priors via memberships. Since the atlas is registered to the subject using affine only, the strong GM prior in the middle of WM (red arrow) introduces non-zero membership to the WM patches. However, the dynamic prior update at each iteration, instead of a fixed prior in most EM based algorithms, reduces the dependence.

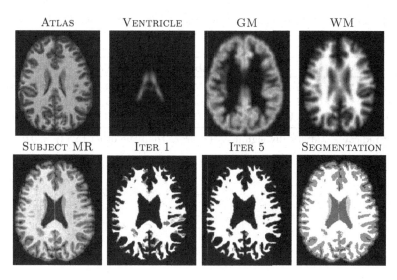

Fig. 2. Top row shows affine registered atlas images, registered to the subject in the bottom row. WM memberships (p_k) for the 1st and 5th iteration of the algorithm (Sec. 2.2) are also shown. The last column shows the max-membership hard segmentation output of our method.

We validated on 12 subjects from CUMC12 database [14], which have manually segmented labels. The manual segmentations do not have any CSF. We segment the images into 4 classes, GM, WM, ventricle and subcortical GM (e.g., caudate, putamen, thalamus). One subject is randomly chosen as atlas. Since they do not have any tissue probability or memberships, Gaussian blurred tissue label-masks ($\sigma = 3$mm) are used as priors $\{a_2, \ldots, a_n\}$. The remaining 11 subjects are segmented using the atlas MR and priors. Dice coefficients comparing three methods on the four tissue classes, as well as the weighted average (W. Ave.) of the four, weighted by the volume of the corresponding tissue, are shown in Table 1. Our method outperforms the other two methods in GM, WM, subcortical GM and in the average ($p < 0.05$ in all cases). Since the ventricle boundary is usually the most robust feature in an MR image, all three methods perform similarly.

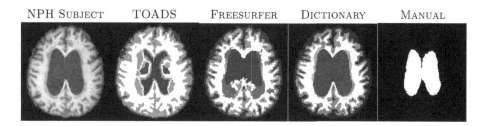

Fig. 3. A subject with NPH is segmented using TOADS, Freesurfer and our dictionary learning method. Rightmost column shows manual delineation of the ventricles.

Table 1. Mean Dice coefficients for four tissue types and their weighted average, averaged over 11 subjects from CUMC12 database are shown

	Ventricle	GM	Subcort. GM	WM	W. Ave.
TOADS	0.778 ±0.089	0.891 ±0.013	0.570 ±0.053	0.853 ±0.011	0.867 ±0.011
Freesurfer	0.759 ±0.082	0.888 ±0.011	0.636 ±0.021	0.853 ±0.008	0.863 ±0.009
Dictionary	0.785±0.055	**0.910±0.012**	**0.755±0.023**	**0.869±0.008**	**0.881±0.008**

bold indicates statistically significantly larger than the other two ($p < 0.05$).

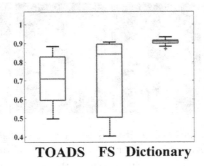

TOADS   FS   Dictionary

Fig. 4. Dice coefficients of between manual ventricle delineation and three automatic methods are shown for 10 subjects with NPH

Next we applied the dictionary learning algorithm on 10 subjects with normal pressure hydrocephalus (NPH), which have enlarged ventricles. Manual segmentations are available only on ventricles. They are segmented with Freesurfer using the -bigventricles flag. Fig. 3 shows one subject with the segmentations and the manual delineation of the ventricles. The atlas is shown in Fig. 2. In this case, 7 tissue classes, cerebellar GM, cerebellar WM, cerebral GM and WM, subcortical GM, CSF and ventricles, are used. Clearly, our method significantly improves the ventricle segmentation. Freesurfer segments part of the ventricles as WM and lesions (red arrow), while TOADS segments part of it as cortical GM. Visually, our method produces better CSF segmentation as well (green arrow). Quantitative improvement is shown in Fig. 4 where Dice coefficients between manually segmented ventricles and automatic segmentations are plotted for the three methods. Our method produces the most consistent Dice coefficient (mean 0.91) across all subjects with very little variance, and it is significantly ($p < 0.05$) larger than TOADS (mean Dice 0.71) and Freesurfer (mean Dice 0.72). Although we used default settings for TOADS or Freesurfer, no amount of parameter tuning would significantly improve the NPH results.

4   Discussion

We have presented a patch based sparse dictionary learning method to segment multiple tissue classes. Contrary to previous binary patch based segmentation methods, we use statistical priors to localize different tissues with similar intensities. We do not require any deformable registration of the subject to the atlas.

References

1. Ashburner, J., Friston, K.J.: Unified segmentation. NeuroImage 26(3), 839–851 (2005)
2. Shiee, N., Bazin, P., Ozturk, A., Reich, D.S., Calabresi, P.A., Pham, D.L.: A Topology-Preserving Approach to the Segmentation of Brain Images with Multiple Sclerosis Lesions. NeuroImage (2009)
3. Dale, A.M., Fischl, B., Sereno, M.I.: Cortical Surface-Based Analysis I: Segmentation and Surface Reconstruction. NeuroImage 9(2), 179–194 (1999)
4. Leemput, K.V., Maes, F., Vandermeulen, D., Suetens, P.: Automated Model-Based Tissue Classification of MR Images of the Brain. IEEE Trans. on Med. Imag. 18(10), 897–908 (1999)
5. Coupé, P., Eskildsen, S.F., Manjón, J.V., Fonov, V.S., Collins, D.L.: The Alzheimer's disease Neuroimaging Initiative: Simultaneous segmentation and grading of anatomical structures for patient's classification: application to Alzheimer's disease. NeuroImage 59(4), 3736–3747 (2012)
6. Tong, T., Wolz, R., Coupe, P., Hajnal, J.V., Rueckert, D.: The Alzheimer's Disease Neuroimaging Initiative: Segmentation of MR images via discriminative dictionary learning and sparse coding: Application to hippocampus labeling. NeuroImage 76(1), 11–23 (2013)
7. Roy, S., Carass, A., Prince, J.: Magnetic Resonance Image Example Based Contrast Synthesis. IEEE Trans. Med. Imag. 32(12), 2348–2363 (2013)
8. Cao, T., Zach, C., Modla, S., Powell, D., Czymmek, K., Niethammer, M.: Registration for correlative microscopy using image analogies. In: Dawant, B.M., Christensen, G.E., Fitzpatrick, J.M., Rueckert, D. (eds.) WBIR 2012. LNCS, vol. 7359, pp. 296–306. Springer, Heidelberg (2012)
9. Aharon, M., Elad, M., Bruckstein, A.M.: K-SVD: An Algorithm for Designing Overcomplete Dictionaries for Sparse Representation. IEEE Trans. Sig. Proc. 54(11), 4311–4322 (2006)
10. Shiee, N., Bazin, P.-L., Cuzzocreo, J.L., Blitz, A., Pham, D.L.: Segmentation of brain images using adaptive atlases with application to ventriculomegaly. In: Székely, G., Hahn, H.K. (eds.) IPMI 2011. LNCS, vol. 6801, pp. 1–12. Springer, Heidelberg (2011)
11. Carass, A., Cuzzocreo, J., Wheeler, M.B., Bazin, P.L., Resnick, S.M., Prince, J.L.: Simple paradigm for extra-cerebral tissue removal: Algorithm and analysis. NeuroImage 56(4), 1982–1992 (2011)
12. Sled, J.G., Zijdenbos, A.P., Evans, A.C.: A non-parametric method for automatic correction of intensity non-uniformity in MRI data. IEEE Trans. on Med. Imag. 17(1), 87–97 (1998)
13. Pham, D.L., Prince, J.L.: An Adaptive Fuzzy C-Means Algorithm for Image Segmentation in the Presence of Intensity Inhomogeneities. Pattern Recog. Letters 20(1), 57–68 (1999)
14. Klein, A., et al.: Evaluation of 14 nonlinear deformation algorithms applied to human brain MRI registration. NeuroImage 46(3), 786–802 (2009)

Multi-atlas Segmentation with Learning-Based Label Fusion

Hongzhi Wang, Yu Cao, and Tanveer Syeda-Mahmood

IBM Almaden Research Center

Abstract. Although multi-atlas segmentation techniques have been producing impressive results for many medical image segmentation problems, most label fusion methods developed so far rely on simple statistical inference models that may not be optimal for inference in high-dimensional feature space. To address this problem, we propose a novel scheme that allows more effective usage of advanced machine learning techniques for patch-based label fusion. Our key novelty is using image registration to guide training sample selection for more effective learning. We demonstrate the power of this new technique in cardiac segmentation using clinical 2D ultrasound images and show superior performance over multi-atlas segmentation and machine learning-based segmentation.

1 Introduction

Multi-atlas segmentation has demonstrated outstanding performance for a wide range of medical image segmentation problems. One key ingredient to its success is that deformable registration can accurately align anatomical structures across subjects for reliable label propagation. With accurate structure alignment, simple label fusion methods such as similarity-based local weighted voting [6,11,15] often can produce state of the art performance.

Although more powerful learning and classification techniques other than weighted voting have been developed in machine learning research, applying advanced machine learning techniques to aid label fusion has not been extensively studied. In some recent work, [13] applies adaboost classification as a postprocessing step to reduce errors produced by multi-atlas segmentation. Similarly, [5] employed random forest classification to reduce ambiguities produced by multi-atlas segmentation. Random forest is also employed in [18] for atlas encoding.

A common limitation of the above mentioned methods is that the classifiers are all trained without taking advantage of registration-based structure alignment, i.e. the key advantage of multi-atlas segmentation. To address this limitation, we explore a new scheme for combining learning techniques with multi-atlas segmentation. Our key novelty lies in an image registration based training sample selection strategy for more effective learning. Similar to the spatially varying image similarity based local weight voting approach, we propose a spatially varying training sample selection strategy that aims to only apply training samples that are anatomically most relevant to the target testing sample for segmenting the target sample. This is achieved by selecting training samples within a

G. Wu et al. (Eds.): MLMI 2014, LNCS 8679, pp. 256–263, 2014.

local neighborhood surrounding the target testing sample after registering and warping atlases into the target image.

We implement our method with random forest and conduct validation in a challenging cardiac segmentation application using clinical four-chamber view 2D echocardiography. We demonstrate promising improvement over the state of the art label fusion method and random forest based segmentation.

2 Method

2.1 Background in Patch-Based Multi-atlas Label Fusion

In this section, we briefly describe multi-atlas segmentation. Let T_F be a target image to be segmented and $A^1 = (A_F^1, A_S^1), ..., A^n = (A_F^n, A_S^n)$ be n atlases, warped to the space of the target image by deformable registration. A_F^i and A_S^i denote the i_{th} warped atlas image and manual segmentation. Each A_S^i is a candidate segmentation for the target image. Label fusion combines these candidate segmentations to produce the final solution.

One simple and highly effective label fusion method is based on weighted voting. For instance, the combined votes for label l are:

$$\hat{p}(l|x, T_F) = \sum_{i=1}^{n} w_x^i p(l|x, A^i) \tag{1}$$

where x indexes through image locations. $\hat{p}(l|x, T_F)$ is the estimated label posterior for the target image. $p(l|x, A^i)$ is the probability that A^i votes for label l at x, with $\sum_{l \in \{1,...,L\}} p(l|x, A^i) = 1$. L is the total number of labels. w_x^i is a local weight assigned to the i_{th} atlas, with $\sum_{i=1}^{n} w_x^i = 1$. The voting weights are typically determined based on the quality of registration produced for each atlas such that more accurately registered atlases are weighted more heavily in producing the final solution.

Patch-based label fusion. For estimating registration/segmentation accuracy, patch-based approaches are among the most effective techniques. For this task, most methods apply similarity metrics typically employed by image-based registration, such as sum of squared distance (SSD) and normalized cross correlation (NCC) computed over local image patches. For instance, when SSD and a Gaussian weighting model are used [11], the voting weights in (1) can be estimated by $w_x^i = \frac{1}{Z(x)} exp\left(-\sum_{y \in \mathcal{N}(x)} \left[A_F^i(y) - T_F(y)\right]^2 / \sigma\right)$, where σ is a model parameter. $\mathcal{N}(x)$ defines the image patch, which is a neighborhood surrounding x, and $Z(x)$ is a normalization constant.

Although the above approach can provide reasonable estimation about registration accuracy for each warped atlas, its contribution for remedying the registration error is limited. To more effectively remedy registration errors, atlas patches within a local searching neighborhood of the registered correspondence could all be considered as the potential corresponding patch for a target patch and are applied for label fusion in patch-based label fusion methods [4,10,15].

2.2   Limitations of Current Patch-Based Label Fusion Methods

Patch-based label fusion could be interpreted as a regression or interpolation problem [9,14], where the goal is to predict the segmentation label for each target voxel given its surrounding image patch. All potential corresponding image patches from the warped atlases provide observed data for this regression task. Given that this regression problem is performed in a high-dimensional feature space, the simple distance metric employed in current patch-based label fusion methods, e.g. the Euclidean metric used above, could be inadequate for accurately characterizing the feature space. This problem is less critical when image registration can be reliably computed. As shown in an empirical study [16], simple metrics such as the Euclidean metric does a good job differentiating small registration errors, however the accuracy of predicting large registration errors quickly drops as the registration error increases. Hence, employing simple metrics in patch-based label fusion becomes more problematic when image registrations are poorly computed.

2.3   Random Forest Based Label Fusion

To address this limitation, we propose to employ more powerful learning techniques for patch-based label fusion. In this paper, we investigate the usage of random forest for this task.

A random forest is an ensemble of decision trees [3]. Each non-leaf node in a decision tree performs a test, e.g. the comparison of a feature value to a given threshold. During training, training data are used to build each decision tree. During testing, a testing data is sent to the root node of each decision tree. Based on the test at the node, the data is sent to either its left or right child node. This process is repeated until a leaf node is reached in a tree. The class distribution of all training samples located in the leaf node is interpreted as the probability that the testing data should be assigned to each class. The final class probability is obtained by averaging the class distributions from all decision trees. Random forest has demonstrated impressive performance in image segmentation [18].

Inspired by the highly successful spatially varying weighted voting scheme, we propose to train spatially varying local random forest classifiers for label fusion. As in patch-based label fusion [4,10], given a target patch, all atlas patches located in a small neighborhood of the registered correspondence are applied for training a local random forest classifier, which is then applied for predicting labels for the target patch. To facilitate our comparison with previous patch-based label fusion, we apply pixel intensity values within each image patch as features to predict the patch's central pixel's label. In our experiment, we apply a $(2r_s + 1) \times (2r_s + 1)$ square-shaped sampling neighborhood specified by the radius r_s for our 2D cardiac ultrasound images. We also use a square-shaped patch specified by a radius r for feature extraction.

Ideally, a distinct random forest classifier should be trained for segmenting each target voxel using warped atlas samples surrounding the target voxel. However, this requirement increases the computational cost. To make our study more practical, we apply the trained classifier to predict segmentation labels for each voxel located in the sampling window in the target image. In addition, we train classifiers on overlapping sampling windows. Centers of the sampling windows are located on a 2D grid with the distance between two neighboring grid nodes in each row and each column equal $\frac{r_s}{2}$. Classification results from overlapping classifiers are averaged to generate the final solution.

2.4 Relation to Training Sample Selection in Machine Learning

In machine learning research, it is well known that not all training samples are always equally important for any given learning task. Choosing the most relevant training samples for any specific classification task is a highly effective technique for improving the learning performance. In general, rules for choosing the most relevant training samples are application dependent. In medical image segmentation, one intuitive rule for choosing relevant training samples is based on their anatomical locations.

Although machine learning methods usually employ more powerful statistical inference techniques than what are employed by current patch-based label fusion methods, existing learning-based segmentation methods still largely ignore the valuable anatomical information encoded in medical images. In contrast, multi-atlas segmentation stands in the opposite extreme in terms of how anatomical information is incorporated for reaching solutions. For instance, it is common that machine learning based methods apply mixed training data sampled from different anatomical area for making segmentation decisions, while multi-atlas segmentation significantly simplifies the problem by applying spatially-varying training data that are anatomically more relevant to the testing data obtained from image registration. Due to this distinction, the best brain segmentation performance achieved by machine learning techniques, e.g. [12,18], are still well below those produced by multi-atlas segmentation [7,1]. In this aspect, *the key advantage of our method lies in combining the complementary advantages of machine learning and multi-atlas segmentation.*

3 Experiments

We conduct experimental study on cardiac segmentation using apical four-chamber view 2D echocardiography. 2D echocardiography is a common modality for diagnosis in clinical practice. Anatomical structure labeling will assist cardiac disease diagnosis by providing geometrical and morphological statistics. This is an ideal application for demonstrating the advantage of our machine learning based label fusion technique. Image registration on echocardiography are challenging as the images are noisy and the anatomical structure deformation among different subjects are large. Hence, label fusion needs to accommodate large registration errors. Furthermore, different anatomical regions often share similar intensity profiles in echocardiography, making image feature based machine learning techniques less effective.

3.1   Data and Experiment Setup

Our dataset consists of a total of 50 patients with a variety of cardiac diseases such as aneurysms, dilated cardiomyopathy and hypertrophies. Each image is manually labeled with the following nine structures: Chamber Junction (CJ), Inter Ventricle Septum (IVS), Left Ventricle (LV), Mitral Valve (MV), Left Atrium (LA), Inter Atrium Septum (IAS), Right Atrium (RA), Tricuspid Valve (TV) and Right Ventricle (RV). We conducted a 5-fold cross-validation. Hence, the dataset is randomly divided into 5 equal size non-overlap groups. Each group is treated as the testing set and the remaining groups are treated as training set in each of the five cross-validation experiments. The results below are summarized over the five cross-validation experiments. In our experiments, we applied sampling windows with $r_s = 5$ for our method.

Deformable image registration. The global image-based registration between each pair of images were performed through sequentially optimizing translation, rigid body, affine and deformable transforms between the registered images. Deformable registration was performed using the greedy diffeomorphic Symmetric Normalization (SyN) algorithm [2] implemented by the Advanced Normalization Tools (ANTs) software package. The Mattes mutual information metric was applied for the registration task. Multi-scale optimization was applied. Three resolution levels with maximum 200 iterations at the coarse and middle levels and 100 iterations at the fine level were applied.

Random Forest setup. We applied the random forest package implemented in R [8] with the default parameter setting, i.e. 500 trees. Using this implementation, our method usually segments each image in about 10 minutes.

Benchmark methods. For comparison, we evaluated joint label fusion (JLF) [15]. This method is one of the state of the art methods for patch-based local weighted voting label fusion and is a consistent top performer in both MICCAI grand challenges on multi-atlas segmentation held in 2012 and 2013 [7,1]. For this study, we applied the authors' implementation that is distributed through the ANTs software package with default parameters, i.e. 5×5 image patches for local image similarity estimation, 7×7 local searching windows and model parameter $\sigma = 2$. As another baseline performance, we also computed the segmentation results produced by majority voting (MV) and by the STAPLE algorithm [17].

In the second comparison, we compare with the segmentation performance produced by the classical usage of random forest for image segmentation (RF). We train a single random forest classifier using the training samples from all atlases without warping them into the target image space and apply this classifier to segment testing images. In addition to the intensity feature extracted from each pixel's surrounding patch, we also include relative spatial location of each training sample with respect to the mass center of the scanned view as an additional feature. To facilitate a direct comparison with other tested methods, we did not include any other features for random forest classification.

Table 1. Segmentation performance of our random forest label fusion (RFLF) method compared with other methods. Results are measured using the Dice similarity coefficient $(2|A \cap B|/|A| + |B|)$.

anatomical regions	MV	STAPLE	RF	JLF	RFLF
CJ	0.53±0.28	0.43±0.21	0.49±0.24	0.57±0.25	0.64±0.18
IVS	0.67±0.27	0.62±0.18	0.72±0.13	0.73±0.19	0.78±0.09
LV	0.77±0.14	0.73±0.17	0.82±0.07	0.80±0.11	0.82±0.08
MV	0.30±0.25	0.34±0.28	0.20±0.10	0.44±0.25	0.50±0.18
LA	0.74±0.20	0.69±0.19	0.73±0.14	0.78±0.17	0.79±0.14
IAS	0.51±0.29	0.38±0.27	0.18±0.14	0.57±0.23	0.59±0.21
RA	0.70±0.21	0.60±0.26	0.69±0.17	0.73±0.20	0.75±0.16
TV	0.07±0.12	0.17±0.21	0.02±0.03	0.17±0.18	0.21±0.19
RV	0.68±0.18	0.53±0.24	0.68±0.17	0.72±0.15	0.72±0.14
Overall	0.55	0.50	0.50	0.61	0.65

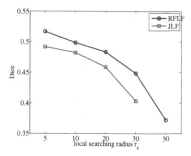

Fig. 1. Segmentation accuracy (in terms of average Jaccard index) of joint label fusion and our random forest based label fusion method with respective to the size of local searching windows

Results. Table 1 summarizes the segmentation performance produced by each method. The performance of the classical machine learning approach that learns a single random forest classifier to assign labels for the entire testing image is clearly below those of multi-atlas segmentation methods. In contrast, applying random forest for local patch-based label prediction produced a significant improvement over the state of the art label fusion method (with $p < 0.05$ on the paired Students t-test compared with JLF and $p < 0.001$ compared with the remaining evaluated methods). This result clearly demonstrates: 1) the simple metric based patch label fusion method is inadequate for our application; 2) the registration based spatially varying sample selection scheme significantly improved the performance of random forest.

Fig. 1 shows the performance of joint label fusion and our random forest based label fusion method with respect to the size of local searching windows. Both methods' performance dropped as the local searching radius increases. This result is expected because larger local searching/sampling windows complicate the label fusion/classification problem by adding more irrelevant samples into

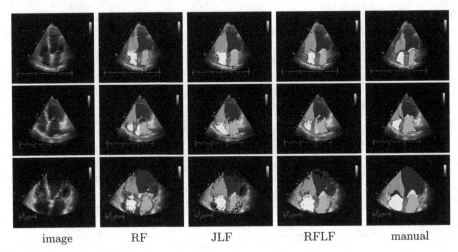

image   RF   JLF   RFLF   manual

Fig. 2. Segmentation results by different methods. Red: CJ; Green: IVS; Blue: LV; Yellow: MV; Sky blue: LA; Pink: IAS; Light brown: RA; Deep blue: TV; Brown: RV.

consideration. This result also indicates that training separate classifiers for distinct anatomical structures, such as in [13,5], is suboptimal because one anatomical structure may still be large enough to include samples that are not strongly relevant with each other for classification purpose. See Fig. 2 for some segmentation examples.

4   Discussion and Conclusions

We introduced a novel scheme for combining the complementary advantages of multi-atlas segmentation with more general machine learning techniques. The key idea is to use image registration to generate spatially varying training sample selection for more effective learning. In our experiments of cardiac segmentation using four chamber view 2D echocardiography, we demonstrated that the registration-based spatially varying sample selection method significantly improves classification accuracy for random forest. By including more descriptive features or by applying postprocessing methods such as [13,5], we expect further prominent improvement in the segmentation performance. In future work, we will also conduct validation on broader applications with different registration accuracy levels.

One common implementation to make multi-atlas segmentation more practical is to preregister all atlases to a common template space. Given a new target image, only one registration from the target image to the template is required. Although it significantly reduces the registration burden, it also compromises the overall registration accuracy. Since our experiments show that our machine learning based label fusion method is more robust to registration errors, it is especially suitable to be implemented through the common template strategy.

References

1. Asman, A., Akhondi-Asl, A., Wang, H., Tustison, N., Avants, B., Warfield, S.K., Landman, B.: Miccai 2013 segmentation algorithms, theory and applications (SATA) challenge results summary. In: MICCAI 2013 Challenge Workshop on Segmentation: Algorithms, Theory and Applications. Springer (2013)
2. Avants, B., Epstein, C., Grossman, M., Gee, J.: Symmetric diffeomorphic image registration with cross-correlation: Evaluating automated labeling of elderly and neurodegenerative brain. Medical Image Analysis 12(1), 26–41 (2008)
3. Breiman, L.: Random forests. Machine Learning 45(1), 5–32 (2001)
4. Coupe, P., Manjon, J., Fonov, V., Pruessner, J., Robles, N., Collins, D.: Patch-based segmentation using expert priors: Application to hippocampus and ventricle segmentation. NeuroImage 54(2), 940–954 (2011)
5. Han, X.: Learning-boosted label fusion for multi-atlas auto-segmentation. In: Wu, G., Zhang, D., Shen, D., Yan, P., Suzuki, K., Wang, F. (eds.) MLMI 2013. LNCS, vol. 8184, pp. 17–24. Springer, Heidelberg (2013)
6. Isgum, I., Staring, M., Rutten, A., Prokop, M., Viergever, M., van Ginneken, B.: Multi-atlas-based segmentation with local decision fusion–application to cardiac and aortic segmentation in CT scans. IEEE Trans. on MI 28(7), 1000–1010 (2009)
7. Landman, B., Warfield, S. (eds.): MICCAI 2012 Workshop on Multi-Atlas Labeling. CreateSpace (2012)
8. Liaw, A., Wiener, M.: Classification and regression by randomforest. R News 2(3), 18–22 (2002), http://CRAN.R-project.org/doc/Rnews/
9. Rohlfing, T., Brandt, R., Menzel, R., Russakoff, D.B., Maurer Jr., C.R.: Quo vadis, atlas-based segmentation? In: The Handbook of Medical Image Analysis–Volume III: Registration Models, pp. 435–486 (2005)
10. Rousseau, F., Habas, P.A., Studholme, C.: A supervised patch-based approach for human brain labeling. IEEE TMI 30(10), 1852–1862 (2011)
11. Sabuncu, M., Yeo, B., Leemput, K.V., Fischl, B., Golland, P.: A generative model for image segmentation based on label fusion. IEEE TMI 29(10), 1714–1720 (2010)
12. Tu, Z., Zheng, S., Yuille, A., Reiss, A., Dutton, R., Lee, A., Galaburda, A., Dinov, I., Thompson, P., Toga, A.: Automated extraction of the cortical sulci based on a supervised learning approach. IEEE TMI 26(4), 541–552 (2007)
13. Wang, H., Das, S., Suh, J.W., Altinay, M., Pluta, J., Craige, C., Avants, B., Yushke-vich, P.: A learning-based wrapper method to correct systematic errors in automatic image segmentation: Consistently improved performance in hippocampus, cortex and brain segmentation. NeuroImage 55(3), 968–985 (2011)
14. Wang, H., Suh, J.W., Das, S., Pluta, J., Altinay, M., Yushkevich, P.: Regression-based label fusion for multi-atlas segmentation. In: CVPR (2011)
15. Wang, H., Suh, J.W., Das, S., Pluta, J., Craige, C., Yushkevich, P.: Multi-atlas segmentation with joint label fusion. IEEE Trans. on Pattern Analysis and Machine Intelligence 35(3), 611–623 (2013)
16. Wang, H., Yushkevich, P.A.: Spatial bias in multi-atlas based segmentation. In: 2012 IEEE Conference on Computer Vision and Pattern Recognition (CVPR), pp. 909–916. IEEE (2012)
17. Warfield, S., Zou, K., Wells, W.: Simultaneous truth and performance level estimation (STAPLE): an algorithm for the validation of image segmentation. IEEE TMI 23(7), 903–921 (2004)
18. Zikic, D., Glocker, B., Criminisi, A.: Atlas encoding by randomized forests for efficient label propagation. In: Mori, K., Sakuma, I., Sato, Y., Barillot, C., Navab, N. (eds.) MICCAI 2013, Part III. LNCS, vol. 8151, pp. 66–73. Springer, Heidelberg (2013)

Interactive Prostate Segmentation
Based on Adaptive Feature Selection
and Manifold Regularization

Sang Hyun Park[1], Yaozong Gao[1], Yinghuan Shi[2], and Dinggang Shen[1]

[1] Department of Radiology, BRIC, University of North Carolina at Chapel Hill, USA
dgshen@med.unc.edu
[2] State Key Laboratory for Novel Software Technology, Nanjing University, China

Abstract. In this paper, we propose a new learning-based interactive editing method for prostate segmentation. Although many automatic methods have been proposed to segment the prostate, laborious manual correction is still required for many clinical applications due to the limited performance of automatic segmentation. The proposed method is able to flexibly correct wrong parts of the segmentation within a short time, even few scribbles or dots are provided. In order to obtain the robust correction with a few interactions, the discriminative features that can represent mid-level cues beyond image intensity or gradient are adaptively extracted from a local region of interest according to both the training set and the interaction. Then, the labeling problem is formulated as a semi-supervised learning task, which is aimed to preserve the manifold configuration between the labeled and unlabeled voxels. The proposed method is evaluated on a challenging prostate CT image data set with large shape and appearance variations. The automatic segmentation results originally with the average Dice of 0.766 were improved to the average Dice 0.866 after conducting totally 22 interactions for the 12 test images by using our proposed method.

Keywords: Interactive segmentation, prostate, feature selection, semi-supervised learning, manifold regularization.

1   Introduction

Prostate cancer is one of the top leading causes of cancer-related death for males. Radiation therapy with high-energy beams or particles is commonly used to cure the early-stage cancers. During the radiotherapy, the high dose radiation should be accurately delivered to the prostate, since the false delivery could lead to under-treatment for the prostate cancer and even severe side effects for the patient. Accordingly, accurate segmentation of the prostate from the surrounding healthy tissues is required, to provide guidance for delivering the radiation beams to the prostate for maximizing the effectiveness of therapy. However, manual segmentation of the prostate in a 3D image is very time-consuming and often causes intra- and inter-variations across clinicians [1].

G. Wu et al. (Eds.): MLMI 2014, LNCS 8679, pp. 264–271, 2014.

Many automatic prostate segmentation methods based on the aligned atlases [1], statistical shape or appearance models [2], or classifiers [3] have been proposed to obtain the reliable prostate segmentation results. Although these automatic methods can largely alleviate the burden of clinicians, inaccurate segmentations are often obtained due to the weak boundary between the prostate and its surrounding tissues, large shape and appearance variations across subjects, and uncertainty of bowel gas and filling. Therefore, heuristic post-processing or manual editing is sometimes needed for correcting the wrong parts after the automatic segmentation process.

Many interactive segmentation methods [4,5], which can provide a fast editing result according to the user interaction, have been proposed in the computer vision field. However, these methods cannot generate flexible correction results with few user interactions, because only the intensity and gradient information are generally used to construct the model without utilizing the high-level knowledge from training data. Recently, interactive methods based on the prior knowledge of training data have been proposed. Barnes *et al.* [6] proposed the image completion and reshuffling methods based on *PatchMatch*, which can seek for the corresponding image patches efficiently by first randomly searching for a similar patch and then expanding correspondences to the adjacent regions. Park *et al.* [7] further enforced the spatial relationships of adjacent patches to constrain the specific shapes of organs. The use of label information of similar patches can improve the editing performance for many applications. However, simple label and intensity information cannot deal with the intra- and inter-subject appearance variations, as well as the weak boundary of prostate in our case of application.

In this paper, we propose a new interactive editing method, which can 1) generate the flexible correction results with a few clinician's interactions, and 2) fast deliver intermediate results to a clinician. The correction result of the proposed method is very robust to the amount and locations of interactions, since possible variations of data have been guided by the training data and incorporated into our algorithm. Unlike the existing interactive methods that directly use the label or intensity histogram as the priors, in the proposed method, informative features are adaptively extracted from each local correction region according to its discriminative characteristics. In addition, the manifold configuration of voxels in the target image is also considered in the semi-supervised regularization formulation. These adaptive features can flexibly deal with both intra- and inter-appearance variations and further represent mid-level cues for identifying the weak boundary beyond the simple image features; also the manifold configuration is learned to reflect the anatomical relationships between the labeled and unlabeled voxels.

2   Interactive Segmentation Framework

The proposed editing procedure is repeated whenever a clinician's interaction is inserted into a wrong part of previous segmentation L^{t-1}, where t is the interaction time. If there are many wrong parts on the segmentation, multiple corrections are repeatedly conducted until obtaining satisfactory result. Each correction consists of the following procedures. First, in a local region near the interaction, appropriate training labels, well matched with the interaction and the previous segmentation, are selected from the training set. Based on the selected training labels, both the confident regions, $e.g.$, the prostate and background, and the unconfident regions are estimated. Then, the informative features, which are important for separating the prostate and the background on the confident regions, are selected. The labels of all voxels are determined by optimizing the semi-supervised regularization formulation which is aimed to preserve the manifold configuration between the labeled and unlabeled voxels. The details are presented in the following sub-sections.

2.1   Initial Segmentation and Preprocessing

The initial segmentation L^0 can be obtained by any kind of automatic or interactive methods. In this paper, we use the regression-based automatic segmentation method [8] to obtain L^0.

All training images and their labels are aligned onto the target image to rapidly search for appropriate training data in the online editing procedure. We use the MRF based non-rigid registration method (Drop) [9] for the alignment. It takes roughly one minute for aligning each training image, but this time-consuming procedure can be done without clinician's effort before the interactive correction. The interactive correction, a main proposed algorithm, starts from the next sub-section.

2.2   Determination of ROI from User Interaction

The proposed method receives foreground and background scribbles or dots as the interactions for a wrong part of previous segmentation L^{t-1}. The correction is conducted on a local region near the interaction with assumption that the regions near the interaction have segmentation errors, while the other parts of L^{t-1} are assumed to be correct temporarily. If there are errors on the other parts, the errors can be sequentially corrected in the next interactions. The local region of interest (ROI) Φ^t is determined as a bounding box which includes the interaction and also has a small margin, so that the possible local variations can be covered. We set the margin as $9 \times 9 \times 2$ voxels, considering the large thickness of our CT images. According to the interaction, a voxel v on Φ^t will be labeled as foreground ($U^t(v) = 1$), background ($U^t(v) = -1$), or unlabeled ($U^t(v) = 0$), where U^t is the label image of tth round interaction.

2.3   Selection of Reference Training Data

To use of prior knowledge included in the training data, the appropriate training data will be selected according to the interaction. Here, we assume that the appropriate training data should have the training label M which is well matched

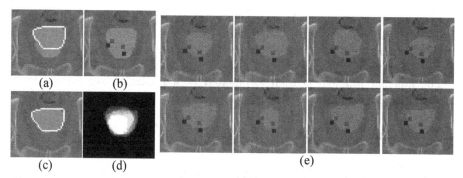

Fig. 1. (a) Initial segmentation (green) and ground truth (white line), (b) foreground (red) and background (blue) user annotations on the initial segmentation, (c) corrected result (green), (d) probabilistic label constructed by averaging the reference labels, and (e) selected reference labels (orange)

with 1) U^t on the annotated voxels and also 2) L^{t-1} on the other voxels. We define the label-based similarity cost $S(M, U^t, L^{t-1})$ as:

$$S(M, U^t, L^{t-1}) = \sum_{\substack{v \in \Phi^t, \\ U^t(v) \neq 0}} (\delta(M(v) - U^t(v)) + w_U \cdot \sum_{\substack{v \in \Phi^t, \\ U^t(v) = 0}} (\delta(M(v) - L^{t-1}(v)),$$

$$(1)$$

where δ is the Kronecker delta. The first term represents the number of voxels which have the same labels in M and U^t, while the second term represents the number of voxels which have the same labels in M and L^{t-1}. The more M is consistent with U^t and L^{t-1}, the higher similarity cost will be obtained. w_U is a parameter used to balance between the two terms. Since the number of annotated voxels $(U^t(v) \neq 0)$ is relatively smaller than that of unlabeled voxels $(U^t(v) = 0)$, w_U is set as a small value (i.e., $w_U = 0.01$) in the experiments below. The similarity costs are computed for all training data, and then totally n_r training labels with the highest costs are selected as the reference training data. The examples of reference labels are shown in Fig. 1 (e).

2.4 Prostate Segmentation by Semi-supervised Labeling

Although the segmentation of target image can be obtained by using the majority voting of the reference labels, the simple label fusion technique could not reflect the meaningful appearance or structures of the target image. Therefore, we first estimate the confident prostate and background regions in Φ^t by using the reference labels. Then, the labels of unconfident voxels are carefully determined by considering the prostate likelihood of the confident voxels and also the manifold configurations between the confident and unconfident voxels in a semi-supervised regularization formulation.

To estimate the confident regions, a probabilistic label P is computed by averaging the reference labels (Fig. 1 (d)). If $P(v)$ is higher than 0.7, v is estimated as a confident prostate voxel ($y(v) = 1$), while if $P(v)$ is lower than 0.1, v is estimated as a confident background voxel ($y(v) = -1$). These confident voxels are regarded as totally n_l labeled voxels and all others are regarded as totally n_u unlabeled voxels ($y(v) = 0$).

The labeling problem is then formulated as a Laplacian regularized least square (LapRLS) equation [10] as:

$$\hat{\mathbf{w}} = \min_{\mathbf{w}}\{||\mathbf{J}(\mathbf{y} - \mathbf{Kw})||_2^2 + \gamma_1 \mathbf{w}^T \mathbf{Kw} + \frac{\gamma_2 n_l}{(n_l + n_u)^2}\mathbf{w}^T \mathbf{KLKw}\}, \qquad (2)$$

where $\mathbf{w} = [w_1, ..., w_{n_l+n_u}]$ is the parameter set to be optimized. The first term represents the prostate likelihood of the labeled voxels, while the second term represents the smoothness regularization of $\mathbf{w}$. The last term represents the relationship between the labeled and unlabeled voxels used for preserving their manifold configuration. $\mathbf{J} = diag(1, ..., 1, 0, ..., 0)$ is a diagonal matrix with the first n_l diagonal entries as 1 and the rest as 0. $\mathbf{y} = [y(v_1), ..., y(v_{n_l}), y(v_{n_l+1}), ..., y(v_{n_l+n_u})]$ is the label set. $\mathbf{K}$ is the $(n_l + n_u) \times (n_l + n_u)$ gram matrix with the elements $K(v_i, v_j)$ defined by the Gaussian RBF kernel as $K(v_i, v_j) = \exp(-\tau||\mathbf{f}(v_i) - \mathbf{f}(v_j)||_2^2)$, where $\mathbf{f}(v)$ is the feature vector of voxel v. $\mathbf{L}$ is the $(n_l + n_u) \times (n_l + n_u)$ Laplacian matrix defined across all labeled and unlabeled voxels. The Gaussian RBF kernel is similarly used to define the voxel relationship. γ_1 and γ_2 are the weighting parameters for the second and third terms.

The optimal parameter $\hat{\mathbf{w}}$ can be computed as:

$$\hat{\mathbf{w}} = (\mathbf{JK} + \gamma_1 n_l \mathbf{I} + \frac{\gamma_2 n_l}{(n_l + n_u)^2}\mathbf{LK})^{-1}\mathbf{y}, \qquad (3)$$

where $\mathbf{I}$ is the identity matrix. After estimating $\hat{\mathbf{w}}$, the likelihood of all voxels can be computed as $\hat{P} = \mathbf{K}\hat{\mathbf{w}}$. If $\hat{P}(v)$ is larger than 0, the voxel v is classified to the prostate ($L^t(v) = 1$), otherwise, classified to the background ($L^t(v) = 0$).

Here, the features $\mathbf{f}(v)$ can be defined by any type of appearance or context features, but the discriminative power of $\mathbf{f}(v)$ is highly related to the final segmentation performance. Since the prostate have very weak boundary and large shape and appearance variations, simple appearance or context features cannot generate the reliable result. We adaptively select the features that have the high discriminative power on each local region. First, various 3D Haar features [11] are randomly extracted from the confident labeled voxels. Then, the discriminative power of a feature is measured by the Fisher separation criterion (FSC) score S_{FSC} [12] as:

$$S_{FSC} = \frac{\mu_f - \mu_b}{\sqrt{\sigma_f - \sigma_b}}, \qquad (4)$$

where μ_f and μ_b denote the mean feature values of prostate and background voxels, respectively. Similarly, σ_f and σ_b denote the variances of prostate and background voxels, respectively. n_f features with the largest FSC scores, i.e., the highest discriminative power, are finally selected and included in $\mathbf{f}(v)$.

Table 1. Mean DSC scores of the separate correction results on local region of interest and on the entire region for 22 interactions, and mean DSC scores of the accumulated results on the entire region for 12 test images

	Initial	Manual	WVA	WVL	LapRLS+RF	LapRLS+SF
Local (separated)	0.548	0.574	0.789	0.848	0.805	**0.854**
Global (separated)	0.757	0.761	0.79	0.804	0.797	**0.805**
Global (accumulated)	0.766	0.773	0.84	0.863	0.854	**0.866**

3 Experimental Evaluation

The proposed method (LapRLS+SF) was evaluated on a challenging prostate CT image dataset which consists of 73 images, scanned from different patients. The image size is $512 \times 512 \times (61 \sim 81)$ with $0.94 \times 0.94 \times 3.00 mm^3$ voxel spacing. The dataset includes various subjects with large shape and appearance variations. The boundary of prostate in each image was manually delineated by a radiation oncologist and used as the ground truth for measuring the segmentation performance. The performance was measured by the Dice similarity coefficient (DSC). We divided the dataset into 19 test images and 54 training images, and applied the regression-based automatic segmentation method [8]. We obtained the satisfactory results for 7 cases, which had more than 0.85 DSC scores. The proposed editing method was applied to correct the results of the remaining 12(=19-7) images. The parameters of the proposed method were empirically set as follows: n_f=1000, $n_r = 7$, $\gamma_1 = 10^{-2}$, $\gamma_2 = 10^{-1}$.

The proposed method was compared with a manual editing method, weighted voting methods, and the LapRLS method with random features (LapRLS+RF). Only the labels of voxels annotated by the user were changed in the manual editing method. To show the effect of label-based similarity (1), we provide both the weighted voting result based on the appearance similarity cost (WVA) and the result based on the label-based similarity cost (WVL). Specifically, the training labels which have the highest intensity-based normalized cross correlation (NCC) are selected for the WVA. The selected training labels are averaged with the weights, which are linearly computed by the NCC cost, and the voxels with the averaged label value more than 0.5 are determined as the prostate. Similarly, the training labels which have the highest label-based similarity are selected for the WVL and the voxels with the averaged label value more than 0.5 are determined as the prostate. We also provide the result of LapRLS method using 1000 random Haar features to present the effect of feature selection. Since the improvement of correction could be relatively small in the entire image even though the improvement on the local region was very large, the DSC were measured both on the ROI and on the entire image for each interaction. The final DSC of accumulated correction results were also measured on the entire image.

The original average DSC score of the automatic results for the 12 test images was 0.766. We input the several dots on wrong parts as shown in Fig 2 until the DSC scores of all results are more than 0.85. The corrections for 12 images were completed within 22 interactions, on average, 1.8 interactions per image.

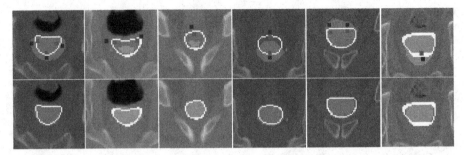

Fig. 2. Editing results for several wrong cases. Initial results (green), ground truth boundary (white), and user interactions (red and blue dots) are shown in the top row. Editing results (green) obtained by the proposed method are shown in the bottom row.

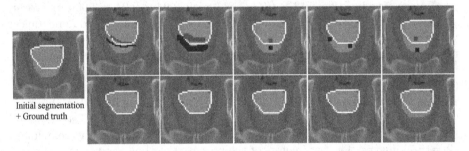

Initial segmentation
+ Ground truth

Fig. 3. Editing results according to the different interactions. Initial segmentation (green) and ground truth (white line) are shown in left. Different user interactions and the corrected results are shown in the upper and bottom rows, respectively.

Table 1 shows the mean DSC performance of each comparison method for the 22 interactions. Since the small numbers of dots were used for the interaction, the result of manual editing method was slightly improved from the automatic segmentation result. On the other hand, the performances of all methods based on training set were largely improved. Among all methods based on training set, the proposed method outperformed both the label fusion based methods.

Fig. 2 shows the qualitative correction results for several cases. Since the training labels constrained the irregular shape variations, the segmentation was flexibly updated even if few interactions were given. Fig. 3 shows the robustness of the proposed method according to the different interactions. The overall corrected results were similar to each other and robust to the placement and quantity of interactions. We note that this property helps reduce the inter-variability between different clinicians and different processing time.

The experiments were implemented on a PC with a 3.5 GHz Intel quad-core i7 CPU, and 16GB of RAM. The computational time was less than 3 seconds for each correction without any specific code optimization. We expect that the computational time will be further reduced to less than a second if code is optimized or the method is parallelized.

4 Conclusion

We have proposed a novel interactive editing method for correcting the prostate segmentation in CT images. The proposed method obtains the robust correction results with very few interactions for various wrong cases, by selecting the location-adaptive features and imposing the manifold configuration. We expect that the proposed method could largely reduce the laborious burdens of manual editing, as well as the intra- and inter-variability between clinicians.

Acknowledgement. This work was supported in part by NIH grant CA140413.

References

1. Davis, B.C., Foskey, M., Rosenman, J., Goyal, L., Chang, S., Joshi, S.: Automatic segmentation of intra-treatment CT images for adaptive radiation therapy of the prostate. In: Duncan, J.S., Gerig, G. (eds.) MICCAI 2005. LNCS, vol. 3749, pp. 442–450. Springer, Heidelberg (2005)
2. Chen, S., Lovelock, D.M., Radke, R.J.: Segmenting the prostate and rectum in ct imagery using anatomical constraints. Medical Image Analysis 15(1), 1–11 (2011)
3. Li, W., Liao, S., Feng, Q., Chen, W., Shen, D.: Learning image context for segmentation of prostate in CT-guided radiotherapy. In: Fichtinger, G., Martel, A., Peters, T. (eds.) MICCAI 2011, Part III. LNCS, vol. 6893, pp. 570–578. Springer, Heidelberg (2011)
4. Boykov, Y., Veksler, O., Zabih, R.: Fast approximate energy minimization via graph cuts. IEEE Transactions on PAMI 23(11), 1222–1239 (2001)
5. Grady, L.: Random walks for image segmentation. IEEE Transactions on PAMI 28(11), 1768–1783 (2006)
6. Barnes, C., Shechtman, E., Finkelstein, A., Goldman, D.B.: PatchMatch: A randomized correspondence algorithm for structural image editing. In: Proceedings of SIGGRAPH (2009)
7. Park, S.H., Yun, I.D., Lee, S.U.: Data-Driven Interactive 3D Medical Image Segmentation Based on Structured Patch Model. In: Gee, J.C., Joshi, S., Pohl, K.M., Wells, W.M., Zöllei, L. (eds.) IPMI 2013. LNCS, vol. 7917, pp. 196–207. Springer, Heidelberg (2013)
8. Anonymous: Learning distance transform for boundary detection and deformable segmentation in ct prostate images. To be submitted (2014)
9. Glocker, B., Komodakis, N., Tziritas, G., Navab, N., Paragios, N.: Dense image registration through MRFs and efficient linear programming. Medical Image Analysis 12(6), 731–741 (2008)
10. Belkin, M., Niyogi, P., Sindhwani, V.: Manifold regularization: A geometric framework for learning from labeled and unlabeled examples. Journal of Machine Learning Research 7, 2399–2434 (2006)
11. Criminisi, A., Shotton, J., Robertson, D., Konukoglu, E.: Regression forests for efficient anatomy detection and localization in CT studies. In: Menze, B., Langs, G., Tu, Z., Criminisi, A. (eds.) MICCAI 2010. LNCS, vol. 6533, pp. 106–117. Springer, Heidelberg (2011)
12. Gao, Y., Liao, S., Shen, D.: Prostate segmentation by sparse representation based classification. Medical Physics 39(10), 6372–6387 (2012)

Feature Selection Based on SVM Significance Maps for Classification of Dementia

Esther Bron[1], Marion Smits[2], John van Swieten[3],
Wiro Niessen[1,4], and Stefan Klein[1]

[1] Biomedical Imaging Group Rotterdam,
Departments of Medical Informatics and Radiology, Erasmus MC,
Rotterdam, The Netherlands
e.bron@erasmusmc.nl
[2] Department of Radiology, Erasmus MC, Rotterdam, The Netherlands
[3] Department of Neurology, Erasmus MC, Rotterdam, The Netherlands
[4] Imaging Physics, Applied Sciences, Delft University of Technology, The Netherlands

Abstract. Support vector machine significance maps (SVM p-maps) previously showed clusters of significantly different voxels in dementia-related brain regions. We propose a novel feature selection method for classification of dementia based on these p-maps. In our approach, the SVM p-maps are calculated on the training set with a time-efficient analytic approximation. The features that are most significant on the p-map are selected for classification with an SVM classifier. We validated our method using MRI data from the Alzheimer's Disease Neuroimaging Initiative (ADNI), classifying Alzheimer's disease (AD) patients, mild cognitive impairment (MCI) patients who converted to AD within 18 months, MCI patients who did not convert to AD, and cognitively normal controls (CN). The voxel-wise features were based on gray matter morphometry. We compared p-map feature selection to classification without feature selection and feature selection based on t-tests and expert knowledge. Our method obtained in all experiments similar or better performance and robustness than classification without feature selection with a substantially reduced number of features. In conclusion, we proposed a novel and efficient feature selection method with promising results.

1 Introduction

Computer-aided diagnosis of neurodegenerative diseases is an emerging research field in which machine learning approaches are used to distinguish for example Alzheimer's disease (AD) patients from normal (CN) controls [1]. For extracting image-based features for classification, many methods have used a voxel-wise approach based on brain morphometry [1]. These voxel-wise approaches give high-dimensional feature vectors which have led to the exploration of feature selection methods for reducing dimensionality and improving performance [1,2].

For the support vector machine (SVM) classifier, a significance map (p-map) can be calculated that shows the regions that consistently influence the classification. In previous work, we showed that these p-maps find clusters of significantly

G. Wu et al. (Eds.): MLMI 2014, LNCS 8679, pp. 272–279, 2014.

different voxels in regions known to be involved in dementia [3]. Based on this, we propose a novel method for feature selection based on these SVM p-maps. The feature selection method is purely data-driven and is from a methodological point of view closely linked to the SVM classifier, giving it a clear interpretation.

Feature selection using SVM p-maps has not been applied before, probably because SVM p-map computation with permutation testing is time-consuming. Instead, we use a fast recently published method for analytic computation [4]. In this work, we validate this feature selection method in a classification experiment of AD, mild cognitive impairment (MCI) and CN based on T1-weighted MR scans and compare it to other feature selection methods.

2   Methods

2.1   Support Vector Machine

SVMs are frequently used for classification in medical imaging including computer-aided diagnosis [1,5,6]. This classifier is based on maximization of the margin around the hyperplane $(\boldsymbol{w}^T\boldsymbol{x} + b)$ that separates samples of the different classes. Each sample $i = 1, ..., m$ consists of an N-dimensional feature vector $\boldsymbol{x}_i$ and a class label $y_i \in \{+1, -1\}$. The maximization of the margin corresponds to:

$$\boldsymbol{w}^*, b^*, \boldsymbol{\xi}^* = \arg\min_{\boldsymbol{w},b,\boldsymbol{\xi}} \frac{1}{2}||\boldsymbol{w}||^2 + C\sum_{i=1}^{m}\xi_i \tag{1}$$

$$s.t. \quad y_i(\boldsymbol{w}^T\boldsymbol{x}_i + b) \geq 1 - \xi_i; \quad \xi_i \geq 0; \quad i = 1, ..., m$$

In this soft-margin SVM, ξ_i is a penalty for misclassification or classification within the margin. Parameter C sets the weight of this penalty. The resulting weight vector $\boldsymbol{w}^*$ encodes the contributions of all features to the classifier.

2.2   SVM Significance Map

The significance value (p-value) is a quantification of how significant the contribution of each feature to the SVM classifier is. To obtain the p-values, permutation testing is needed to estimate a null distribution on the weight vector $(\boldsymbol{w})$ [5,6]. For permutation testing however, a large number of SVM classifiers needs to be trained making it very time-consuming for high-dimensional feature vectors.

A faster solution for permutation testing is presented by *Gaonkar et al.* [4] who derived an analytic approximation of the null distribution of $\boldsymbol{w}$. For this approximation, the SVM classifier is simplified by making two assumptions. First, under the assumption that the classes are separable which is true if many features and a relatively small number of samples are used, the soft-margin SVM can be simplified by using a hard-margin SVM, which does not use the misclassification penalties ξ_i. Second, under the assumption that for most permutations most samples will be support vectors, the hard-margin SVM can be further simplified to a least-squares SVM, which has a closed-form solution $\boldsymbol{w} = \boldsymbol{K}\boldsymbol{y}$, with:

$$\boldsymbol{K} = \boldsymbol{X}^T[(\boldsymbol{X}\boldsymbol{X}^T)^{-1} + (\boldsymbol{X}\boldsymbol{X}^T)^{-1}\boldsymbol{J}(-\boldsymbol{J}^T(\boldsymbol{X}\boldsymbol{X}^T)^{-1}\boldsymbol{J})^{-1}\boldsymbol{J}^T(\boldsymbol{X}\boldsymbol{X}^T)^{-1}] \tag{2}$$

where $\boldsymbol{J}$ is a column matrix of ones and the matrix $\boldsymbol{X}$ contains one feature vector in each row. Given a sufficiently high number of subjects, the probability density function of every feature (j) can be approximated with a Gaussian distribution:

$$w_j \overset{d}{\to} \mathcal{N}\left((2q-1)\sum_{i=1}^{m}K_{ij}, (4q-4q^2)\sum_{i=1}^{m}K_{ij}^2\right) \tag{3}$$

where q is the fraction of the data with class label $y_i = +1$. A p-value for each feature is obtained by testing $\boldsymbol{w}^*$ against the analytic null distribution in (3). As every feature is a voxel, the p-values can be combined into a p-map image. The experiments of *Gaonkar et al.* [4] show that p-maps obtained with this approximation are very similar to those obtained with permutation testing.

2.3   P-Map for Feature Selection

In this work, we propose to perform feature selection based on the p-map. Since the p-map provides information on which features contribute most to the classifier, feature selection based on this p-map is expected to reduce features in a meaningful way. Intuitively, using such an SVM-based feature selection method prior to SVM-based classification is an attractive approach, as in this way the feature selection and the classification use the same multivariate decision model on the same training data. Since the p-map can be used for feature selection in a non-iterative way, it is more efficient than some other feature selection methods (e.g. recursive feature elimination based on $\boldsymbol{w}^*$ [2]).

For feature selection, the p-map is calculated for the training set using the efficient method described in section 2.2. All features with a p-value below $\alpha = 0.05$ are selected. Given the low false positive detection rate of permutation testing, no further correction for multiple comparisons is performed [4]. After feature selection, a linear hard-margin SVM classifier is trained and tested.

3   Experiments

3.1   Data

Data from the Alzheimer's disease Neuroimaging Initiative (ADNI) was used. The cohort is adopted from [1] and consists of AD patients, MCI patients that converted to AD within 18 months (MCIc), MCI patients that did not convert to AD within 18 months (MCInc), and CN. The participants were 137 AD patients (67 male, age: 76.0 ± 7.3 yrs, MMSE: 23.2 ± 2.0), 76 MCIc (43 male, 74.8 ± 7.4 yrs, MMSE: 26.5 ± 1.9), 134 MCInc (84 male, 74.5 ± 7.2 yrs, MMSE: 27.2 ± 1.7), and 162 CN (76 male, 76.3 ± 5.4 yrs, MMSE: 29.2 ± 1.0). T1w imaging was acquired at 1.5T with a voxel size of ~1mm^3 [7].

3.2   Image Processing

Probabilistic tissue segmentations were obtained for white matter, gray matter (GM) and cerebrospinal fluid using SPM8 (Statistical Parametric Mapping, UK).

For construction of a template space, the coordinate transformations from the template space to the subject's space were derived from pairwise image registration [8] of a subset of 150 T1w images (81 CN, 69 AD [1]). We performed pairwise registrations with consecutively a rigid (including isotropic scaling), affine, and non-rigid B-spline transformation model. The non-rigid B-spline registration used a three-level multi-resolution framework with isotropic control-point spacing of 24, 12, and 6 mm at the three resolutions respectively. A template image was created by averaging the deformed individual images. To transform the other subjects' images to template space, coordinate transformations were derived from pairwise registrations to the subset. The registrations to the template space were visually inspected to check if they were correct.

3.3   Classification

For classification [9], features were based on voxel-based morphometry, which means that we use GM probabilistic segmentations in the template space that are modulated by the Jacobian determinant of the deformation field. To correct for head size, the features were divided by intracranial volume. The features were normalized to zero mean and unit variance.

Four classification settings were defined: 1) AD-CN, 2) AD-MCI, 3) MCI-CN, and 4) MCIc-MCInc. For each setting, classification performance was quantified by the accuracy and the area under the ROC-curve (AUC) with two-fold cross-validation. The cross-validation was iterated 100 times with random splits of the participants into a training and test set of the same size while preserving class priors. We tested differences between classifiers with a paired t-test. To address the robustness of the classification, the coefficient of variation (CV) was calculated, which is the standard deviation of performance divided by the mean.

The visualization of the selected features was based on one specific training and test set in which the age and sex distributions were preserved [1]. To identify clusters of features selected by the p-map method, visual inspection was performed by counting the number of selected features in every atlas region [10] after removal of the smallest clusters by morphological opening.

3.4   Experimental Set-Up

We compared 4 classifiers: I) Classification on all features (No feature selection), II) proposed p-map feature selection (P-map), III) univariate t-test for each voxel ($\alpha = 0.05$, T-test), and IV) ROI selection based on expert knowledge (ROI).

For IV), the following ROIs were included (Figure 1) [2]: 1) Cingulate gyrus (CG), 2) Hippocampus including amygdala (HC), 3) Parahippocampal gyrus (PHG), 4) Fusiform gyrus (FG), 5) Superior parietal gyrus (SPG), 6) Middle/inferior temporal gyrus (MITG), 7) Temporal lobe (TL) including FG and MITG, 8) HC + PHG, and 9) TL + HC + PHG. The ROIs were segmented with a multi-atlas segmentation for every subject individually and subsequently transformed to template space. The labels were fused using majority voting. For the individual multi-atlas segmentations, 30 labeled T1w images containing 83

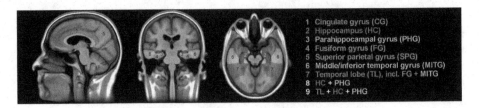

Fig. 1. ROIs for feature selection based on previous knowledge, adapted from [2]

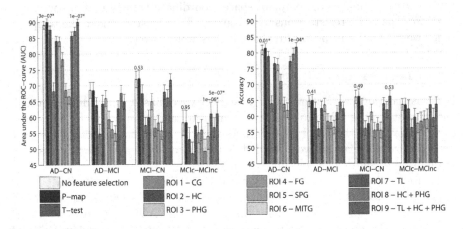

Fig. 2. Classification performance: the separate panels show mean and standard deviation of AUC and accuracy over 100 cross-validations. Paired t-test p-values are shown for results better than classification without feature selection, marked by * if significant.

ROIs each were used [10]. The atlas images were registered to the subjects image using a rigid, affine, and non-rigid B-spline transformation model consecutively.

For each cross-validation run with feature selection (II-IV), features were selected based on the training set. Using the selected features, an SVM was trained on the training set and applied to the test set.

3.5 Results

Fig. 2 shows the classification performances for the original classification without feature selection (white bars) and the different feature selection methods. For the AD-CN and MCI-CN classification settings, the mean AUC of the p-map method (black bars) is slightly higher than that of the original classification. On average the improvement in AUC is 0.2%. For all classification settings except MCIc-MCInc, the p-map method improves accuracy. The t-test method (blue bars) never improves performance. For the p-map and t-test methods, all differences with the original classification are rather small. The AUC of the p-map method was on average 4.3% higher than that of the t-test method. The performances of the ROI selection methods vary. The best performing ROI,

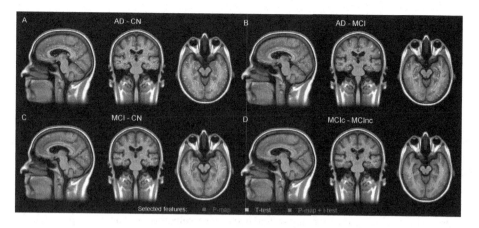

Fig. 3. A cross-section of the template space image showing features that are selected by the p-map method (red), t-test method (blue), or both methods (purple)

Table 1. Coefficient of variation (CV) defined for the AUC and the Accuracy as the standard deviation divided by the mean. *Original* shows the classification without feature selection. The CVs in the green cells are smaller than without feature selection.

Groups	Original	P-map	T-test	ROI1 CG	ROI2 HC	ROI3 PHG	ROI4 FG	ROI5 SPG	ROI6 MITG	ROI7 TL	ROI8 HC+ PHG	ROI9 TL+HC +PHG
CV [%] for Area under the curve (AUC)												
AD-CN	**1.4**	1.3	1.5	3.9	1.7	1.8	3.0	3.6	3.6	1.7	1.4	1.2
AD-MCI	**3.7**	3.8	4.9	3.9	3.9	4.9	5.7	5.3	3.6	3.7	3.4	4.0
MCI-CN	**3.7**	3.5	4.2	4.6	3.9	4.1	4.1	4.7	5.1	3.4	3.9	2.9
MCIc-MCInc	**6.9**	6.7	7.2	7.7	5.6	6.7	7.1	7.8	7.5	5.7	6.1	5.9
CV [%] for Accuracy												
AD-CN	**1.9**	1.8	2.0	3.7	2.2	2.5	3.5	4.1	4.0	2.2	2.2	1.9
AD-MCI	**2.7**	2.9	4.1	3.5	3.6	4.1	3.9	3.9	3.1	3.5	3.4	3.2
MCI-CN	**3.2**	3.5	3.7	4.0	3.7	3.4	4.0	4.0	4.7	3.4	4.2	3.0
MCIc-MCInc	**3.0**	3.3	4.5	5.5	4.3	5.4	5.0	4.8	5.0	3.7	4.9	3.6

which consists of the hippocampus, parahippocampal gyrus and the temporal lobe (ROI 9), improves AUC in three and accuracy in two settings.

The paired t-test shows that the p-map method and ROI 9 gave a significantly better performance than classification without feature selection in the AD-CN setting (Fig. 2). For the MCIc-MCInc, the AUC is significantly improved by two ROI methods that include the temporal lobe. The p-map is the only feature selection method that never significantly decreases classification performance. In addition, the performance differences between the p-map and the t-test methods were significant in all settings as tested with the paired t-test ($p < 0.001$). The p-map feature selection took on average 10 minutes (range: 6-13 min) and is performed once for every training set.

The most robust methods were (Table 1): no feature selection, p-map feature selection, and ROI9. In all settings except MCI-CN, the CV of AUC of latter two was slightly smaller than using no feature selection.

Table 2. Regions containing main clusters of features selected with the p-map method

AD-CN	AD-MCI	MCI-CN	MCIc-MCInc
Hippocampus	Hippocampus	Hippocampus	Mid./inf. temporal gyrus
Parahippocampal gyrus	Parahippocampal gyrus	Parahippocampal gyrus	Superior parietal gyrus
Lateral occipital lobe	Lateral occipital lobe	Lateral occipital lobe	Fusiform gyrus
Thalamus	Thalamus	Insula	Frontal gyri
	Mid./inf. temporal gyrus	Cingulate gyrus	Anterior orbital gyrus
	Superior parietal gyrus	Caudate nucleus	Remainder parietal lobe
	Frontal gyri	Mid./inf. temporal gyrus	Remainder temporal lobe

From the $1.4 \cdot 10^6$ features, the p-map method selected a substantially smaller subset: the mean number of selected features over 100 iterations in four settings was $5.5 \cdot 10^4$. The t-test method selected on average $1.1 \cdot 10^5$ features. An overview of features selected by the p-map and t-test method is shown in Fig. 3. Table 2 lists the regions in which most features were selected by the p-map method. Except for MCIc-MCInc, we found the most clusters of selected features in the hippocampus, parahippocampal gyrus, lateral occipital lobe and thalamus.

4 Conclusion and Discussion

We proposed feature selection using SVM significance maps and compared this method to classification using no feature selection, and feature selection based on t-tests and expert knowledge ROIs. The proposed method yielded in most cases a similar or higher performance than using no feature selection.

Chu et al. [2] concluded that feature selection only improves performance if expert knowledge is used. For the AD-CN and MCI-CN settings, our accuracies without feature selection were similar to those of Chu et al. Both studies found that selecting the temporal lobe, hippocampus and parahippocampal gyrus (ROI 9) slightly improved performance. Our p-map selection method showed an improvement similar to that of ROI 9, which was significant for AD-CN. The p-map method never significantly decreased performance. It should be noted that the performance improvements compared to using no feature selection were modest.

Atrophy of the hippocampus (including amygdala) and parahippocampal gyrus is well known to play an important role in AD [11,12,13]. Additionally, atrophy in the cingulate gyri [12,13,14], caudate nucleus [11,12], insula [11,12], thalamus [11,14], superior parietal gyrus (precuneus) [12,14], temporal gyri [12,14] and frontal cortex [12] were reported in AD and MCI. These regions correspond very well to the regions in which the p-map method selected clusters of voxels (Table 2). Two exceptions are: 1) the p-map method found features in the lateral occipital lobe, which have not previously been reported, and 2) although atrophy in the hippocampi and mediotemporal lobe is also considered a predictor for conversion of MCI patients to AD [11], this was not identified by the p-map feature selection in the MCIc-MCInc setting. For the regions found with the p-map method, the main difference between the four classification settings was how clustered the selected voxels are to specific regions. For the AD-CN classification, the selected features were very clustered to specific regions, while for the other settings the selected features were more spread over the temporal, frontal and parietal lobes. We conclude that the overall correspondence between the findings and the literature confirms the validity of the p-map method.

A future direction of this work is to investigate the influence of the selection threshold (α) and its optimal setting. In addition, we will compare other feature selection methods, i.e. randomized t-tests and recursive feature elimination [2].

In conclusion, we presented a feature selection method that in most cases showed a slight improvement in classification performance and robustness. Three advantages of this p-map method are that: 1) the reduction of the number of features never decreases performance, 2) without using expert knowledge the method selects features in regions corresponding to those previously implicated in AD and MCI, and 3) processing time may be drastically reduced because the method is fast as feature selection takes only 10 minutes and the classification is performed on a smaller feature set.

References

1. Cuingnet, R., Gerardin, E., Tessieras, J., et al.: Automatic classification of patients with Alzheimer's disease from structural MRI: A comparison of ten methods using the ADNI database. Neuroimage 56(2), 766–781 (2011)
2. Chu, C., Hsu, A., Chou, K., et al.: Does feature selection improve classification accuracy? Impact of sample size and feature selection on classification using anatomical magnetic resonance images. Neuroimage 60, 59–70 (2012)
3. Bron, E., Steketee, R., et al.: Diagnostic classification of arterial spin labeling and structural MRI in presenile early stage dementia. Hum. Brain Mapp. 35(9) (2014)
4. Gaonkar, B., Davatzikos, C.: Analytic estimation of statistical significance maps for support vector machine based multi-variate image analysis and classification. Neuroimage 78, 270–283 (2013)
5. Mourão Miranda, J., Bokde, A.L.W., Born, C., et al.: Classifying brain states and determining the discriminating activation patterns: Support Vector Machine on functional MRI data. Neuroimage 28(4), 980–995 (2005)
6. Wang, Z., Childress, A.R., Wang, J., Detre, J.A.: Support vector machine learning-based fMRI data group analysis. Neuroimage 36(4), 1139–1151 (2007)
7. Jack, C., Bernstein, M., Fox, N., et al.: The Alzheimer's Disease Neuroimaging Initiative (ADNI): MRI methods. J. Magn. Reson. Imaging 27(4), 685–691 (2008)
8. Seghers, D., D'Agostino, E., Maes, F., Vandermeulen, D., Suetens, P.: Construction of a brain template from MR images using state-of-the-art registration and segmentation techniques. In: Barillot, C., Haynor, D.R., Hellier, P. (eds.) MICCAI 2004. LNCS, vol. 3216, pp. 696–703. Springer, Heidelberg (2004)
9. Chang, C.C., Lin, C.J.: LIBSVM: A library for support vector machines. ACM TIST 2(3), 27 (2011)
10. Gousias, I., Rueckert, D., Heckemann, R., et al.: Automatic segmentation of brain MRIs of 2-year-olds into 83 regions of interest. Neuroimage 40, 672–684 (2008)
11. Bastos Leite, A., Scheltens, P., Barkhof, F.: Pathological aging of the brain: an overview. Top Magn. Reson. Imaging 15(6), 369–389 (2004)
12. Frisoni, G., et al.: Detection of grey matter loss in mild Alzheimer's disease with voxel based morphometry. J. Neurol. Neurosurg. Psychiatry 73, 657–664 (2002)
13. Chételat, G., et al.: Mapping gray matter loss with voxel-based morphometry in mild cognitive impairment. Neuroreport 13, 1939–1943 (2002)
14. Pennanen, C., Testa, C., Laakso, M.P., et al.: A voxel based morphometry study on mild cognitive impairment. J. Neurol. Neurosurg Psychiatry 76(1), 11–14 (2005)

Prediction of Standard-Dose PET Image by Low-Dose PET and MRI Images

Jiayin Kang, Yaozong Gao, Yao Wu, Guangkai Ma,
Feng Shi, Weili Lin, and Dinggang Shen

Department of Radiology and BRIC, University of North Carolina at Chapel Hill

Abstract. Positron emission tomography (PET) is a nuclear medical imaging technology that produces 3D images of tissue metabolic activity in human body. PET has been used in various clinical applications, such as diagnosis of tumors and diffuse brain disorders. High quality PET image plays an essential role in diagnosing diseases/disorders and assessing the response to therapy. In practice, in order to obtain the high quality PET images, standard-dose radionuclide (tracer) needs to be used and injected into the living body. As a result, it will inevitably increase the risk of radiation. In this paper, we propose a regression forest (RF) based framework for predicting standard-dose PET images using low-dose PET and corresponding magnetic resonance imaging (MRI) images instead of injecting the standard-dose radionuclide into the body. The proposed approach has been evaluated on a dataset consisting of 7 subjects using leave-one-out cross-validation. Moreover, we compare the prediction performance between sparse representation (SR) based method and our proposed method. Both qualitative and quantitative results illustrate the practicability of our proposed method.

1 Introduction

Positron emission tomography (PET) is a molecular imaging technique which produces 3D images reflecting tissue metabolic activity in human body. Since developed in the early 1970s, PET has been widely used in oncology for diagnosing a variety of cancers [1]. Moreover, it was also widely used for clinically diagnosing brain disorders [2], monitoring the therapy response and guiding the treatment planning in radiation therapy [3].

High-quality PET image plays an essential role in diagnosing diseases/disorders and assessing the response to therapy. However, due to the constraint on injected radioactivity, low-dose PET images are widely obtained in clinical applications with a compromised quality in comparison to those of the standard-dose PET images. Moreover, the quality of low-dose PET image will be further decreased due to various factors during the process of acquisition, transmission and reconstruction. Consequently, it will affect the accurate diagnosis of diseases/disorders. In practice, in order to obtain the high quality PET images, standard-dose radionuclide (tracer) needs to be used and injected into the living body. As a result, it will inevitably increase the risk of radiation and also lengthen the imaging time.

G. Wu et al. (Eds.): MLMI 2014, LNCS 8679, pp. 280–288, 2014.

Although many methods have been proposed for improving the PET image quality, most of them focused on low-dose/standard-dose PET itself, such as partial volume correction, motion volume correction [3]. To the best of our knowledge, no previous studies have been reported to predict standard-dose PET image by using low-dose PET and MRI images.

In this paper, we propose a regression-forest-based framework for predicting standard-dose PET image using both low-dose PET and MRI images. Our method mainly consists of **two steps**: **1)** the prediction of initial standard-dose PET image by tissue-specific regression forests with image appearance features from both low-dose PET and MRI images; **2)** incremental refinement of the predicted standard-dose PET image by iteratively estimating the image difference between the current prediction and the target standard-dose PET. By incrementally adding the estimated image difference towards the target standard-dose PET, our proposed method is able to gradually improve the quality of predicted standard-dose PET. Fig. 1 gives a flowchart of our method.

The reminder of the paper is organized as follows: Section 2 briefly introduces the regression forest, followed by the elaboration of our proposed method in two steps. Then, Section 3 presents both qualitative and quantitative results of our method, and also compares it with the sparse representation technique. Finally, Section 4 presents the conclusion.

2 Method

As aforementioned, our method consists of two major steps, initial standard-dose PET prediction and incremental refinement. Both steps adopt regression forest as the non-linear prediction model. In this section, we will first briefly introduce the regression forest. Then, we will explain the two steps in detail.

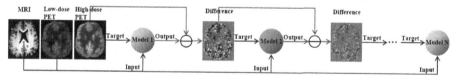

Fig. 1. The flowchart of our proposed framework

2.1 Regression Forest

Random forest [4] consists of multiple binary decision trees, with each tree trained independently with random features and thresholds. The final prediction of a random forest is the average over the predictions of all its individual trees. As an ensemble method, it has recently gained much popularity on both classification and regression problems [5,6]. Note that, when applied to the non-linear regression task, random forest is often called as regression forest.

Similar to other supervised models, the use of regression forest consists of both training and testing stages. **In the training stage**, given a set of training data

$\{(\mathbf{f}_i, t_i) | i = 1, \cdots, N\}$, where $\mathbf{f}_i$ and t_i indicate the feature vector and regression target of the i-th training sample, regression forest aims to learn a non-linear model for predicting the target t based on the input features $\mathbf{f}$. In the regression forest, each binary decision tree is trained independently. A decision tree consists of two types of nodes, namely split nodes (non-leaf nodes) and leaf nodes. The split node is often associated with a decision stump function $g(\mathbf{f}|j, \theta) = \pi_j(\mathbf{f}) \leq \theta$, where $\pi_j(\mathbf{f})$ indicates the response of the j-th feature in the input feature vector $\mathbf{f}$, and θ is a threshold. The optimal combination of feature j and threshold θ is learned by maximizing the average variance decrease in each dimension of the regression target after splitting. The leaf node stores the average regression target of training samples falling into this node. The training of decision tree starts with finding the optimal split at the root node, and recursively proceeds on child nodes until either the maximum tree depth is reached or the number of training samples is too small to split. **In the testing stage**, a new testing sample is pushed through each learned decision tree, starting at the root node. At each split node, the associated decision stump function is applied to the testing sample. If the result is false, then this testing sample is sent to the left child; otherwise, it is sent to the right child. Once the testing sample reaches a leaf node, the average regression target stored in that leaf node will be taken as the output of this binary decision tree. The final prediction value of the entire forest is the average of outputs from all decision trees.

2.2   Prediction of Initial Standard-Dose PET Image by Tissue-specific Regression Forests

Due to large volume of human brain (e.g., usually with millions of image voxels), it is difficult to learn a global regression model for accurately predicting the standard-dose PET image over the entire brain. Many studies [7] have shown that learning multiple local models would improve the prediction performance compared with a single global model. Therefore, in this paper we learn one regression forest for each brain tissue, i.e., white matter (WM), gray matter (GM) and cerebrospinal fluid (CSF). Since the appearance variation within each brain tissue is much less than that across different brain tissues, our tissue-specific regression forest can yield more accurate predictions than a global regression forest model (trained for the entire brain). As similar to most learning-based methods, the proposed method consists of training stage and testing stage as follows:

In the training stage, our training data consists of MRI, low-dose PET, and standard-dose PET from different training patients (or called as training subjects). Each training subject has MRI image, low-dose PET image and the corresponding standard-dose PET image. Before learning the tissue-specific regression forests, the three images of all training subjects are linearly aligned onto a common space by FLIRT [8]. Then, a brain segmentation method [9] is adopted to segment the brain region into WM, GM and CSF for each training subject based on the respective MRI image. To train the regression forest for one tissue type, we first randomly sample a set of points $\{(\mathbf{f}_i, t_i) | i = 1, \cdots, N\}$

within this tissue region for every training subject. For the i-th point/sample at position $v \in \mathbb{R}^3$, we extract the local intensity patches from both MRI and low-dose PET images centered at position v for serving as the input features $\mathbf{f}_i$ in the regression forest. The voxel intensity of the corresponding standard-dose PET image at the position v is taken as the regression target t_i. In this way, we can learn three tissue-specific regression forests in the training stage, which will be in charge of predicting standard-dose PET image within their respective tissue region.

In the Testing Stage, given a testing subject with both MRI and low-dose PET, we first linearly align these MRI and low-dose PET images onto the common space (as defined in the training stage) by using FLIRT [8], and automatically segment the MRI image into three brain tissues by [9]. Then, the standard-dose PET image can be predicted in a voxel-wise manner by using the local image appearance information from the aligned MRI and low-dose PET images. Specifically, for each voxel in the unknown standard-dose PET image, we can extract the local intensity patches at the same location from both MRI and low-dose PET images. Based on the extracted intensity patches and the tissue label at this location, we can apply the corresponding tissue-specific regression forest to predict the standard-dose PET value for this voxel. By iterating all image voxels, a standard-dose PET image can be predicted.

2.3   Incremental Refinement by Image Difference Estimation

Motivated by the success of ensemble models [4], we further propose an incremental refinement framework for iteratively improving the quality of the predicted standard-dose PET image. To accomplish this, we learn a sequence of tissue-specific regression forests for gradually minimizing the image difference between the predicted and the target standard-dose PET images during the training stage. In particular, the tissue-specific regression forests at iteration k aims to estimate the image difference between the predicted standard-dose PET image by the previous k-1 iterations and the target standard-dose PET image.

Similar to training tissue-specific regression forests (as described in the above Subsection 2.2) for predicting initial standard-dose PET image, we first randomly sample a set of training samples/points $\{(\mathbf{f}_i, t_i^{diff}) | i = 1, \cdots, N\}$ within each tissue region for every training subject. Specifically, for the i-th sample/point at position $v \in \mathbb{R}^3$, we extract the local intensity patches from both MRI and low-dose PET images centered at position v for serving as the input features $\mathbf{f}_i$ in the regression forest; The voxel value of the real difference map (computed between ground truth and standard-dose PET image predicted in previous step)at the position v is taken as the regression target t_i^{diff}. In this way, we can learn three tissue-specific regression forests during the training stage, which will be in charge of predicting (estimating) the image difference within their respective tissue region. By adding the estimated image difference on top of previously predicted standard-dose PET image, the new updated prediction could be closer to the target standard-dose PET image, thus improving the prediction accuracy.

In the testing stage, given a new testing subject with MRI and low-dose PET images, the learned tissue-specific regression forests can be applied sequentially to obtain a final predicted standard-dose PET image. Specifically, in the first iteration, only the technique described in Section 2.2 is adopted to predict an initial standard-dose PET image. Then, the tissue-specific regression forests in the next iterations will be used to sequentially estimate the image difference between the current prediction and the target standard-dose PET image. The estimated image differences by the later regression forests will be sequentially added onto the initially predicted standard-dose PET image for incremental refinement. As will be validated in the experiments, our proposed incremental refinement framework can further boost the prediction accuracy of tissue-specific regression forests.

3   Experimental Results

Data Description: Our method was evaluated on a dataset consisting of 7 subjects. Each subject has three images: MRI, low-dose PET, and standard-dose PET. After aligned onto the PET image space, each image has the size of $344 \times 344 \times 127$, and the voxel size of $2.09 \times 2.09 \times 2.03 \text{mm}^3$. It is worth noting that for each subject, the low-dose PET sets are the completely separate acquisitions from the standard-dose PET sets, and the low-dose PET are 180-second reconstructions whereas the standard-dose PET are 720-second reconstructions.

Preprocessing: All images were preprocessed by following steps. **1)** *Linear alignment*: three images (MRI, low-dose PET, and standard-dose PET) of each subject were linearly aligned onto a common space; **2)** *Skull stripping*: non-brain parts were removed from the aligned images; **3)** *Intensity normalization*: each modality image was normalized via histogram matching; **4)** *Tissue segmentation*: WM, GM and CSF were segmented from each skull-stripped MR image.

Parameter Setting: In this paper, we choose the following parameters for all experiments—patch size: $9 \times 9 \times 9$; the number of trees in a forest: 10; the number of randomly selected features: 1000; the maximum tree depth: 15; the minimum number of samples at each leaf: 5; and the number of iterations in incremental refinement: 2.

For the purpose of evaluating our proposed method, a leave-one-out cross-validation method was adopted in our experiments. In each cross-validation step, six of seven subjects were used to build the prediction models, and the remaining one subject was used as the testing image to be predicted by the learned models.

Fig 2 presents the qualitative results of our method on two subjects, and also compares our proposed method with sparse representation technique [10]. Similar to our method, sparse representation technique can also be adopted to voxel-wisely predict the standard-dose PET image by utilizing information from both MRI and low-dose PET images. In the sparse representation technique, to estimate the standard-dose PET intensity t for a voxel $v \in \mathbb{R}^3$, a sparse coefficient $\boldsymbol{\alpha}_v$ needs to be first computed by solving the following problem:

$$\min_{\boldsymbol{\alpha}_v \geq 0} \frac{1}{2} \|D_v \boldsymbol{\alpha}_v - \mathbf{f}(v)\|_2^2 + \lambda_1 \|\boldsymbol{\alpha}_v\|_1 + \frac{\lambda_2}{2} \|\boldsymbol{\alpha}_v\|_2^2, \tag{1}$$

where $\mathbf{f}(v)$ is the feature vector of voxel v, defined as the vector of concatenated intensity of local patches from both MRI and low-dose PET; $\boldsymbol{\alpha}_v$ is the sparse coefficient of voxel v to be estimated; D_v is the dictionary of voxel v, consisting of feature vectors of voxels within a small neighborhood of voxel v in all training subjects; λ_1 and λ_2 control the sparsity and smoothness of the estimated sparse coefficient $\boldsymbol{\alpha}_v$. Once $\boldsymbol{\alpha}_v$ is obtained, it can be used as weights to average the corresponding voxel intensities in the standard-dose PET training images for prediction. For fair comparison, we optimize both λ_1 and λ_2 for the best performance of the sparse representation technique. In the experiments, λ_1 and λ_2 are set to be 0.1 and 0.01, respectively. The neighborhood size is set to $5 \times 5 \times 5$, and the patch size is set to $9 \times 9 \times 9$.

From Fig. 2, we can see that our proposed method (RF) achieves more accurate predictions than sparse representation technique (SR) (i.e., with smaller difference magnitudes and more similar image appearance with the ground-truth). The limited prediction accuracy of sparse representation might be due to two reasons: 1) both MRI and low-dose PET modalities are treated equally in the sparse representation; 2) only linear prediction models are adopted, which might be insufficient to capture the complex relationship among MRI, low-dose PET, and standard-dose PET images. In contrast, our proposed method adopts regression forest to simultaneously identify informative features from MRI and low-dose PET images for standard-dose PET image prediction, and learn the non-linear relationship among MRI, low-dose PET and standard-dose PET images.

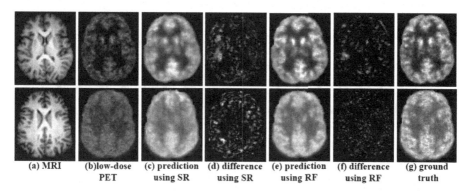

| (a) MRI | (b)low-dose PET | (c) prediction using SR | (d) difference using SR | (e) prediction using RF | (f) difference using RF | (g) ground truth |

Fig. 2. Comparison between sparse representation (SR) and our proposed method (RF) on two different subjects as shown in the first and second rows, respectively

To quantitatively evaluate the quality of predicted standard-dose PET images, we adopt two commonly used metrics, normalized mean squared error (NMSE) and peak signal-to-noise ratio (PSNR), which are defined as:

$$\text{NMSE} = \frac{\|H - \hat{H}\|_2^2}{\|H\|_2^2}, \quad \text{PSNR} = 10\log_{10}(\frac{L^2}{\frac{1}{M}\|H - \hat{H}\|_2^2}) \tag{2}$$

where H is the ground-truth standard-dose PET image, $\hat{H}$ is the predicted standard-dose PET image, L is the maximal intensity range of images H and $\hat{H}$, and M is the total number of voxels in the image. In general, a good algorithm provides lower NMSE and higher PSNR.

Table 1 and Fig. 3 quantitatively compare the sparse representation technique (SR) with our proposed method using one iteration (Model1) and two iterations (Model1+Model2). In order to demonstrate the improvement of predicted standard-dose PET image over the low-dose PET image, we also calculate the NMSE and PSNR for low-dose PET image with respect to the ground-truth.

Table 1. Performance comparison in terms of NMSE and PSNR (Note that $Model_{1+2}$ means Model1+Model2)

Sub. No.	Low-dose PET		SR		RF(Model1)		RF($Model_{1+2}$)	
	NMSE	PSNR	NMSE	PSNR	NMSE	PSNR	NMSE	PSNR
1	0.360	13.394	0.108	18.634	0.073	20.339	**0.058**	**20.797**
2	0.278	10.713	0.034	20.023	0.013	24.056	**0.010**	**24.875**
3	0.289	10.243	0.026	20.778	0.016	22.800	**0.013**	**23.456**
4	0.268	11.204	0.041	19.461	0.033	20.780	**0.030**	**21.176**
5	0.251	15.013	0.103	18.926	0.044	22.672	**0.038**	**22.900**
6	0.301	12.001	0.075	18.059	0.046	20.187	**0.040**	**20.308**
7	0.276	12.884	0.066	19.160	0.040	21.429	**0.034**	**22.009**
Mean	0.289	12.207	0.065	19.292	0.038	21.752	**0.032**	**22.217**

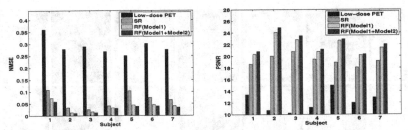

Fig. 3. Average NMSE and PSNR of 7 subjects using SR and proposed method (RF)

From Both Table 1 and Fig. 3, we can see that our method achieves better accuracy than the SR technique (with lower NMSE and higher PSNR). In addition, compared with NMSE and PSNR of low-dose PET images, our method is able to significantly improve the quality of original low-dose PET images.

Moreover, in order to illustrate the performance improvement by further using Model2, Fig. 4 gives a comparison between Model1 and Model1+Model2 on a sequence of voxels with maximal prediction errors using Model1. From Table 1 and Fig. 3, we can know that the overall performance for the entire brain is improved slightly by further using Model2. However, as shown in Fig. 4, for those

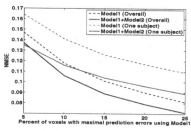
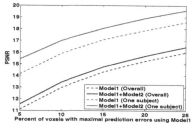

Fig. 4. Performance comparison between proposed Model1 and Model1+Model2. Blue lines denote for the results from all subjects, while red lines denote for the results from a selected subject.

voxels with maximal prediction errors by Model1, the performances by further using Model2 are improved obviously, especially for some subjects as shown in red lines in Fig. 4. The main reason for this phenomenon should be that for the most voxels in the brain, Model1 already achieves very good performance, thus affecting the calculation of overall improvement amount by Model2.

4   Conclusion

In this paper, we propose a regression-forest-based framework for predicting standard-dose PET images using low-dose PET and MRI images without increasing the radiation burden. Experimental results show that our proposed method can well predict brain standard-dose PET images. Moreover, the proposed method outperforms the sparse representation technique under comparison. This is the first time in the literature to show that standard-dose PET image can be predicted using low-dose PET and MRI images without directly injecting the standard-dose radionuclide into the living body. In our future work, we will include more subjects to further improve the prediction performance.

References

1. Rohren, E.M., Turkington, T.G., Coleman, R.E.: Clinical Applications of PET in Oncology. Radiology 231, 305–332 (2004)
2. Zhang, D., Wang, Y., Zhou, L., Yuan, H., Shen, D.: Multimodal Classification of Alzheimer's Disease and Mild Cognitive Impairment. NeuroImage 55, 856–867 (2011)
3. Bai, W., Brady, M.: Motion Correction and Attenuation Correction for Respiratory Gated PET Images. IEEE TMI 30, 351–365 (2011)
4. Breiman, L.: Random Forests. Machine Learning 45, 5–32 (2001)
5. Lindner, C., Thiagarajah, S., Wilkinson, J.M., arcOGEN Consortium, Wallis, G.A., Cootes, T.F.: Fully Automatic Segmentation of the Proximal Femur using Random Forest Regression Voting. IEEE TMI 32, 1462–1472 (2013)
6. Fanelli, G., Dantone, M., Gall, J., Fossati, A., Van Gool, L.: Random Forests for Real Time 3D Face Analysis. IJCV 101, 437–458 (2013)

7. Gao, Y., Liao, S., Shen, D.: Prostate Segmentation by Sparse Representation Based Classification. In: Ayache, N., Delingette, H., Golland, P., Mori, K. (eds.) MICCAI 2012, Part III. LNCS, vol. 7512, pp. 451–458. Springer, Heidelberg (2012)
8. Fischer, B., Modersitzki, J.: FLIRT: A Flexible Image Registration Toolbox. In: Gee, J.C., Maintz, J.B.A., Vannier, M.W. (eds.) WBIR 2003. LNCS, vol. 2717, pp. 261–270. Springer, Heidelberg (2003)
9. Zhang, Y., Brady, M., Smith, S.: Segmentation of Brain MR Images through a Hidden Markov Random Field Model and the Expectation-maximization Algorithm. IEEE TMI 20, 45–57 (2001)
10. Yang, J., Wright, J., Huang, T.S., Ma, Y.: Image Super-resolution via Sparse Representation. IEEE TIP 19, 2861–2873 (2010)

Solutions for Missing Parameters
in Computer-Aided Diagnosis
with Multiparametric Imaging Data

Hussam Al-Deen Ashab, Piotr Kozlowski, S. Larry Goldenberg,
and Mehdi Moradi*

University of British Columbia, Vancouver, BC, Canada
moradi@ece.ubc.ca

Abstract. Multiparametric MRI (mpMRI) is becoming widely used as
a means of determining the need for prostate biopsy and also for targeting prostate biopsies. One problem with the mpMRI approach is that not
all MRI modalities might be available for each patient. For example, the
use of gadolinium-based contrast agents in dynamic contrast enhanced
MRI (DCE-MRI) results in allergic reactions in some patients with reported reaction rates as high as 19.8% which results in missing DCE-MRI
parametric maps. The process of modifying a classifier to work on incom-
plete dataset is challenging and time consuming. This modification may
require a time consuming retraining or having multiple classifiers for each
missing data type. Therefore, the objective of the work presented here
is to develop an image-based classification technique for the detection
of prostate cancer with the capability of handling missing DCE parameters. We propose four different methods and show their effectiveness in
maintaining high Area Under Curve (AUC) while handling missing parameters without the requirement of any modifications to the classifier
models.

1 Introduction

Prostate cancer (PCa) is one of the leading causes of morbidity and mortality
for North American men with an estimated mortality rate of 33,620 deaths and
262,190 diagnosis in 2013 [1]. Prostate cancer diagnosis is confirmed by transrectal ultrasound (TRUS) guided biopsy, followed by histopathologic evaluation of
the extracted samples. While capable of delineating the prostate itself, due to
low image quality and low tumour contrast in B-mode images, TRUS has positive predictive values in the range of 30-60% [2]. To improve cancer detection
rates, researchers studied other imaging modalities extensively.

Magnetic resonance imaging (MRI) techniques such as diffusion weighted
imaging (DWI) and dynamic contrast-enhanced (DCE) MRI have shown to be
highly accurate for the detection and staging of PCa particularly when used
in combination [3–5]. This has elevated multiparametric MRI, which combines
DCE and diffusion MRI, and could include MR spectroscopy, to be the most
reliable imaging tool for prostate cancer detection [3]. Many researchers have

G. Wu et al. (Eds.): MLMI 2014, LNCS 8679, pp. 289–296, 2014.
© Springer International Publishing Switzerland 2014

used the combinations of the features extracted from these imaging modalities in a supervised machine learning framework [5–7].

However, the use of contrast agents in DCE MRI such as gadolinium-based contrast agents shows adverse reactions including headaches, nausea, unresponsiveness, and cardiopulmonary arrest in a relatively small group of patients. The reaction rate is reported to be as high as 19.8% [8] for different types of gadolinium-based contrast agents. Additionally, Marckmann et al. [9] found that gadolinium-based contrast agents may play a causative role in nephrogenic systemic fibrosis (NSF). These reactions prevent the acquisition of DCE MRI data from some patients which will lead to missing DCE features and reducing cancer detection capability of the proposed methods. Therefore, in this work we aim to develop machine learning methods, to classify regions of interest of the tissue in prostate using the DCE and DTI data, with the capability to handle missing features from DCE MRI in some cases. The goal is to achieve high detection rate at least as good as using DTI data alone for classification when the DCE parameter maps are missing. We use the biopsy result as the reference label for the classified regions of interest. The developed frameworks can be applied to other imaging applications. For example, in the absence of mpMRI, different groups have used a combination of ultrasound methods such as B-mode, elastography, and contrast-enhanced Doppler to maximize the performance of ultrasound in prostate cancer imaging. An effective method for handling the missing parameters, without the need to build and train new classification models for every subset of features, could make such multiparametric methods accessible for institutions where one of these technologies is unavailable.

This paper is organized as follows: Section 2 describes the Materials and Methods used for handling missing features and description of the available data. In particular, it includes (2.1) Description of the available data and type of features used, (2.2) Description of the techniques used to handle missing features, (2.3) description of the approach to simulate the missing data and cross validation. Section 3 presents the results and discusses the experiments performed. Section 4 provides concluding remarks, and future work.

2   Materials and Methods

2.1   Data

DTI and DCE MRI data, at 3T, of patients (n = 29) with elevated prostate specific antigen (PSA) and/or palpable prostatic nodule (PSA range from 0.94 to 15 ng/mL) were used in this study. The data was obtained with the approval of the Research Ethics Board of the University of British Columbia with informed consent of the patients. All MRI examinations were performed on a 3T MRI scanner (Achieva, Philips Healthcare, Best, the Netherlands). DCE MRI was performed using a 3D T1-weighted (T1W) spoiled gradient echo sequence (TR/TE = 3.4/1.06 ms, flip angle = 15°, FOV = 24 cm, 256×163 matrix, 2 averages). The DCE data per slice consisted of 75 T1-weighted images (three pre-injection and 72 post-injection images) obtained at a temporal resolution of 10.6

s. The DTI data were processed off-line to calculate fractional anisotropy (FA) and average diffusivity $< D >$ values. DCE MRI data were processed off-line with software procedures developed in house using Matlab (Mathworks, Natick, MA, USA) and Igor Pro (WaveMetrics, Portland, OR, USA). Pharmacokinetic parameters: volume transfer constant, k^{trans}, fractional volume of extravascular extracellular space, v_e, and fractional plasma volume v_p were calculated by fitting the extended Kety model to the contrast agent concentration curves [10]. Fitting was carried out in every pixel of every slice within a region of interest (ROI) encompassing the prostate gland to generate maps of the pharmacokinetic parameters. Each ROI, constructed based on the location of a biopsy core, was represented by the five-dimensional feature vector $<$FA,D,k^{trans}, v_e, $v_p >$. These were the mean values of the corresponding parameters in all pixels within the ROI which represents one biopsy core. The dataset included 240 normal, and 29 cancerous ROIs. To map the biopsy locations to parametric maps we followed the methodology reported in both [5] and [6]. While we have designed methods, described below, for handling potentially missing DCE data, within this dataset all the five features were available for all ROIs.

2.2 Handling Missing Features

One simple approach to handling missing DCE data is to estimate the missing DCE features, from the nearest neighbors in the DTI space with available DCE data and replace the missing features with their estimations. We have tried this independently and in combination with voting and in combination with clustering and classification frameworks. An entirely different approach is the use of Bayesian likelihood ratio estimation which does not include the estimation of missing features. We have described these approaches in this section. This is followed by the description of the method used to compare the performance of these methods in handling missing DCE features in our dataset. In the descriptions below, all support vector machine (SVM) classifiers were built using the radial basis function (RBF) kernel.

KNN Imputation with SVM: In this approach, we trained one SVM classifier for mpMRI classification with the five features. We imputed the missing data using k-nearest-neighbourhood (KNN) approach. The KNN method finds the k nearest training samples in the DTI space based on Euclidean distance, to the data point with missing DCE data and imputes the DCE features for that data point with a weighted mean of the DCE features of the nearest neighbours. This approach practically fills in the missing values to enable using the same classifier on cases with missing DCE features. k was determined with cross-validations.

KNN Imputation with Majority Voting (MV) on Several Classifiers: In this approach, we trained nine different classifiers on the data. These were (we use the term multi-feature to refer to the classifier that uses all five features): 1) multi-feature SVM, 2) DTI-SVM, 3) DCE-SVM, 4) multi-feature quadratic classifier, 5) DCE quadratic classifier, 6) DTI quadratic classifier, 7) multi-feature linear classifier, 8) DCE linear classifier, and 9) DTI Linear classifier. Multi-feature classifiers were built using all mpMRI features, DTI classifiers were built using mpMRI DTI features (FA,$< D >$), and DCE classifier were built using DCE features (k^{trans}, v_e, v_p). The implementation of linear and quadratic classifiers were based on linear discriminant analysis (LDA) and quadratic discriminant analysis (QDA).

Given this pool of classifiers, there are a number of combining techniques to follow. The simplest is to choose the best performing classifier on the training data which does not guarantee the optimal performance on the test data set. Instead, we imputed the missing data using KNN approach and combined the results of nine classifiers by a majority voting mechanism to achieve a better performance.

KNN Imputation with Clustering and Selection: Another technique is the clustering and selection which was adopted from Kuncheva [11]. In clustering and selection, the training data is clustered and a separate classifier is trained on each cluster. The test samples are first assigned to one of the clusters based on distance from the center of the training clusters and then classified using the corresponding classifier. During the training phase, k-means clustering technique was followed (optimal $k = 3$), based on Euclidean distance. Then a leave-one-patient-out cross validation on the training data from the 28 patients were used to choose the best classifier performing in each cluster. In the testing phase, we used the best performing classifier in each cluster to assign the label to the test data belonging to each cluster.

Bayesian Likelihood Ratio Method: This approach is different entirely from the first three, in that it does not include estimation of the missing features. In this method, two separate SVM classifiers were fused. The first classifier (DTI-SVM) was built using DTI MRI features (FA, $< D >$) and the second classifier (DCE-SVM) using DCE MRI features (k^{trans}, v_e, v_p). Leave-one-patient-out cross-validation was performed for setting the parameters of each classifier. Those two classifiers were fused using the Bayesian likelihood ratio fusion technique [12]. In this method, a test sample is considered cancerous, if the decision rule in equation 1 below holds.

$$\frac{f_{cancer}^{DCE}(n_0)}{f_{normal}^{DCE}(n_0)} * \frac{f_{cancer}^{DTI}(n_0)}{f_{normal}^{DTI}(n_0)} \geq \frac{f_{cancer}^{DTI}(n)}{f_{normal}^{DTI}(n)} * \frac{f_{cancer}^{DCE}(n)}{f_{normal}^{DCE}(n)} \forall n = 1, ..., N \quad (1)$$

f_{cancer} and f_{normal} are the densities of tissue classification scores, estimated using Gaussian mixture models, output by DTI-SVM and DCE-SVM classifiers, N is the number of training samples, and n_0 is the query sample. In case of missing data, the corresponding likelihood ratio is equal to one. As a result, only the DTI classifier contributes to the decision.

2.3   Removing DCE Features and Cross-Validation to Compare the Four Approaches

In our data, all five parameters were available from all cases. We simulated the effect of missing DCE components of the feature vector by removing them from an increasing number (m) of cases (m = 1,....,29) in the test step. In each step, m patient cases were randomly chosen and their corresponding DCE features were removed from the test set of the leave-one-patient-out cross validation scheme. The cross validation was repeated 50 times for each value of m (in case of clustering and selection, and Majority voting the cross validation was repeated 29 times due to time constraints), with missing DCE features to get a robust estimate of the effect of missing DCE features on the classification outcome. Note that in the training step of each leave-one-patient-out iteration, DCE features from 28 cases were included.

3   Results and Discussion

We first report the results of our analysis without missing data. Fig 1 summarizes these results based on area under ROC curve (AUC). For SVM classifier, the top left graph shows the performance of DTI, DCE and DTI-DCE (multi-feature) classifiers. These have resulted in AUC of 0.91, 0.83 and 0.95. In comparison, when two separate SVMs are trained and the combined using the likelihood ratio method, the AUC is 0.92. The other three graphs show the performance of LDA and QDA for DCE, DTI, and DTI-DCE (multi-feature) combinations. In the DTI-DCE combination, the LDA and QDA result in an AUC of 0.93 and 0.91 respectively. The SVM was then used with the KNN method to test the drop of the classifier performance, based on the drop in AUC, with missing features as shown in Fig 2. The results of the KNN approach and the Likelihood ratio fusion approach were compared as shown in Fig 2. The cross-validation yielded a mean AUC of 0.95 using KNN imputation with SVM when DCE features of one patient were removed, showing almost no decline compared to the situation without missing data. It was noted that using $k = 8$ neighbours provided the best results based on the AUC. In other words, we found that if we have one case with missing DCE and if we estimate the DCE parameters of that case, as the average of the DCE parameters of its eight closest neighbors in the DTI space, we observe no decline in AUC. In a similar cross-validation, the likelihood ratio fusion method resulted in a mean AUC of 0.93 when DCE features of one patient were removed. As shown in Fig 2, as the number (m) of cases with missing DCE features was increased, the imputation technique performed consistently better than the DTI-SVM classifier (AUC=0.91). For the likelihood ratio method, the performance dropped below that of DTI-SVM for m=13.

As described above, we also considered majority voting with KNN to improve the performance of PCa detection. The KNN imputation was used to impute the missing data and then all the classifiers provide a decision regarding the test data. The class with majority vote was assigned to the test data. The cross-validation yielded a mean AUC of 0.95 using majority voting when DCE features of one

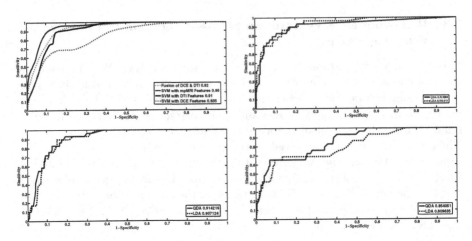

Fig. 1. ROCs and AUCs without missing features: (a) Top left - ROC curve of four classifier models. Likelihood ratio classifier that fuses two SVM classifiers DTI-SVM and DCE-SVM (green), multi-feature SVM which uses all five features (Blue) $< FA, D, k^{trans}, v_e, v_p >$, DTI-SVM (Black) that uses DTI features (FA, $< D >$), and DCE-SVM (Red) $< k^{trans}, v_e, v_p >$, (b) Top right - Quadratic classifier (blue) and Linear classifier (Dashed Black) using all five features, (c) Low left -Quadratic classifier (blue) and Linear classifier (Dashed Black) using DTI features and (d) Low right - Quadratic classifier (blue) and Linear classifier (Dashed Black) using DCE features.

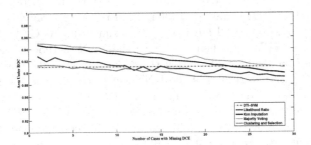

Fig. 2. AUC reduction as the number (m) of missing DCE cases increases for the four proposed methods: KNN with SVM, Likelihood Ratio fusion, majority voting with KNN imputation, and clustering and selection with KNN. The red dashed line marks the AUC of the DTI-SVM without missing data.

patient were removed, showing almost no decline compared to the situation without missing data. As the number (m) of cases with missing DCE features was increased, the fused classifiers performed consistently better than the DTI-SVM (AUC=0.91), for up to m=29 when all cases were removed as shown in Fig 2. Even though the majority voting method outperform the multi-features SVM with KNN imputation, it is more complicated and required the training of more than one classifier. In a similar cross-validation, the clustering and selection method resulted in a mean AUC of 0.91 when DCE features of one patient were removed. As shown in Fig 2, as the number (m) of cases with missing DCE features was increased, the fused classifiers performed better than the DTI-SVM (AUC=0.91), for up to m=2.

4   Conclusion

In this work, we reported several methods that successfully handle missing DCE features in computer-aided diagnosis using mpMRI. It is important to note that our effort towards avoiding the process of training and maintaining multiple classifiers is driven by the recent interest in multimodality methods. While the data in this work came from only two different MRI technologies, efforts for the simultaneous use of multiparametric ultrasound [13] and multiparametric MRI for prostate cancer imaging could introduce several new modalities.

We showed that as an increasing number of cases with missing DCE features are presented to the classifiers, KNN imputation of missing features outperforms the fusion of two classifiers using Bayesian likelihood ratio in terms of AUC. An interesting result was the good performance of the KNN imputation method. This method was able to impute the missing DCE features using SVM to consistently achieve a performance better than the DTI-SVM (AUC=0.91) for up to m=22 whereas the likelihood ratio fusion technique did not achieve as good performance as the KNN method. Moreover, we showed how using KNN imputation with majority voting outperform the use of KNN imputation alone or clustering and selection method. Majority voting method can handle missing data and achieve high detection performance at least as good as using DTI-SVM alone when all the DCE features were removed from the testing data. Even though the majority voting technique provides better performance than all the other techniques, it requires multiple classifiers built. It should be noted that the relatively low performance of the clustering and selection approach could be due to our choice of the number of clusters. We will work on optimizing this approach using cross-validation in an independent dataset.

It is curious that DCE features can be estimated from nearest neighbors in DTI space. In general DTI looks at cellular density and morphology of the tissue at the cellular level, whereas DCE looks at the blood supply and permeability of the blood vessels. Thus, in principle the two sets of parameters should be mostly independent. However, the extra-cellular extra-vascular space measured in v_e will likely depend on the cellular density as well. Therefore, there may be some relationship between v_e and the average diffusivity $< D >$. Also, the vessel density will have some effect on the average diffusivity. Despite these potential relationships, our method should be considered as a data-driven approach. In all our experiments, the training data within the leave-one-out process included the DCE parameters. In other words, our ability to estimate the DCE parameters relies on the availability of a relatively rich training dataset. This is typically the case in clinical practice where the CAD system is built on a large dataset. Our methods enable the use of the CAD system on a new case with missing features.

Acknowledgement: Funding from Canadian Institutes for Health Research (CIHR) and Natural Sciences and Engineering Research Council of Canada.

References

1. Siegel, R., Naishadham, D., Jemal, A.: Cancer statistics, 2013. CA: a Cancer Journal for Clinicians 63, 11–30 (2013)
2. Benchikh El Fegoun, A., El Atat, R., Choudat, L., El Helou, E., Hermieu, J.F., Dominique, S., Hupertan, V., Ravery, V.: The learning curve of transrectal ultrasound-guided prostate biopsies: Implications for training programs. Urology 81, 12–16 (2013)
3. de Rooij, M., Hamoen, E.H.J., Futterer, J.J., Barentsz, J.O., Rovers, M.M.: Accuracy of multiparametric mri for prostate cancer detection: A meta-analysis. AJR Am. J. Roentgenol. 202(2), 343–351 (2014)
4. Chan, I., Wells III, W., Mulkern, R.V., Haker, S., Zhang, J., Zou, K.H., Maier, S.E., Tempany, C.M.: Detection of prostate cancer by integration of line-scan diffusion, T2-mapping and T2-weighted magnetic resonance imaging; a multichannel statistical classifier. Medical Physics 30, 2390 (2003)
5. Moradi, M., Salcudean, S.E., Chang, S.D., Jones, E.C., Buchan, N., Casey, R.G., Goldenberg, S.L., Kozlowski, P.: Multiparametric mri maps for detection and grading of dominant prostate tumors. Journal of Magnetic Resonance Imaging 35, 1403–1413 (2012)
6. Kozlowski, P., Chang, S.D., Meng, R., Mädler, B., Bell, R., Jones, E.C., Goldenberg, S.L.: Combined prostate diffusion tensor imaging and dynamic contrast enhanced MRI at 3T quantitative correlation with biopsy. Magnetic Resonance Imaging 28(5), 621–628 (2010)
7. Ozer, S., Langer, D.L., Liu, X., Haider, M.A., van der Kwast, T.H., Evans, A.J., Yang, Y., Wernick, M.N., Yetik, I.S.: Supervised and unsupervised methods for prostate cancer segmentation with multispectral MRI. Med. Phy. 37, 1873 (2010)
8. Kirchin, M.A., Pirovano, G., Venetianer, C., Spinazzi, A.: Safety assessment of gadobenate dimeglumine (multihance®): Extended clinical experience from phase i studies to post-marketing surveillance. Journal of Magnetic Resonance Imaging 14(3), 281–294 (2001)
9. Marckmann, P., et al.: Nephrogenic systemic fibrosis: suspected causative role of gadodiamide used for contrast-enhanced magnetic resonance imaging. Journal of the American Society of Nephrology 17(9), 2359–2362 (2006)
10. Tofts, P., et al.: Estimating kinetic parameters from dynamic contrast-enhanced T1-weighted MRI of a diffusable tracer: standardized quantities and symbols. Journal of Magnetic Resonance Imaging 10(3), 223–232 (1999)
11. Kuncheva, L.I.: Switching between selection and fusion in combining classifiers: An experiment. IEEE Transactions on Systems, Man, and Cybernetics, Part B: Cybernetics 32(2), 146–156 (2002)
12. Nandakumar, K., Jain, A.K., Ross, A.: Fusion in multibiometric identification systems: What about the missing data? In: Tistarelli, M., Nixon, M.S. (eds.) ICB 2009. LNCS, vol. 5558, pp. 743–752. Springer, Heidelberg (2009)
13. Moradi, M., et al.: Detection of prostate cancer from RF ultrasound echo signals using fractal analysis. In: IEEE EMBC, pp. 2400–2403 (2006)

Online Discriminative Multi-atlas Learning for Isointense Infant Brain Segmentation

Xuchu Wang[1,2], Li Wang[2], Heung-Il Suk[2], and Dinggang Shen[2]

[1] Key Laboratory of Optoelectronic Technology and Systems of Ministry
of Education, College of Optoelectronic Engineering,
Chongqing University, Chongqing 400044, China
seadrift.wang@gmail.com
[2] Department of Radiology and Biomedical Research Imaging Center (BRIC),
University of North Carolina at Chapel Hill, Chapel Hill, NC 27599, USA
{li_wang,hsuk,dgshen}@med.unc.edu

Abstract. Multi-atlas labeling in a non-local patch manner has emerged as an important approach to alleviate both the possible misalignment and mis-match among patches for guiding accurate image segmentation. However, the relationship among candidate patches and their intra/inter-class variability are less investigated, which limits the discriminative power of these patches. To address these issues, we present a new online discriminative multi-atlas learning method for labeling the target patch by the best representative candidates in a sparse sense. Specifically, the online multi-kernel learning is firstly adopted to map the patches into a cascade of discriminative kernel spaces for producing corresponding probability maps to model a label of each sample in these spaces. Then the online discriminative dictionary learning is proposed to build the atlas that handles the intra-class compactness and inter-class separability simultaneously. Finally, sparse coding is used to select patches in the dictionary for label propagation. In this way, the multi-atlas information dynamically learned with the context probability maps is iteratively incorporated to build the atlas dictionary, for gradually excluding the misleading candidate patches. The proposed method is validated by experiments on isointense infant brain tissue segmentation, and achieves promising results in comparison with several different labeling strategies.

1   Introduction

Accurate tissue segmentation of infant brain images into white matter (WM), gray matter (GM) and cerebrospinal fluid (CSF) is fundamental work in measuring and understanding the early brain development. These images usually consist of reduced tissue contrast, increased noise, and severe partial volume effect due to the ongoing maturation and WM myelination. Especially in the isointense images ($6 \sim 12$ months old), the tissue contrast is extremely low in MR modality, and the intensity distributions of WM and GM are largely overlapped in both T1 and T2 images [1, 2], which becomes a challenge for traditional brain tissue segmentation methods.

G. Wu et al. (Eds.): MLMI 2014, LNCS 8679, pp. 297–305, 2014.
© Springer International Publishing Switzerland 2014

Multi-atlas patch-based labeling methods have recently emerged as an attractive direction for brain MRI segmentation [3–9]. Early work uses the deformable registration to establish the point-based correspondence between each atlas with known labels and the target. After that, the label fusion is applied on this target by using the context of all warped atlas [3, 4]. Recent studies [5–9] have moved forward by less emphasizing explicit registration while using more complicated models that incorporates flexible configurations such as the network among patch-based features. These methods assume that the similar image patches should have the similar anatomical label [6] and then transfer labels from the atlas to the target image by modeling those strongly correlated patches. Although these multi-atlas labeling methods have shown their effectiveness, there are still some limitations in practice:

1) The relationship among the candidate atlases is less investigated [5, 6]. Traditionally they are independently measured their similarity to the target patch. More recent works explore the labeling error among them by imposed some constraints (e.g. spatial bias [7], sparsity [9], Bayesian framework [10]). These improvements alleviate the influences from possible mis-registration and structural dissimilarity between the atlas and the target image. However, the relationship among the patches is still not thoroughly discovered in a transformed space. Furthermore, the computational burden will increase dramatically along with the increasing templates, and if candidate patches are mis-labeled to certain amount, they will dominate the label fusion process and lead to wrong result [7].

2) Intrinsically, the patch dictionary for label fusion is collected in an unsupervised way, i.e., making the combination of candidate patches close to the target patch [10]. This dictionary is optimal for patch representation but not necessarily optimal for label fusion. Although recent work has explored the dictionary learning for hippocampus labeling [11], the intra-class and inter-class variability is less considered, which probably limits the discriminative power of learned atoms. Furthermore, the context information that reveals the anatomical correspondences in probability sense is less incorporated to improve the accuracy of label fusion [5].

To address these limitations, we aim to learn a discriminative multi-atlas dictionary adaptively for labeling the target patch by the best representative candidates in a sparse sense. Specifically, the online multi-kernel learning is used to map the patches into discriminative kernel spaces for producing corresponding probability maps to model a label of each sample in these spaces. Then the online discriminative dictionary learning is proposed to build the atlas that handles the intra-class compactness and inter-class separability simultaneously. Finally, sparse coding is used to select only a small number of candidate patches that best represent the target patch. In this way, the multi-atlas information is dynamically learned by controlling the sizes of the kernels and the atlas dictionary. We applied the proposed method for the isointense infant brain tissue segmentation and achieved promising results compared to the state-of-the-art labeling methods, which shed light on the applicability of the proposed method in these scenarios.

2   Methodology

Fig. 1 presents a schematic diagram of our proposed method. Here, we formulate
the tissue segmentation as a multi-class classification problem. In the training
stage, we linearly align the training multi-modality images to the atlas space,
and then extract the normalized intensities to build training patches associated
to a voxel position. These patch samples are then inputted to the online multi-
kernel learner to train a classifier to produce a tissue probability map for each
class (i.e., WM, GM, CSF). This learning module repeats to produce a set of
probability maps with different precision until the stop criteria are satisfied. In
each iteration, the maps are feed-backed to the trainer as context information
to assist further purifying the kernel space. Then the set of the probability maps
and the appearance features from image patches are combined with the label set,
and fed into the online discriminative dictionary learning module. In the testing
stage, a target image works in the similar way. The details are given below.

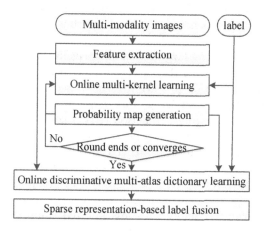

Fig. 1. Diagram of the training procedure of the proposed method

2.1   Online Multi-Kernel Learning

To handle the multiple features in the different modality images (e.g. T1, T2,
and FA), we use a multi-kernel learning (MKL) method to fuse the hyperplanes
modeling the different features. The MKL methods are theoretically solid in the
minimization of an upper bound of the generalization error. It solves a joint
optimization problem while also learning the optimal weights for combining the
kernels. For a multi-class classification problem, given a set of N training in-
stances $\{\mathbf{x}_i, y_i\}_{i=1}^{N}$, where $\mathbf{x}_i \in \mathbb{R}^D$ is an input vector and $y_i \in \{1, \cdots, c\}$ is a
class label, the generic convex optimization of MKL [12] in primal is

$$\min_{\overline{\mathbf{w}}} \frac{\gamma}{2} \|\overline{\mathbf{w}}\|_{2,p}^2 + \frac{1}{N} \sum_{i=1}^{N} \xi_i$$
$$\text{s.t. } \overline{\mathbf{w}} \cdot (\overline{\phi}(\mathbf{x}_i, y_i) - \overline{\phi}(\mathbf{x}_i, y)) \geq 1 - \xi_i, \forall i, y \neq y_i \tag{1}$$

where $\overline{\phi}(\mathbf{x}, y) = \left[\phi^1(\mathbf{x}, y), \cdots, \phi^k(\mathbf{x}, y), \cdots \phi^K(\mathbf{x}, y)\right]$, K is the number of kernels[1]; $\phi^k(\mathbf{x}, y)$ denotes a joint feature mapping function of the k-th kernel; $\overline{\mathbf{w}} = [\mathbf{w}^1, \cdots, \mathbf{w}^k, \cdots, \mathbf{w}^K]$ is a concatenation of the weight coefficients, $\|\overline{\mathbf{w}}\|_{2,p} = \left\| \left[\|\mathbf{w}^1\|_2, \cdots, \|\mathbf{w}^k\|_2, \cdots, \|\mathbf{w}^K\|_2\right] \right\|_p$ is the p-norm of the vector of K elements, each of which is formed by ℓ_2-norm of the vectors $\{\mathbf{w}^k\}_{k=1}^K$, $\{\xi_i\}_{i=1}^N$ is a set of slack variables, and γ is a regularization control parameter.

This optimization problem can be solved in the framework of stochastic subgradient descent algorithms for any strongly convex function [13]. At each step, the algorithm takes a random sample of the training set and calculates a subgradient of the objective function evaluated on the sample. Then, it performs a sub-gradient descent step with a decreasing learning rate, followed by a projection inside the space where the solution lies.

The MKL in our approach works in an online way. Specifically, for sequential training samples, the algorithm receives the next instance and makes a prediction. Once the algorithm makes its prediction, it observes the correct label and then updates its current model. The goal is to minimize the cumulative loss obtained from the sequence of observations, thus improving the chances of making accurate predictions in the subsequent rounds. In this way, the computational prohibition of storing large kernel matrices in the batch framework can be efficiently tackled. Following [14], we use Mercer kernels without introducing explicitly the dual formulation to learn a kernel-based prediction function from a pool of predefined kernels (or kernel functions) in the optimization problem. In this work, we use a radial basis function (RBF) kernel with a self-tuned parameter, i.e. the distance among k-th nearest neighbors in the training set. In practice, we store the original data rather than the kernel evaluations, at the expense of the computational cost per iteration. Once the hyperplane is found, we use a logistic function to produce the probability map of each class. Fig. 2 shows an intermediate result of the learning under different training strategies. Since the under-learning strategy with less iterated training (≤ 3) easily outputs the obscure details in the cortex region, and the over-learning one with too much iterated training (≥ 12) captures the clean but over-fitted details in these regions, we set a small iteration (8) or once the probability of a class is larger than 0.5, we regard the learner converged.

2.2   Online Discriminative Dictionary Learning

The atlas dictionary in many existing investigations is regarded to contain features as much as possible, but a large size dictionary increases a computational burden and results in error summarization to replace the right label [7]. In this paper, motivated by [15], we propose an improved Fisher discriminant dictionary learning that constructs dictionary with less atoms but good representational ability. Specifically, in the dictionary learning stage, we construct a structured dictionary $\mathbf{D} = [\mathbf{D}_1, \mathbf{D}_2, \cdots, \mathbf{D}_c]$, where $\mathbf{D}_i$ denotes the sub-dictionary associated with the i-th class. Each column in $\mathbf{D}$ denotes the input sample features, i.e. the vectorized re-arrangement of the intensities patches and their cor-

---

[1] In this work, it is equal to the number of modalities.

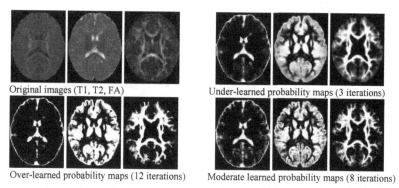

Original images (T1, T2, FA)   Under-learned probability maps (3 iterations)

Over-learned probability maps (12 iterations)   Moderate learned probability maps (8 iterations)

Fig. 2. Probability maps of tissues (CSF,GM,WM) under different training iterations

responding probability patches. For simplicity, let $\mathbf{Y} = [\mathbf{Y}_1, \mathbf{Y}_2, \cdots, \mathbf{Y}_c]$ and $\mathbf{X} = [\mathbf{X}_1, \mathbf{X}_2, \cdots, \mathbf{X}_c]$ denote, respectively, training samples and the coding coefficient matrix over dictionary, i.e., $\mathbf{Y} \simeq \mathbf{DX}$. Then, we build the model as

$$J(\mathbf{D}, \mathbf{X}) = \min_{\mathbf{D}, \mathbf{X}}\{r(\mathbf{Y}, \mathbf{D}, \mathbf{X}) + \lambda_1||\mathbf{X}||_1 + \lambda_2 f(\mathbf{X})\}, \qquad (2)$$

where $||\mathbf{X}||_1$ measures the sparsity, $f(\mathbf{X}) = tr(S_{lw}(\mathbf{X}) - S_{lb}(\mathbf{X})) - \eta||\mathbf{X}||_F^2$ is a discriminative constraint imposed on $\mathbf{X}$ to guide $\mathbf{D}$ to be discriminative for samples in $\mathbf{Y}$, $S_{lw}(\mathbf{X})$ and $S_{lb}(\mathbf{X})$ are the local within-class and between-class scatter of $\mathbf{X}$, respectively, λ_1, λ_2, and η are tuning parameters, $r(\mathbf{Y}, \mathbf{D}, \mathbf{X}) = \sum_i^c r(\mathbf{Y}_i, \mathbf{D}, \mathbf{X}_i)$ is the discriminative fidelity term, i.e.

$$r(\mathbf{Y}_i, \mathbf{D}, \mathbf{X}_i) = ||\mathbf{Y}_i - \mathbf{DX}_i||_F^2 + ||\mathbf{Y}_i - \mathbf{D}_i\mathbf{X}_i||_F^2 + \sum_{j=1, j\neq i}^c ||\mathbf{D}_j\mathbf{X}_i^j||_F^2, \qquad (3)$$

where $||\cdot||_F$ is the Frobenius norm. The first two terms in Eq. (3) guarantee that $\mathbf{Y}_i$ can be represented by $\mathbf{D}$ and $\mathbf{D}_i$ approximately with $\mathbf{X}$ and $\mathbf{X}_i$, respectively, and the third one ensures that the representation of $\mathbf{Y}_i$ over $\mathbf{d}_i^j(i \neq j)$ is small. $\mathbf{X}_i^j$ is the coding coefficient of $\mathbf{Y}_i$ over the sub-dictionary $\mathbf{D}_j$. The solution of $\mathbf{D}$ can be obtained by iteratively updating $\mathbf{X}$ and $\mathbf{D}$ while fixing the other until $J(\mathbf{D}, \mathbf{X})$ converges or changes small. Hence, by incorporating the label and the scatter information, the learned dictionary is capable of estimating the subtle structure around ambiguous voxels in the original result. In practice, we can use clustering or sampling technique to reduce the original size. Fig. 3 presents an example of the projecting coefficients of three testing voxels of different classes on the cortex region. It is seen that their coefficients on the dictionary are sparse and separable. In the online dictionary updating stage, we employ the method in [16] to update the sub-dictionary that directly corresponds to the input feature with the known class label.

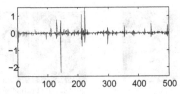

Fig. 3. Projecting coefficients of three voxels in different classes on a learned dictionary with 500 atoms. (color preferred)

2.3 Sparse Representation-Based Label Fusion

Once the trained feature dictionary is obtained, it can be applied into the typical multi-atlas segmentation methods, e.g., nonlocal major voting [5], joint label fusion [7][9], and sparse representation [1]. This segmentation category considers the contribution of each atlas to the final label according to a nonnegative weight. In this study, our focus is to combine the strengths of context and the discriminative dictionary learning for exacting tissue segmentation, so we use a sparse representation technique to find the weight [1, 9]. The final label probability is a simply weighted sum of the sparse coefficients, that is, given a set of T atlas coefficients and their segmentation ground truth $\{(I_t, L_t)\}_{t=1:T}$ registered to a common image, after extracting coefficients, the label of a patch $\mathbf{x}$ in a target image I_{new} is computed by $L_{new}(\mathbf{x}) = \frac{1}{Z}\sum_{t=1}^{T}\sum_{\mathbf{y}\in\mathcal{N}_t(\mathbf{x})} w_t(\mathbf{x},\mathbf{y})L_t(\mathbf{y})$, where $Z = \sum_{t=1}^{T}\sum_{\mathbf{y}\in\mathcal{N}_t(\mathbf{x})} w_t(\mathbf{x},\mathbf{y})$ and $\mathcal{N}_t(\mathbf{x})$ denotes the neighborhood intensity and probability maps patch set of $\mathbf{x}$, $w_t(\mathbf{x},\mathbf{y})$ is the weight of the contribution of the patch $\mathbf{y}$ in I_t to estimate the tissue label of $\mathbf{x}$. The final structure segmentation result is thresholded at the isosurface according to the maximum coefficient.

3   Experimental Results

To validate the proposed method, we apply it to segment a group of 22 isointense infants images. The study has been approved by the ethics committee of our institute and the written informed consent forms were obtained. T1-weighted images were acquired on a Siemens head-only 3T scanners with a circular polarized head coil for 144 sagittal slices with a resolution of $1\times1\times1$ mm^3. T2-weighted images were obtained for 64 axial slices with a resolution of $1.25\times1.25\times1.95$ mm^3. Diffusion tensor images (DTI) consisted of 60 axial slices with a resolution of $2\times2\times2$ mm^3, TR/TE=7680/82 ms, 42 non-collinear diffusion gradients, and diffusion weighting b=-1000 s/mm^2. The DTI were reconstructed and the respective FA images were computed. T2 and FA images were linearly aligned to their corresponding T1 images and resampled with $1\times1\times1$ mm^3. We performed preprocessing for bias correction, skull stripping, and cerebellum removal.

The main parameters in our experiments were set as: modality number $F = 3$, norm $p = 1.05$, $\gamma = 1/(CN)$ with $C \in \{0.001, 0.1, 1, 10, 100, 1000\}$ by leave-one-out cross-validation in the online MKL training. $\lambda_1 = 0.005$, $\lambda_2 = 0.05$, and within-class and between-class neighbors were fixed to 5 in the dictionary learning. In sparse representation package [17], the regularization parameters in

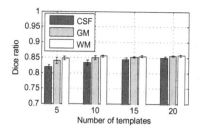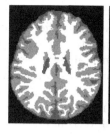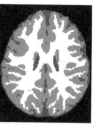

Fig. 4. Classification accuracy under different training templates and examples of ground-truth image (middle), along with our segmentation results (right)

Table 1. Comparison of segmentation accuracies in Dice ratio (mean± std %)

Method	MajorVot.	LevelSet	Nonlocal	SparseRep.	Proposed
Registration	Nonlinear	Nonlinear	Nonlinear	Nonlinear	Linear
WM	73.4±2.8	77.5±1.75	85.8±1.0	82.0±1.4	85.6±0.8
GM	73.7±1.3	77.7±1.42	82.5±1.0	81.9±1.1	84.9±0.9
CSF	68.9±1.2	84.2±1.4	83.5±1.9	84.2±1.4	85.3 ±1.0

sparsity and smooth terms were set to 0.05 and 0.5 respectively. The patch size were $5\times5\times5$ and searching neighbor size were $7\times7\times7$. Fig. 4(left) shows three tissue classification accuracies of our method under 5, 10, 15, 20 templates, from which we can see that the accuracy becomes stable after 10. A segmentation example is also shown in Fig. 4(right). Our method clearly distinguishes the main tissues, and the most errors occur near the high curvature regions.

To quantitatively evaluate our method, we compare it with the methods of majority voting, coupled level sets [18], nonlocal patch-based method [5], and patch-based sparse method [1] on 22 isointense infant brain images. We employ the Dice ratios (DR) to measure the overlapping rate of the segmentation results with the ground-truth. Due to the computation burden of nonlinear registration in other methods, we conducted our method using only linear registration to obtain atlas with leave-one-out cross validation prototype. The experimental results on 10 slices with fixed vertical-index in each subject are reported in Table 1, from which it is seen that the different method performed differently on segmenting WM/GM/CSF, and our method consistently showed better performance thanks to the nolocal patch-based and sparse representation-based approaches. Furthermore, it uses multi-kernel learning to obtain the discriminative features of the multi-source images.

4   Conclusions

We have presented a novel online discriminative multi-atlas learning method for isointense infant brain tissue segmentation. Our method maps the atlas to a cascade of kernel space for handling the intra-class compactness and inter-class separability simultaneously. The probability maps serve as context information, and are iteratively incorporated to build an atlas dictionary by gradually excluding the misleading candidate patches in label fusion. The discriminative dictionary learning is further adopted to group the most representative atlas in sparsity constraints. Experimental results show that combining multi-kernel learning, discriminative dictionary learning, and context information can improve gradually the segmentation accuracy. It is noteworthy that we use only the intensity feature under linear registration, and does not incorporate anatomical structure constraints. They will be considered in our future work.

References

1. Wang, L., Shi, F., Li, G., Lin, W., Gilmore, J.H., Shen, D.: Integration of sparse multi-modality representation and geometrical constraint for isointense infant brain segmentation. In: Mori, K., Sakuma, I., Sato, Y., Barillot, C., Navab, N. (eds.) MICCAI 2013, Part I. LNCS, vol. 8149, pp. 703–710. Springer, Heidelberg (2013)
2. Wang, L., Shi, F., Li, G., Gao, Y., Lin, W., Gilmore, J.H., Shen, D.: Segmentation of neonatal brain MR images using patch-driven level sets. NeuroImage 84, 141–158 (2014)
3. Warfield, S.K., Zou, K.H., Wells III, W.M.: Simultaneous truth and performance level estimation (STAPLE): an algorithm for the validation of image segmentation. IEEE Trans. Med. Imaging 23(7), 903–921 (2004)
4. Heckemann, R.A., Hajnal, J.V., Aljabar, P., Rueckert, D., Hammers, A.: Automatic anatomical brain MRI segmentation combining label propagation and decision fusion. NeuroImage 33(1), 115–126 (2006)
5. Coupé, P., Manjón, J.V., Fonov, V., Pruessner, J.C., Robles, M., Collins, D.L.: Patch-based segmentation using expert priors: Application to hippocampus and ventricle segmentation. NeuroImage 54(2), 940–954 (2011)
6. Rousseau, F., Habas, P.A., Studholme, C.: A supervised patch-based approach for human brain labeling. IEEE Trans. Med. Imaging 30(10), 1852–1862 (2011)
7. Wang, H., Suh, J.W., Das, S.R., Pluta, J., Craige, C., Yushkevich, P.A.: Multi-atlas segmentation with joint label fusion. IEEE Trans. PAMI 35(3), 611–623 (2013)
8. Wu, G., Wang, Q., Liao, S., Zhang, D., Nie, F., Shen, D.: Minimizing joint risk of mislabeling for iterative patch-based label fusion. In: Mori, K., Sakuma, I., Sato, Y., Barillot, C., Navab, N. (eds.) MICCAI 2013, Part III. LNCS, vol. 8151, pp. 551–558. Springer, Heidelberg (2013)
9. Wu, G., Wang, Q., Zhang, D., Nie, F., Huang, H., Shen, D.: A generative probability model of joint label fusion for multi-atlas based brain segmentation. Medical Image Analysis 18(6), 881–890 (2014)
10. Bai, W., Shi, W., O'Regan, D.P., Tong, T., Wang, H., Jamil-Copley, S., Peters, N.S., Rueckert, D.: A probabilistic patch-based label fusion model for multi-atlas segmentation with registration refinement: Application to cardiac MR images. IEEE Trans. Med. Imaging 32(7), 1302–1315 (2013)
11. Tong, T., Wolz, R., Coupé, P., Hajnal, J.V., Rueckert, D.: Segmentation of MR images via discriminative dictionary learning and sparse coding: Application to hippocampus labeling. NeuroImage 76, 11–23 (2013)
12. Orabona, F., Luo, J., Caputo, B.: Multi kernel learning with online-batch optimization. J. Mach. Learn. Res. 13, 227–253 (2012)
13. Shalev-Shwartz, S., Srebro, N.: SVM optimization: inverse dependence on training set size. In: ICML, pp. 928–935 (2008)

14. Jie, L., Orabona, F., Fornoni, M., Caputo, B., Cesa-Bianchi, N.: OM-2: An online multi-class multi-kernel learning algorithm. In: CVPRW, pp. 43–50 (2010)
15. Yang, M., Zhang, L., Feng, X., Zhang, D.: Fisher discrimination dictionary learning for sparse representation. In: ICCV, pp. 543–550 (2011)
16. Mairal, J., Bach, F., Ponce, J., Sapiro, G.: Online dictionary learning for sparse coding. In: ICML, p. 87 (2009)
17. Liu, J., Ji, S., Ye, J.: SLEP: Sparse Learning with Efficient Projections. Arizona State University (2009)
18. Wang, L., Shi, F., Lin, W., Gilmore, J.H., Shen, D.: Automatic segmentation of neonatal images using convex optimization and coupled level sets. NeuroImage 58(3), 805–817 (2011)

Persistent Reeb Graph Matching
for Fast Brain Search*

Yonggang Shi, Junning Li, and Arthur W. Toga

Laboratory of Neuro Imaging (LONI), Institute for Neuroimaging and Informatics,
Keck School of Medicine, University of Southern California
yshi@loni.usc.edu

Abstract. In this paper we propose a novel algorithm for the efficient
search of the most similar brains from a large collection of MR imaging
data. The key idea is to compactly represent and quantify the differences
of cortical surfaces in terms of their intrinsic geometry by comparing
the Reeb graphs constructed from their Laplace-Beltrami eigenfunctions.
To overcome the topological noise in the Reeb graphs, we develop a
progressive pruning and matching algorithm based on the persistence
of critical points. Given the Reeb graphs of two cortical surfaces, our
method can calculate their distance in less than 10 milliseconds on a PC.
In experimental results, we apply our method on a large collection of 1326
brains for searching, clustering, and automated labeling to demonstrate
its value for the "Big Data" science in human neuroimaging.

1 Introduction

With the advance of MR imaging techniques and the availability of large scale
data from multi-site studies such as the Alzheimer's Disease Neuroimaging Initiative (ADNI) [1] and Human Connectome Project (HCP) [2, 3], brain imaging
is now entering the era of "Big Data" research [4]. To fully take advantage of
the rich source of imaging data, one key challenge is to efficiently organize these
data and provide search tools with real-time performance that can quickly find
the most similar brains to a *query* brain. For example, comparing the brain of a
patient with a control group of most similar brains has the potential of allowing
us to factor out structural differences and improve the signal to noise ratio in
disease diagnosis and the detection of treatment effects in drug trials.

Besides simple measures such as intra-cranial volume, sophisticated comparisons that can take into account more elastic brain differences usually involve
nonlinear warping techniques, which can take at least minutes to compute a
pairwise registration. To overcome this difficulty, it is essential to develop rich
characterizations of the brain with a small footprint to enable efficient calculation. In this work, we propose a novel method to compare the similarity of
cortical surfaces based on their intrinsic geometry. We use the Reeb graphs constructed from the Laplace-Beltrami (LB) eigenfunctions of the cortical surfaces

---

* This work was supported by NIH grants K01EB013633 and P41EB015922.

G. Wu et al. (Eds.): MLMI 2014, LNCS 8679, pp. 306–313, 2014.

as the compact, yet informative, description of the brain [5, 6]. Due to the presence of noise in the Reeb graph, we develop a progressive pruning and matching process based on the persistence of critical points [7, 8]. With our novel method, a similarity measure of two cortical surfaces can be calculated in less than 10 milliseconds in our MATLAB implementation. In our experiments, we demonstrate the potential of our method for "Big Data" problems by applying it to find the most similar brains from a collection of 1326 brains. The similarity measure also allows the clustering of cortical surfaces to reveal brain asymmetry in terms of intrinsic geometry. We also demonstrate the potential of our method in automated cortical labeling via intrinsic mapping between a brain and its nearest neighbor.

The rest of the paper is organized as follows. In section 2, we introduce the LB eigenfunctions of cortical surfaces and the construction of their Reeb graphs. The persistent Reeb graph matching process is developed in section 3 to compute the similarity between cortices. Experimental results are presented in section 4. Finally, conclusions and future work are discussed in section 5.

2   Reeb Graph of LB Eigenfunctions

Given a cortical surface $\mathcal{M}$, the LB eigen-system is defined as

$$\Delta_{\mathcal{M}} f_n = -\lambda_n f_n \quad (n = 0, 1, 2, \cdots) \tag{1}$$

where $\Delta_{\mathcal{M}}$ is the LB operator on the surface, and the pair (λ_n, f_n) are the n-th eigenvalue and eigen-function, respectively. The set of eigen-functions $\Phi = \{f_0, f_1, f_2, \cdots, \}$ form an orthonormal basis on the surface. Using the LB eigen-system, an embedding $I_{\mathcal{M}}^{\Phi} : \mathcal{M} \to \mathbb{R}^{\infty}$ was proposed in [9]:

$$I_{\mathcal{M}}^{\Phi}(x) = (\frac{f_1(x)}{\sqrt{\lambda_1}}, \frac{f_2(x)}{\sqrt{\lambda_2}} \cdots, \frac{f_n(x)}{\sqrt{\lambda_n}}, \cdots) \quad \forall x \in \mathcal{M}, \tag{2}$$

where intrinsic surface analysis can be performed such as mapping and automated labeling [10].

For surfaces with salient geometric profiles, the LB eigenfunctions have been used successfully as feature functions for the construction of Reeb graphs [6]. Given a Morse function f on a surface $\mathcal{M}$, its Reeb graph is defined as follows [11].

Definition 1. *Let $f : \mathcal{M} \to \mathbb{R}$. The Reeb graph $R(f)$ of f is the quotient space with its topology defined through the equivalent relation $x \simeq y$ if $f(x) = f(y)$ for $\forall x, y \in \mathcal{M}$.*

Various approaches were developed for the numerical construction of Reeb graphs. In this work, we use the algorithm proposed in [6] to build the Reeb graph as a graph of critical points. Given an eigenfunction f_n of $\mathcal{M}$, we first calculate its critical points $C_n = \{C_n^1, C_n^2, \cdots, C_n^K\}$, which include maximum, minimum, and saddle points, and sort them according to their function value such that $f_n(C_n^1) < f_n(C_n^2) < \cdots < f_n(C_n^K)$. Using the level contours in the neighborhoods of the critical points, a parcellation of the surface can be obtained and region growing can then be applied to connect neighboring nodes in the Reeb graph. In the end, the Reeb graph is represented as $R(f_n) = (C_n, E_n)$, where C_n is the nodes of the graph, and $E_n = \{E_n^1, E_n^2, \cdots\}$ is the

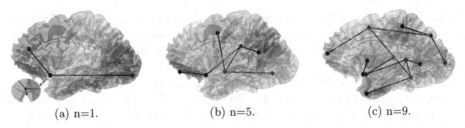

(a) n=1.   (b) n=5.   (c) n=9.

Fig. 1. The Reeb graphs of the 1st, 5th, 9th eigenfunction of a cortical surface. In (a)-(c), the surface is color-coded with the corresponding eigenfunction. A zoomed view of a spurious critical point was shown (a).

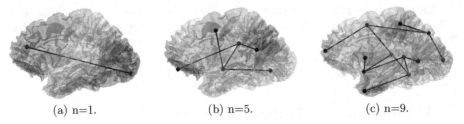

(a) n=1.   (b) n=5.   (c) n=9.

Fig. 2. The pruned Reeb graphs

set of edges, where each edge connects two nodes. Following the Morse theory, the Reeb graph encodes the topology of the surface. Cortical surfaces are generally reconstructed with genus zero topology, thus all of their Reeb graphs have tree structures.

As an example, we plot in Fig. 1 the Reeb graphs of a cortical surface, which is represented as a mesh of 200K triangles. With the increase of the order, the eigenfunction becomes more oscillatory. This means they will have more critical points and thus a more complicated structure in the computed Reeb graph. The complexity of the Reeb graph, however, is not solely determined by the order of the eigenfunction. Because we use a discrete representation of the surface and eigenfunction, numerical approximations will sometimes create spurious critical points as shown in Fig. 1(a). To use the Reeb graph for brain indexing and search, it is critical to robustly detect and remove such spurious structures without compromising the representation power of the Reeb graph.

3   Persistent Reeb Graph Matching

Based on the concept of *persistence* in discrete topology, we develop in this section a Reeb graph pruning and matching algorithm. This provides the core step for efficient brain search by comparing the intrinsic geometry of cortical surfaces.

For an edge $E_n^k = (C_n^i, C_n^j)$ of the Reeb Graph $R(f_n) = (C_n, E_n)$, its weight is defined according to its persistence:

$$w(E_n^k) = |f_n(C_n^i) - f_n(C_n^j)| \tag{3}$$

which is the difference of the LB eigenfunction value of the two critical points C_n^i and C_n^j. Using the weight on edges, we also have a matrix representation R_n of the Reeb

Table 1. Persistent Reeb Graph Match Algorithm

Set $D_{min}^n = \infty$. Repeat the following steps until the minimal edge weight of R_n^1 and R_n^2 are above the persistence threshold δ.
1. Calculate the cost matrix D^+.
2. Calculate the cost matrix D^-.
3. Compute the distance D at the current pruning level. If $D < D_{min}^n$, set $D_{min}^n = D$ and record the correspondence.
4. Prune the minimal edge in both Reeb graphs, and update the pruning cost P_n^1 and P_n^2. Go back to step 1.

---

graph with its entries defined as $R_n(i, j) = |f_n(C_n^i) - f_n(C_n^j)|$ if there exists an edge between the node C_n^i and C_n^j. By using the persistence to define the edge weights, we not only have a natural way for outlier pruning but also an efficient mechanism to model the distribution of the critical points on the surface. By comparing the Reeb graphs of different surfaces, we can thus quantify their differences in terms of intrinsic geometry.

For Reeb graph pruning, an intuitive approach can be developed for the selection of a persistence threshold. Because the LB eigenfunctions have oscillatory patterns similar to Fourier basis functions, their peak values are essentially the expected persistence of the maximum and minimum. Based on this observation, we choose the persistence threshold based on the maximum of the eigenfunction as $\delta = max(|f_n|)/5$ in our experiments. To remove spurious edges, we sort all edges according to their persistence. At each step, we find the edge E_n^k with the smallest weight. If $w(E_n^k) < \delta$, we remove it from the edge set by collapsing the two nodes $C_n^i, C_n^j \in E_n^k$. For a node C_n^i, we calculate its total weight $S(C_n^i)$ as

$$S(C_n^i) = \sum_{C_n^i \in E_n^k} w(E_n^k). \tag{4}$$

We collapse the two nodes by removing the node with the smaller total weight and adding all its connections to the other node. For example, if $S(C_n^i) < S(C_n^j)$, we remove C_n^i from the node set of the Reeb graph $R(f_n)$. Except for the edge E_n^k to be removed, for all other edges that were connected to C_n^i, we update them by replacing C_n^i with C_n^j. We then check if the degree of any node becomes two. If so, we add an edge to connect its two neighbors and remove this node and its two edges from the graph. For all new edges, their weights are calculated according to (3) with the function values of the nodes. The above steps can be repeated until the persistence threshold is reached. For the example shown in Fig. 1, we applied the pruning process and the new results are shown in Fig. 2.

For fast brain search, the core step is to efficiently compute a similarity measure between two cortical surfaces. The solution we develop here is based on comparing the Reeb graphs of their corresponding LB eigenfunctions. Let $\mathcal{M}_1$ and $\mathcal{M}_2$ denote two surfaces we want to compare. We denote their corresponding eigenfunctions as f_n^1 and $f_n^2(n = 1, ..., N)$. For the n-th eigenfunction f_n^1 and f_n^2, we first compute their Reeb graphs $R(f_n^1)$ and $R(f_n^2)$. Let $R(f_n^1) = (C^1, E^1)$ with $C^1 = (C_1^1, ..., C_{K_1}^1)$, $R(f_n^2) = (C^2, E^2)$ with $C^2 = (C_1^2, ..., C_{K_2}^2)$. To start the iterative pruning and matching algorithm, we first prune both graphs to have the same number of K nodes with $K \leq min(K_1, K_2)$. We define the pruning cost P as the total edge weights between the original and pruned Reeb graph. The pruning cost of both graphs are denoted as P_n^1 and P_n^2. After that, an iterative process as summarized in Table 1 is applied to match the Reeb graphs of the two surfaces. Next we describe the details of each step.

Let K denote the number of nodes in the Reeb graphs at the start of each iteration. We define the cost matrix of size $K \times K$ for matching the nodes of $R(f_n^1)$ to $R(f_n^2)$ as

$$A^+(i,j) = |(S(C_i^1) - S(C_j^2)| + |f_n^1(C_i^1) - f_n^2(C_j^2)| \tag{5}$$

Using the cost matrix A^+, we run the Hungarian algorithm and find the one-to-one correspondences ϕ^+ from the nodes of $R(f_n^1)$ to $R(f_n^2)$. We compute the distance between the Reeb graphs as:

$$D^+ = \sum_{i=1}^{K} \sum_{j=1}^{K} |R_n^1(i,j) - R_n^2(\phi^+(i), \phi^+(j))| + \sum_{i=1}^{K} |f_n^1(i) - f_n^2(\phi^+(i))| \tag{6}$$

where R_n^1 and R_n^2 are the matrix representation of the Reeb graphs.

Because of the sign ambiguity of the eigenfunction, we flip the sign of the eigenfunction f_n^2 and compute the cost matrix as

$$A^-(i,j) = |(S(C_i^1) - S(C_j^2)| + |f_n^1(C_i^1) + f_n^2(C_j^2)| \tag{7}$$

With the cost matrix A^-, the correspondence computed with the Hungarian algorithm is denoted as ϕ^-, and the distance between the Reeb graphs is:

$$D^- = \sum_{i=1}^{K} \sum_{j=1}^{K} |R_n^1(i,j) - R_n^2(\phi^-(i), \phi^-(j))| + \sum_{i=1}^{K} |f_n^1(i) + f_n^2(\phi^-(i))| \tag{8}$$

The overall cost of the matching at the current iteration is then

$$D = \min(D^+, D^-) + P_n^1 + P_n^2 \tag{9}$$

which is the sum of the graph distance and pruning costs. If convergence is not reached, we continue the above steps after pruning the minimal edges from both graphs as described in Table 1. Otherwise, the optimal match and the distance D_{min}^n is recorded.

By applying the persistence Reeb graph matching algorithm for eigenfunctions up to the order N, we have the overall distance between $\mathcal{M}_1$ and $\mathcal{M}_2$ for brain search:

$$d(\mathcal{M}_1, \mathcal{M}_2) = \sum_{n=1}^{N} D_{min}^n. \tag{10}$$

4   Experimental Results

In our experiments, we applied our method to T1-weighted MR images from three publicly available datasets. The first dataset consists of the 225 subjects released by the HCP up to date. The second dataset is composed of the 101 MR images of the Mindboggle atlas [12]. The third dataset includes 1000 MR images from all baseline visits of the ADNI2 project. Overall we have a total of 1326 T1-weighted images from a diverse population. Cortical surfaces were automatically reconstructed with the method in [6]. The white matter (WM) surfaces of all subjects were used in our experiments for persistent Reeb graph matching (PRGM), which is currently implemented in MATLAB. Before we perform PRGM, the first 9 LB eigenfunctions and their Reeb graphs were computed for all subjects.

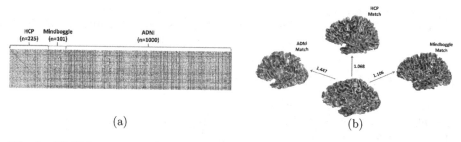

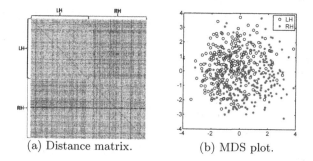

(a)   (b)

Fig. 3. PRGM results of HCP cohorts versus the HCP, Mingboggle, and the ADNI cohorts. (a) The distance matrix. (b) The closest match of an HCP subject in the three cohorts. Distance to each matched brain is plotted alongside the arrow.

(a) Distance matrix.   (b) MDS plot.

Fig. 4. The use of persistent Reeb graph matching for brain asymmetry analysis on the HCP cohort

4.1   Fast Brain Search

To demonstrate the capability of our method in finding the most similar brains from a large brain collection, we applied PRGM between the HCP cohorts and all brains from the three cohorts. For the left WM surface of a HCP subject, a PRGM is applied against the left WM surface of each of the 1326 subjects and the distance is computed as in (10). On a PC with a 2.7GHz CPU, every pair of PRGM takes less than 10 milliseconds. As shown in Fig. 3 (a), we obtain a distance matrix of size 225 × 1326. Among the 225 HCP subjects, the closest match for 116 of them are from the HCP collection, 15 of them are from the Mindboggle collection, and 94 of them are from the ADNI collection. As an example, we show in Fig. 3(b) the left WM surface of one HCP subject and the nearest brains we found via PRGM from all three datasets.

4.2   Brain Asymmetry

In our second experiment, we applied pairwise PRGM to all the left hemisphere (LH) and right hemisphere (RH) WM surfaces of the HCP cohort. The distances are saved into a matrix of size 450 × 450 as shown in Fig. 4(a), which exhibits a clear pattern: the (LH,LH) and (RH,RH) blocks of the matrix have smaller distance values than the (LH,RH) block. This suggests that we could use the PRGM distance to evaluate brain asymmetry on a large scale. To further illustrate this point, we applied multidimensional scaling (MDS) to the distance matrix and plotted the results in Fig. 4(b). While there are overlaps, it is clear that the LH and RH surfaces form very distinct clusters. A t-test was applied to the projection of the MDS embedding coordinates onto the diagonal line, i.e., the vector $(-1, 1)$, and a highly significant p-value 9.4e−34 was obtained.

4.3   Fast Resolution of Sign Ambiguity in LB Embedding

To compare two surfaces with their LB embeddings as defined in (2), it is usually a challenging and computationally expensive task to resolve the ambiguities including the sign of the eigenfunctions, switching of the order of the eigenfunctions, and possible splitting of the eigenspaces due to multiplicity. With PRGM matching, we find the nearest surface from a large brain collection such that the risk of order switching is greatly reduced. For lower order eigenfunctions, multiplicity is uncommon for cortical comparisons in our experience. Thus the focus is on resolving the sign ambiguity of LB embeddings for two very similar surfaces. Using the corresponding critical points provided by PRGM, we show here that this can be achieved extremely efficiently.

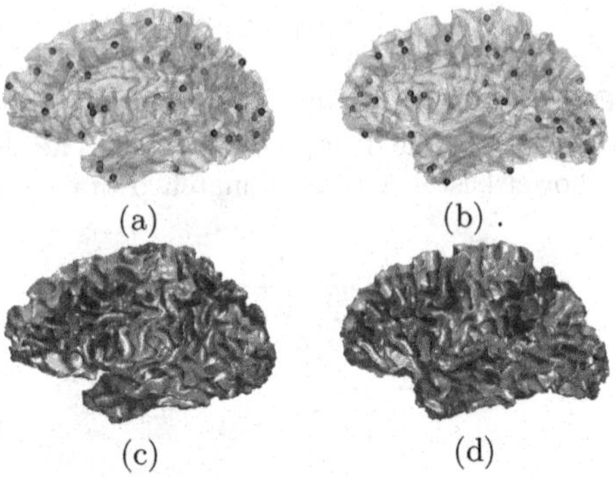

For the HCP subject and its closest Mindboggle match shown in Fig. 3(b),

(a)   (b) .

(c)   (d)

Fig. 5. Reeb graph matching for fast sign ambiguity resolution and cortical labeling. Critical point set on the HCP (a) and Mindboggle subject (b). (c) Automatically generated labels on the HCP subject. (d) Manually delineated labels on the Mindboggle subject.

the PRGM applied to the first 9 eigenfunctions generates a set of 48 corresponding critical points as shown in Fig. 5 (a) and (b). For the n−th eigenfunction of the first

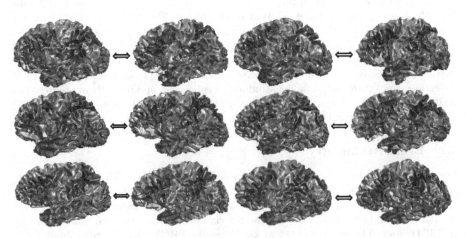

Fig. 6. Cortical labeling results of six HCP subjects paired with their nearest match from the Mindboggle cohort. In each pair of surfaces: Left: HCP; Right: Mindboggle.

surface $f_n^1(n = 1, \cdots, 9)$, we calculate its difference with f_n^2 or $-f_n^2$ on the corresponding point set and use the one with the smaller difference to construct the embedding of the second surface. This process can also be done in less than 10 milliseconds in our MATLAB implementation. After that, we can compute the nearest point map in the embedding space between the surfaces and pull back the manually delineated labels on the Mindboggle surface to the HCP subject [10]. The resulting labels are plotted in Fig. 5(c) and (d). For further demonstration, we plotted the cortical labeling results of six more HCP surfaces with the same strategy. These results show that excellent cortical labeling can be done efficiently with PRGM-based search. For future work, these results also lay the foundation for further improved labeling performance with the fusion of labels from multiple neighbors [10].

5 Conclusions

In this paper we developed a novel approach for brain search based on persistent Reeb graph matching. For future work, we will investigate different graph matching techniques and compare their speed and search performance with the Hungarian algorithm used in our current work. We will also incorporate other geometric features such as the skeletons of the sulci and gyri of the cortex for more informative comparisons.

References

1. Mueller, S., Weiner, M., Thal, L., Petersen, R.C., Jack, C., Jagust, W., Trojanowski, J.Q., Toga, A.W., Beckett, L.: The Alzheimer's disease neuroimaging initiative. Clin. North Am. 15, 869–877, xi–xii (2005)
2. Essen, D.V., Ugurbil, K., et al.: The human connectome project: A data acquisition perspective. NeuroImage 62(4), 2222–2231 (2012)
3. Toga, A., Clark, K., Thompson, P., Shattuck, D., Van Horn, J.: Mapping the human connectome. Neurosurgery 71(1), 1–5 (2012)
4. Van Horn, J.D., Toga, A.: Human neuroimaging as a "Big Data" science. Brain Imaging and Behavior, 1–9 (2013)
5. Reuter, M., Wolter, F.E., Shenton, M., Niethammer, M.: Laplace-beltrami eigenvalues and topological features of eigenfunctions for statistical shape analysis. Computer-Aided Design 41(10), 739–755 (2009)
6. Shi, Y., Lai, R., Toga, A.: Cortical surface reconstruction via unified Reeb analysis of geometric and topological outliers in magnetic resonance images. IEEE Trans. Med. Imag. (3), 511–530 (2013)
7. Edelsbrunner, Letscher, Zomorodian: Topological persistence and simplification. Discrete Comput. Geom. 28(4), 511–533 (2002)
8. Lee, H., Kang, H., Chung, M., Kim, B.N., Lee, D.S.: Persistent brain network homology from the perspective of dendrogram. IEEE Trans. Med. Imag. 31(12), 2267–2277 (2012)
9. Rustamov, R.M.: Laplace-beltrami eigenfunctions for deformation invariant shape representation. In: Proc. Eurograph. Symp. on Geo. Process., pp. 225–233 (2007)
10. Shi, Y., Lai, R., Toga, A.W.: Conformal mapping via metric optimization with application for cortical label fusion. In: Gee, J.C., Joshi, S., Pohl, K.M., Wells, W.M., Zöllei, L. (eds.) IPMI 2013. LNCS, vol. 7917, pp. 244–255. Springer, Heidelberg (2013)
11. Reeb, G.: Sur les points singuliers d'une forme de Pfaff completement integrable ou d'une fonction nemérique. Comptes Rendus Acad. Sciences 222, 847–849 (1946)
12. Klein, A., Tourville, J.: 101 labeled brain images and a consistent human cortical labeling protocol. Frontiers in Neuroscience 6(171) (2012)

In Vivo MRI Based Prostate Cancer Identification with Random Forests and Auto-context Model

Chunjun Qian[1], Li Wang[1], Ambereen Yousuf[2], Aytekin Oto[2], and Dinggang Shen[1]

[1] Department of Radiology and BRIC, University of North Carolina at Chapel Hill, NC
dgshen@med.unc.edu
[2] Department of Radiology, Section of Urology, University of Chicago, Chicago, IL

Abstract. Prostate cancer is one of the major causes of cancer death for men. Magnetic Resonance (MR) image is being increasingly used as an important modality to detect prostate cancer. Therefore, identifying prostate cancer in MRI with automated detection methods has become an active area of research, and many methods have been proposed to identify the prostate cancer. However, most of previous methods only focused on identifying cancer in the peripheral zone, or classifying suspicious cancer ROIs into benign tissue and cancer tissue. In this paper, we propose a novel learning-based multi-source integration framework to directly identify the prostate cancer regions from *in vivo* MRI. We employ the random forest technique to effectively integrate features from multi-source images together for cancer segmentation. Here, the multi-source images include initially only the multi-parametric MRIs (T2, DWI, eADC and dADC) and later also the iteratively estimated and refined tissue probability map of prostate cancer. Experimental results on 26 real patient data show that our method can accurately identify the cancerous tissue.

Keywords: Prostate cancer, MRI segmentation, Random forests, Auto-context.

1 Introduction

Prostate cancer is the most commonly diagnosed non-skin cancer and the second leading cause of cancer death among U.S. men [1]. Current clinical practice for the diagnosis of prostate cancer is using a transrectal ultrasound (TRUS) biopsy, when finding a positive prostate specific antigen (PSA) in blood test. A large screening trial using PSA and TRUS has shown that it is possible to reduce prostate cancer mortality by 20-30% [2]. However, these studies have also shown that PSA testing in combination with TRUS biopsies has a relatively low specificity. Additionally, cancers are often under-graded in TRUS biopsies [3]. These problems lead to over-diagnosis and over-treatment of patients for prostate cancer. Alternatively, multi-parametric high-contrast magnetic resonance (MR) imaging provides a powerful and noninvasive imaging tool for detecting suspicious cancerous tissues [4], as shown in Fig. 1. However, it requires a high level of expertise from the radiologist to read prostate MRI and suffers from observer variability [5]. Additionally, reading prostate MR is quite time-consuming.

G. Wu et al. (Eds.): MLMI 2014, LNCS 8679, pp. 314–322, 2014.

Automated computer-aided detection and diagnosis (CAD) of prostate cancer could help reduce both of these problems and open the door to prostate cancer screening using multi-parametric MRI. Many methods have been proposed to identify or detect prostate cancer regions in MR images [6,7,8]. For example, Sedat et al. [6] proposed a computer-aided diagnosis system to identify the suspicious cancer ROIs in peripheral zone (PZ). They also found that multispectral MRI provides better information about cancer and normal regions in the prostate when compared to the methods using single MRI techniques. Similarly, Niaf et al. [7] proposed a CAD system based on supervised learning to assess the presence of prostate cancer in the PZ based on three MR sequences with promising results. However, there are two limitations for the previous work: 1) They only focused on classifying suspicious cancer ROIs, which were often pre-outlined by the radiologists, into benign tissue and cancer tissue. 2) Instead of identifying cancer ROIs in the whole prostate, they only focused on the peripheral zone, which usually have to be manually labeled from prostate by the experts.

To deal with these limitations, in this paper, we propose a novel learning-based multi-source integration framework for accurate identification of the prostate cancer. To the best of our knowledge, our work is the first one to directly identify the cancer from the prostate MRI. Specifically, in our method, we first employ the random forests [9] to train a classifier based on the training subjects with multi-parametric MRIs (T2-weighted, DWI, dADC, and eADC, as shown in Fig. 1). The trained classifier provides the initial cancer probability map for each training subject. Inspired by the auto-context model [10,11], the estimated tissue probability map is further used as additional source to train the next classifier, which combines the high-level context features from the estimated cancer probability map with the appearance features from multi-parametric MRIs for refining cancer classification. By iteratively training the classifiers based on the updated cancer probability map, we can finally obtain a sequence of classifiers. Similarly, in the testing stage, given a target subject, the learned classifiers are sequentially applied to iteratively refine the estimation of cancer probability map by combining multi-parametric MRI information with the previously-estimated cancer probability map. We have validated the proposed method on 26 patient subjects with promising performance.

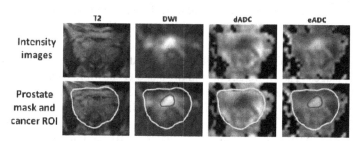

Fig. 1. T2, DWI, dADC, and eADC images are used for cancer identification. In the second row, the prostate boundary and cancer region are indicated by the yellow curve and red curve, respectively.

2   Method

2.1   Data and Image Preprocessing

The dataset consists of a series of multi-parametric MR (T2, DWI, ADC) images from 26 patients [19]. Since the generated ADC images are calculated from DWI by adjusting b-value, two kinds of ADC images are provided: dADC and eADC, eADC is the inverted form of dADC. All MR images were acquired with an endorectal coil and a phased-array surface coil with a Philips MR scanner. Immediately before MR imaging, 1 mg of glucagon was injected intramuscularly to decrease peristalsis of the rectum. For all of the subjects, the data acquisition parameters are shown in Table 1, and 1-3 cancer delineations on MRI of each subject were done manually by a radiologist by cooperating with a pathologist who sliced each prostate and identified all distinct tumors. These cancer ROIs were mostly outlined on T2-weighted images, and some were outlined on DWI. We resampled all images into the size 512×512 with the resolution 0.3125×0.3125×3(mm³), and aligned DWI, dADC and eADC images to T2 image for each subject by using the FLIRT tool [20]. Histogram matching was also performed on each type of MRI across different subjects.

Table 1. MR Image Acquisition Parameters

Multi-parametric MRI	Sequence Type	Repetition Time (msec)	Echo Time (msec)	Resolution (mm³)	Flip Angle (degree)
T2-weighted	Fast spin echo	3166-6581	90-120	0.3125×0.3125×3	90
DWI	Fast spin echo, echo planar imaging	2948-8616	71-85	1.406×1.406×3	90

2.2   Prostate Cancer Identification with Random Forests and Auto-context Model

In our method, we formulate the identification of prostate cancer as a two-class classification problem. To solve such a classification problem, we proposed a novel learning-based multi-source integration framework by employing the random forests [9] and auto-context model [10,11]. For simplicity, let N be the total number of the training subjects and let $I = \{I_{T2}^i, I_{DWI}^i, I_{dADC}^i, I_{eADC}^i, i = 1, ..., N\}$ be a set of multi-parametric MRIs. As a supervised learning method, our method consists of training and testing stages. The flowchart of training stage is shown in Fig. 2. In the training stage, we will train a sequence of classification forests, each with the input of multi-source images/maps. In the first iteration, the classification forest takes only the multipara-metric MRIs I as input, and learn the image appearance features from different multi-parametric MRIs for voxel-wise classification. By applying the trained forest in the first iteration, each i-th training subject will produce tissue probability maps for prostate cancer I_{PC}^i and non-prostate cancer I_{nPC}^i, as shown in the second column of Fig. 2. In the later iterations, inspired by the auto-context model [10,11], the tissue probability maps $\bar{I} = \{I_{PC}^i, I_{nPC}^i, i = 1, ..., N\}$ obtained from the previous iteration will act as additional source images for training. Specifically, high-level context features are extracted from the tissue probability maps to assist the classification, along with appearance features from the multi-parametric MRIs. Since context features are informative about the nearby tissue structures for each voxel, they encode the spatial constraints into the classification, thus improving the quality of the estimated tissue probability maps, as also demonstrated in Fig. 2. Then, the tissue probability maps are iteratively updated and fed into the next training iteration. Finally, a sequence of classifiers will be obtained.

Similarly, in the testing stage, given a target subject with multi-parametric MRIs, we can obtain the initial tissue probability map by applying the trained classifier in the first iteration using only multi-parametric MRIs. In the later iterations, along with multi-parametric MRIs, the tissue probability maps resulted from previous iteration are fed into the next classifier for refinement. Fig. 3 shows an example by applying a

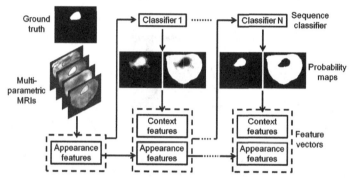

Fig. 2. Flowchart of the training procedure for our proposed method with multi-source images, including T2, DWI, dADC and eADC images, along with cancer probability maps. The appearance features from multi-parametric MR images are used for training the first classifier, and then both appearance features and the context features from probability maps are employed for training the subsequent classifiers.

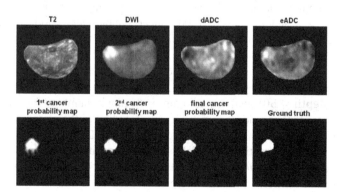

Fig. 3. A typical example by applying our method on an unseen target subject. We use the trained classifier in the first iteration from multi-parametric MRIs to obtain the initial tissue probability maps. In the later iterations, the tissue probability maps resulted from previous iteration are fed into the next classifier for refinement.

sequence of learned classifiers on an unseen target subject. As we can see from Fig. 3, the cancer probability maps are updated with iterations and becoming more and more accurate.

In our implementation, we use Haar-like features [13] for both appearance features and context features due to its efficiency. Specifically, for each voxel x, its Haar-like features are computed as the local mean intensity of any randomly displaced cubical region R_1 or the mean intensity difference over any two randomly displaced, asymmetric cubical regions (R_1 and R_2) within the image patch R [14]:

$$f(x, I) = \frac{1}{|R_1|} \sum_{u \in R_1} I(u) - b \frac{1}{|R_2|} \sum_{v \in R_2} I(v), \quad R_1 \in R, \ R_2 \in R, b \in \{0,1\} \quad (1)$$

where R is the patch centered at voxel x, I is any kind of source image, and the parameter $b \in \{0,1\}$ indicates whether one or two cubical regions are used (as shown in Fig. 4, $b = 1$). In theory, for each voxel we can determine an infinite number of such features.

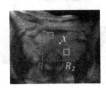

Fig. 4. Computation of Haar-like features. The red rectangle indicates the patch centered at x. Haar-like features are computed as the local mean intensity of any randomly displaced cubical region R_1, or the mean intensity difference over any two randomly displaced, asymmetric cubical regions (R_1 and R_2) within the image patch R.

3   Experimental Results and Analysis

We validate the proposed method via a leave-one-out strategy, i.e., for each target image, we train the random forests based on the remaining 25 subjects. For each training subjects, we randomly select 1000 cancer samples and 1000 normal samples. Then, for each sample with the patch size of $7 \times 7 \times 7$, 10000 random Haar-like features are extracted from all source images: T2, DWI, dADC, eADC images, and tissue/cancer probability maps in every iteration. We set the total iteration as 10. In each iteration, we train 20 classification trees. We stop the tree growth at a certain depth (i.e., depth = 50), with a minimum of 8 sample numbers for each leaf node. The parameters for the random forests are set according to the previous work [18]. In our evaluation, we employ section-based evaluation (SBE) [12], which is defined as a ratio of *the number* of sections in which both the automatic method and expert identify the prostate cancer to *the number* of total sections that the automatic method identifies the prostate cancer. The SBE is typically used for evaluation the performance for prostate cancer diagnoses. According to the prostate size of each subject, the prostate is usually divided into 4-9 sections [12]. For example, Fig. 5 shows the divided sections for a typical prostate.

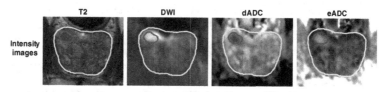

Fig. 5. The divided sections for a typical prostate. The prostate is divided by pink dash lines. The red curve indicates the manual segmentation of cancer ROI, and yellow curve outlines the prostate boundary.

3.1   Importance of context features

Fig. 6 shows the SBEs on 26 patient subjects by sequentially applying the learned classifiers based on the multi-source. It can be seen that the SBEs are improved with the iterations and become stable after a few iterations (i.e., 2 iterations). Specially, in the second iteration, the SBEs are improved greatly due to the integration of the previously-estimated tissue probability maps for guiding classification. These results demonstrate the importance of using context features for cancer segmentation.

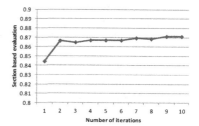

Fig. 6. Change of SBEs with the iterations. The SBEs are improved with the iterations.

3.2   Comparison with Conventional Method

It is difficult to make comparisons with the other methods due to unavailability of their algorithms and their testing subjects. Thus, we currently only compared with the conventional classification method (AdaBoost [17]). AdaBoost is also a machine learning method. In training stage, it generates a series of weak learners by updating the weight on every training sample. These weak learners converge to a final strong learner. In AdaBoost method, we extract Haar-like features, Gabor features, HOG, LBP and gradient features, and set the maximum number of iterations as 100 in the weak learner refining process and also the boosting iterations is set as 2. Fig. 7 shows the qualitative comparison results on the same patient subject in Fig. 5. In the images, the red curves indicate the cancer ROIs, and yellow curves indicate the boundaries of the prostate mask. The results of AdaBoost and our proposed method are shown in the 1st and 2nd rows, and indicated by the green and blue curves, respectively. It can be observed that our result is more consistent with the manual ground truth. For quantitative evaluation, the SBEs on 26 subjects are shown in Fig. 8(a). It can be seen that our proposed method outperforms the AdaBoost method.

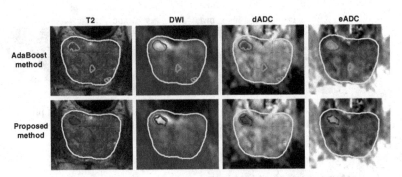

Fig. 7. Qualitative comparison of the proposed method with the AdaBoost method on a patient subject with multi-parametric MRIs. The yellow curve indicates the prostate region. The red curve indicates the manual segmentation, while the automated segmentation by AdaBoost and our proposed method are indicated by green curves and blue curves, respectively.

In addition, we further employ Dice ratios to evaluate the accuracy. The results on 26 patient subjects are shown in Fig. 8(b). It can be also observed that our method achieves a higher accuracy, with average dice ratios 67.06%, compared with 50.58% by the AdaBoost.

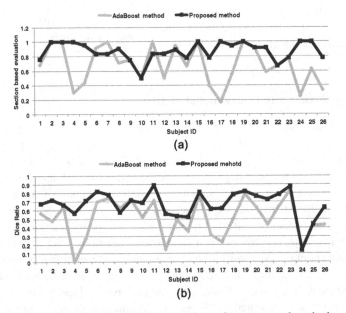

Fig. 8. (a): Section-based evaluation (SBE) comparison of our proposed method and the Ada-Boost method on 26 patients. The average SBE of our method is 87.11%, which is significantly better than AdaBoost method (p-value<0.01). **(b):** Dice ratios of the proposed method and the AdaBoost method on 26 patients. The performance of our proposed method is significantly better than that of AdaBoost method (p-value<0.01).

4   Conclusion

We have proposed a novel framework to identify prostate cancer regions in the *in vivo* MR images. Our proposed method can directly identify cancerous regions from the whole prostate. Specially, we employ the random forests and auto-context model to effectively integrate features from multi-parametric MRIs and tentatively-estimated probability maps for cancer identification. Experimental results on 26 real patient data show that our method can accurately identify the cancerous regions. In our future work, we will validate the proposed method on more patient subjects.

References

1. Siegel, R., et al.: Cancer statistics, 2012. CA: A Cancer Journal for Clinicians 62(1), 10–29 (2012)
2. Schröder, F.H., et al.: Screening and Prostate-Cancer Mortality in a Randomized European Study. NEJM 360(13), 1320–1328 (2009)
3. Hambrock, T., et al.: Prospective Assessment of Prostate Cancer Aggressiveness Using 3-T Diffusion-Weighted Magnetic Resonance Imaging–Guided Biopsies Versus a Systematic 10-Core Transrectal Ultrasound Prostate Biopsy Cohort. European Urology 61(1), 177–184 (2012)
4. Hoeks, C.M.A., et al.: Prostate Cancer: Multiparametric MR Imaging for Detection, Localization, and Staging. Radiology 261(1), 46–66 (2011)
5. Lim, H.K., et al.: Prostate Cancer: Apparent Diffusion Coefficient Map with T2-weighted Images for Detection—A Multireader Study. Radiology, 145–151 (2009)
6. Sedat, O., et al.: Supervised and unsupervised methods for prostate cancer segmentation with multispectral MRI. Medical Physics 37(4), 1873–1883 (2010)
7. Niaf, E., et al.: Computer-aided diagnosis of prostate cancer in the peripheral zone using multiparametric MRI. Phys. Med. Biol. 57(12), 3833–3851 (2012)
8. Litjens, G., et al.: Computer-Aided Detection of Prostate Cancer in MRI. T-MI 33(5), 1083–1092 (2014)
9. Breiman, L.: Random Forests. Machine Learning 45(1), 5–32 (2001)
10. Tu, Z., Bai, X.: Auto-Context and Its Application to High-Level Vision Tasks and 3D Brain Image Segmentation. PAMI 32(10), 1744–1757 (2010)
11. Loog, M., Ginneken, B.: Segmentation of the posterior ribs in chest radiographs using iterated contextual pixel classification. T-MI 25(5), 602–611 (2006)
12. Mohsen, F., et al.: Detection and Localization of Prostate Cancer: Correlation of ^{11}C-Choline PETCT with Histopathologic Step-Section Analysis. JNM 46(10), 1642–1649 (2005)
13. Viola, P., et al.: Robust Real-Time Face Detection. IJCV 57(2), 137–154 (2004)
14. Han, X.: Learning-Boosted Label Fusion for Multi-atlas Auto-Segmentation. In: Wu, G., Zhang, D., Shen, D., Yan, P., Suzuki, K., Wang, F. (eds.) MLMI 2013. LNCS, vol. 8184, pp. 17–24. Springer, Heidelberg (2013)
15. Cheng, H., et al.: Sparsity induced similarity measure for label propagation. In: ICCV, pp. 317–324 (2009)
16. Wright, J., et al.: Sparse Representation for Computer Vision and Pattern Recognition. Proceedings of the IEEE 98, 1031–1044 (2010)

17. Yoav, F., et al.: A decision-theoretic generalization of on-line learning and an application to boosting. JCSS 55(1), 119–139 (1997)
18. Zikic, D., Glocker, B., Criminisi, A.: Atlas Encoding by Randomized Forests for Efficient Label Propagation. In: Mori, K., Sakuma, I., Sato, Y., Barillot, C., Navab, N. (eds.) MICCAI 2013, Part III. LNCS, vol. 8151, pp. 66–73. Springer, Heidelberg (2013)
19. Peng, Y., et al.: Quantitative Analysis of Multiparametric Prostate MR Images: Differentiation between Prostate Cancer and Normal Tissue and Correlation with Gleason Score—A Computer-aided Diagnosis Development Study. Radiology 267(3), 787–796 (2013)
20. Greve, D.N., Fischl, B.: Accurate and robust brain image alignment using boundary-based registration. NeuroImage 48(1), 63–72 (2009)

Learning of Atlas Forest Hierarchy for Automatic Labeling of MR Brain Images

Lichi Zhang[1], Qian Wang[1], Yaozong Gao[2,3],
Guorong Wu[3], and Dinggang Shen[3]

[1] Med-X Research Institute, School of Biomedical Engineering,
Shanghai Jiao Tong University
{lichizhang,wang.qian}@sjtu.edu.cn
[2] Department of Computer Science, University of North Carolina at Chapel Hill
yzgao@cs.unc.edu
[3] Department of Radiology and BRIC, University of North Carolina at Chapel Hill
{grwu,dgshen}@med.unc.edu

Abstract. We propose a multi-atlas-based framework to label brain anatomies in magnetic resonance (MR) images, by constructing a hierarchical structure of atlas forests. We start by training the atlas forests in accordance to individual atlases, and then cluster atlas forests with similar labeling performances into several groups. For each group, a new representative forest is re-trained, based on all atlas images associated with the atlas forests in the group, as well as the tentative label maps output by the clustered atlas forests. This clustering and re-training procedure is conducted iteratively to obtain a hierarchical structure of atlas forests. When applied to an unlabeled image for testing, only the suitable trained atlas forests will be selected from the hierarchical structure. Hence the labeling result of the test image is fused from the outputs of selected atlas forests. Experimental results show that the proposed framework can significantly improve the labeling performance compared to the state-of-the-art method.

1 Introduction

Labeling individual neuro-anatomical regions is important for quantitative analysis of magnetic resonance (MR) brain images. However, due to the complexity of brain structures and their blurred boundaries in the MR data, it is labor-intensive to manually label the MR brain images into different regions. To address this issue, many automatic methods have been proposed. Among them, multi-atlas-based labeling methods are widely used, due to their robustness and simplicity in incorporating prior labeling information from the atlases. Wolz *et al.* [1] implemented the label estimation by learning an image manifold, and thus the labels can be effectively propagated to the test image from the atlases that can provide relatively more reliable label information. Jia *et al.* [2] introduced an iterative multi-atlas-based multi-image segmentation (MABMIS) approach, which utilized sophisticated registration scheme for spatial alignment and determined the labels of all test images simultaneously in the common space.

G. Wu et al. (Eds.): MLMI 2014, LNCS 8679, pp. 323–330, 2014.

Coupé *et al.* [3] proposed a non-local patch-based method for incorporating the priors from the expert manual segmentations. The method relaxes the demanding requirement of accurate image registration. Instead, after aligning all atlases with the test image via affine registration, each voxel in the test image then computes its similarities to the non-local voxels in all linearly-aligned atlases. The labels in the atlases are then adaptively fused for the to-be-labeled voxels under consideration. Continuous efforts (e.g., [4]) have been devoted to further boost the labeling accuracy of the non-local methods. However, these methods require high computation cost in the labeling process. The situation is further deteriorated when the dataset under study includes a large number of atlas images.

Recently Zikic *et al.* [5] proposed to encode each individual atlas by a randomized classification forest [6]. Given an atlas image with its corresponding label map, a randomized classification forest is trained, denoted here as the "atlas forest", to differentiate voxels inside and out of the individual regions based on the voxelwise visual features. Each of the atlas forest can produce a probabilistic labeling result for the test image. Therefore it computes the final labeling by simply averaging all the probability estimates. It was proved experimentally that the performance can be compared favorably with the alternatives (e.g., the non-local method [3]).

However, there are several drawbacks for this method [5]. *First*, each atlas forest is trained using only a single atlas image. Such strategy can have efficient experimentation as claimed, but also negatively influences its performance as the atlas forest may over-fit the single atlas image. *Second*, after labeling result is generated from each trained atlas forest, no feedback is considered by the atlas forests, for further improving the labeling result. *Third*, the final labeling in their work is the average of the probabilities estimated from all atlas forests, while the simple averaging may not necessarily be the optimal for the input test image.

To overcome the aforementioned limitations, we propose a novel framework which utilizes the atlas forest techniques for labeling the MR brain images. We divide the proposed framework into the training stage and the testing stage. During the training stage, a hierarchical structure is built by hierarchically clustering similar atlas forests. Specifically, in the bottom level, one atlas forest only encodes one atlas image. Then, atlas forests are clustered together, from which a new atlas forest is trained in the next higher level. In this way, atlas forests in the higher level are capable of using not only more comprehensive atlases than the lower-level atlas forests, but also the augmented features including outputs calculated from the lower level. This atlas forest clustering and training procedure is performed iteratively to build a hierarchical structure of atlas forests in the end.

In the testing stage, we utilize the trained hierarchical structure of atlas forests to label the input images for testing. *First*, All atlas forests in the bottom level are invoked. Based on their outputs, we *then* identify atlas forests that can potentially contribute the most accurate labeling results to the test image. *Next*, in the higher level, the atlas forests corresponding to the selected lower-level atlas forests are activated, while the rest in the current level are left inactive. *Finally, the labels of the test image is determined by fusing output of the active atlas forests selected from the hierarchical structure, after all levels of the hierarchy are exhausted.*

The main contributions of this work include:

- A hierarchical learning framework is proposed for clustering similar atlas forests together, and thus the re-trained atlas forests can reduce the risk of over-fitting;
- A novel atlas forest selection strategy is proposed, which can boost the labeling accuracy by selecting the most effective atlas forests for the labeling of the new test image.

2 Method

In this section, we present the details of the proposed hierarchical framework, consisting of the training stage and testing stage. In the training stage, we organize a set of atlas forests into a hierarchical structure. In the testing stage, we go through all levels in the hierarchy to obtain the final labeling result for the test image. The two stages are elaborated in Section 2.1 and Section 2.2, respectively.

2.1 Hierarchical Learning of Atlas Forests

Fig. 1 shows an example of a two-level hierarchical structure of atlas forests developed in the training stage. The block of F_j^i in the figure represents the j-th atlas forest learned in the i-th level. $A_j = \{I_j, L_j\}$ is the j-th atlas, where I_j and L_j are the intensity image and the label map of A_j, respectively. We also have two notations M_j^i and C_j^i. M_j^i is the set of atlas forests that are the children nodes of F_j^i in the hierarchical structure, and C_j^i denotes the set of atlas images utilized by the subtree rooted at F_j^i. For example, it can be written as $C_0^1 = \{A_0\}$, $M_0^1 = \emptyset$, $C_1^2 = \{A_4, A_5\}$ and $M_1^2 = \{F_4^1, F_5^1\}$ following Fig. 1. Note that the atlas forest is considered as the classification forest trained with a single or multiple atlas images.

During the training stage, we build a hierarchical structure from the set of atlas images. Initially, we follow the single-atlas encoding approach in [5] to train the atlas forests in the bottom level. The forests obtained from the single-atlas encoding method may over-fit their corresponding training images, which will lead to their classifiers with poor generalization power. We resolve this issue by developing a hierarchical structure of atlas forests. In particular, the atlas forests that are similar in terms of their labeling capabilities are clustered together, and the representative forest of each cluster is re-trained upon all atlases in each cluster.

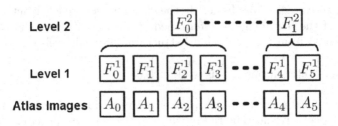

Fig. 1. An example of hierarchical atlas forest structure built during the training process

Atlas Forest Clustering. Here we propose a novel metric to measure the similarity of the labeling capabilities between two atlas forests as

$$S(F_m^i, F_n^i) = \frac{1}{2|C_m^i|} \sum_{A_j \in C_m^i} \text{DSC}(A_j \mid F_n^i) + \frac{1}{2|C_n^i|} \sum_{A_l \in C_n^i} \text{DSC}(A_l \mid F_m^i) , \quad (1)$$

where $S(F_m^i, F_n^i)$ denotes the similarity between two atlas forests in level i, C_m^i and C_n^i are the sets of atlas images utilized by F_m^i and F_n^i respectively, and $\text{DSC}(A_j \mid F_n^i)$ represents the labeling accuracy (measured by the Dice overlapping ratio with respect to the ground-truth) of the atlas A_j by using F_n^i. Given the similarity measure between any pair of atlas forests, we can construct an affinity/similarity matrix, which is used by affinity propagation [7] for atlas forest clustering.

Atlas Forest Training. After atlas forests are clustered based on the similarity defined in Eq. 1, we re-train a new atlas forest in the higher level corresponding to each lower-level cluster. The atlas forests in the higher level utilize the outputs from the clustered atlas forests in the lower level for improving the labeling accuracy. Specifically, to train the higher-level F_j^i, all the atlases within the set C_j^i are used as the training data. Before learning the higher-level atlas forest, we first generate an initial labeling map for every training image by utilizing all the clustered atlas forests (i.e., $F_k^{i-1} \in M_j^i$) in the $(i\text{-}1)$-th level. In particular, the initial labeling map of the training image A_l in the set C_j^i is obtained by averaging all the labeling results of A_l from the clustered atlas forests in the $(i\text{-}1)$-th level, except the one that is trained with the atlas image A_l itself (i.e., using atlas forests in the set $\{F_k^{i-1} \mid F_k^{i-1} \in M_j^i \text{ and } A_l \notin C_k^{i-1}\}$).

After obtaining the initial label map of A_l, we can extract probability features from the initial label map, in addition to the original image features extracted from atlas image A_l. For each voxel, abundant Haar-like operators are used for efficient feature extraction. With both the new probability features and the original image features, the higher-level atlas forest F_j^i is learned to classify the labels of individual voxels. After the new atlas forests are obtained in the high level, they are clustered again according to the similarity defined in Eq. 1. Afterwards, the clustered atlas forests also help to learn new atlas forests in the next higher level. This iterative clustering and re-training procedure continues until the number of the existing atlas forests is below a certain threshold.

Generally speaking, compared to the lower-level atlas forests, a certain higher-level atlas forest is capable of accessing more comprehensive training atlases and features. The outputs of the lower-level atlas forests are refined by the higher-level atlas forests. Meanwhile, context features are directly computed from the lower-level output maps, thus enabling the higher-level atlas forest to generate a robust and accurate labeling result. The construction of the hierarchical structure of atlas forests is implemented using an iterative strategy following the method of auto-context [8]. It is noted that there is an exception occurred when computing the context features in the bottom level, due to the lack of the tentative labeling results from lower level. We intend to calculate the spatial prior of each label instead, by averaging the ground-truth labeling results of all training images, and then regard the probabilistic prior as the source of the probability features for each atlas.

2.2   Image Labeling with the Atlas Forest Hierarchy

In this section, we present how the constructed multi-level hierarchical structure of atlas forests is applied for the labeling process. Similar to the training stage, the process also goes from the bottom level to the top level following an iterative manner. Instead of using all of the learned classifiers for labeling as described in [5], the proposed method selects only the potentially *optimal* atlas forests. Therefore, the labeling process can avoid the possible negative influence from certain atlas forests, which are not suitable for labeling the test image.

Different from the traditional atlas selection approaches such as the work in [9], the novel atlas forest selection method is developed based on the clustering information obtained in the training stage. For a test image, we first compute the *consistency* across labeling outputs from individual atlas forests in each cluster, and then use the consistency measure to gauge the cluster as well as its member classifiers. Our main reason is that, if a cluster of atlas forests could well handle the test image, their outputs should be similar to its actual labeling information, and thus are highly consistent. On the contrary, if the classifiers are more likely to generate incorrect labeling results with respect to the *unknown* ground-truth labels of the test image, their outputs are more inconsistent due to unpredictable and uncontrollable error patterns in the labeling process.

Our goal in forest selection is to find the optimal cluster(s), whose member atlas forests are consistent for labeling the test image. Let $\hat{I}$ be the test image, we commence by applying all of forests F_k^{i-1} in the cluster M_j^i, and comparing their labeling outputs with each other using the Dice overlapping ratio in the $(i\text{-}1)$-th level. The mean value of the pairwise Dice ratios is regarded as the *absolute* labeling consistency coefficient for the cluster M_j^i, which is denoted as $D(\hat{I}, M_j^i)$.

It is worth noting that $D(\hat{I}, M_j^i)$ only depends on the specific cluster M_j^i. Thus the measures cannot be directly compared across individual clusters. To this end, we further convert the *absolute* consistency coefficient into a *relative* measure, by dividing over the population-level consistency indicator of each cluster. Then, the relative consistency measures can be utilized for the selection of optimal atlas forests.

The population-level consistency indicator is computed by utilizing the information contributed by the training images. In particular, the consistency between any pair of atlas forests of the same cluster is calculated and averaged upon all training images. Then the population-level consistency indicator of the cluster $\bar{D}(M_j^i)$ is defined as the mean value of all pairwise consistency measures within the cluster. Finally, we have the metric $W(\hat{I}, M_j^i)$ regarded as the *relative* labeling consistency coefficient, which is written as

$$W(\hat{I}, M_j^i) = \frac{D(\hat{I}, M_j^i)}{\bar{D}(M_j^i)} \ . \tag{2}$$

When the atlas forests with the top W scores are selected, each selected atlas forest can produce one labeling result. The overall labeling map in the current level is computed from those labeling estimates using the majority voting approaches. This obtained map will be used as the initial label map for the next higher level. In the next higher level, we only consider clusters that contain the selected atlas forests in the lower level. By iteratively performing atlas selection and brain labeling in the new level, the labeling result of the test image will be gradually refined. This iterative process ends when reaching the top-most level.

3   Experimental Results

In this section, we evaluate the proposed framework for anatomical region labeling on MR brain images. In particular, the Alzheimer's Disease Neuroimaging Initiative (ADNI) dataset[1] is adopted. The ADNI dataset provides rich brain images using 1.5 T MR scans, with two annotated regions representing the left and the right hippocampi in the adult brains. Before labeling, we perform a series of standard pre-processing works as introduced in [3] to ensure the validity of the estimation.

To demonstrate the robustness of the proposed framework, we use 5-fold cross-validation in the evaluation. Stated succinctly, we randomly select 50 images from the normal control subjects of ADNI dataset to serve as the experimental dataset, which are equally divided into 5 groups. In each fold, we select one group containing 10 images for testing, and the rest for training. Settings for training the forests are identical in all 5-fold cross validation experiment. There are 8 trees measured in each forest, the number of tree depths is 30, and each leaf has at least 8 samples. The voxelwise features are calculated from the 3D patches with the maximal size of $10 \times 10 \times 10$ voxels.

Two levels of the hierarchical structure of atlas forests are adopted for efficient computations. We follow the recommended setting in affinity propagation by

---

[1] http://adni.loni.ucla.edu

associating parameters in clustering atlas forests to their similarity measures. In the bottom level, we consider each atlas forest as the individual cluster, thus there are 40 small clusters. Using the clustering method, we can group the atlas forests into several larger clusters in the second level.

The experiments conducted present the overall improvements when the proposed framework is implemented. Table 1 compares the baseline method (following the strategy of single-atlas encoding in [5]) with the proposed framework. It is shown that the proposed framework improves the estimation by more than 10% compared with the single-atlas encoding method [5].

Table 1. Quantitative comparison between the single-atlas encoding method and the proposed method in labeling the left and right hippocampi

DSC (%)	Single-atlas Encoding	Proposed Method
Left Hippocampus	64.94 ± 2.20	**76.25 ± 2.40**
Right Hippocampus	67.15 ± 1.04	**76.86 ± 1.21**
Overall	66.05 ± 1.62	**76.64 ± 1.81**

Next we break down two techniques for evaluation, which are: 1) hierarchical clustering and re-training of atlas forests, and 2) atlas forest selection (AFS). Fig. 2 shows the comparison results between the ground-truth and the estimates using the Dice overlapping ratio. The left panel of the figure shows the results of labeling the left hippocampus, while the other one is for the right hippocampus. It can be observed that all results in the higher level are better than those in the lower level, indicating the effectiveness of clustering and re-training atlas forests. Besides, the labeling accuracies of the proposed framework with (optimal) atlas selection (blue plots) are always better than that without atlas selection (red plots). This demonstrates the effectiveness of the AFS module in the proposed framework.

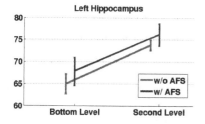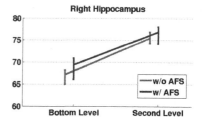

Fig. 2. Left and right panels show the labeling accuracies of different configurations on the left and the right hippocampi, respectively. The blue plots indicate the labeling accuracies **with** AFS by using different hierarchical levels, and the red plots indicate the labeling accuracies **without** AFS by using different hierarchical levels.

4   Conclusion

In this paper, we propose a novel hierarchical framework for iteratively clustering and learning the atlas forests. Besides, a novel atlas forest selection is also presented to filter out the potentially negative influences from atlas images. Experimental results on the ADNI dataset indicate that the proposed framework significantly outperforms the state-of-the-art single-atlas encoding method [5]. Future research will validate the proposed framework by constructing much deeper and more complex hierarchical structure of atlas forests. We will also conduct comprehensive evaluations by employing more datasets containing multiple anatomical labels.

References

1. Wolz, R., Aljabar, P., Hajnal, J.V., Hammers, A., Rueckert, D.: Leap: Learning embeddings for atlas propagation. NeuroImage 49(2), 1316–1325 (2010)
2. Jia, H., Yap, P.T., Shen, D.: Iterative multi-atlas-based multi-image segmentation with tree-based registration. NeuroImage 59(1), 422–430 (2012)
3. Coupé, P., Manjón, J.V., Fonov, V., Pruessner, J., Robles, M., Collins, D.L.: Patch-based segmentation using expert priors: Application to hippocampus and ventricle segmentation. NeuroImage 54(2), 940–954 (2011)
4. Wu, G., Wang, Q., Zhang, D., Nie, F., Huang, H., Shen, D.: A generative probability model of joint label fusion for multi-atlas based brain segmentation. Medical Image Analysis 18(6), 881–890 (2014)
5. Zikic, D., Glocker, B., Criminisi, A.: Atlas encoding by randomized forests for efficient label propagation. In: Mori, K., Sakuma, I., Sato, Y., Barillot, C., Navab, N. (eds.) MICCAI 2013, Part III. LNCS, vol. 8151, pp. 66–73. Springer, Heidelberg (2013)
6. Breiman, L.: Random forests. Machine Learning (2001)
7. Frey, B.J., Dueck, D.: Clustering by passing messages between data points. Science 315(5814), 972–976 (2007)
8. Tu, Z., Bai, X.: Auto-context and its application to high-level vision tasks and 3D brain image segmentation. IEEE Transactions on Pattern Analysis and Machine Intelligence 32(10), 1744–1757 (2010)
9. Aljabar, P., Heckemann, R.A., Hammers, A., Hajnal, J.V., Rueckert, D.: Multi-atlas based segmentation of brain images: atlas selection and its effect on accuracy. NeuroImage 46(3), 726–738 (2009)

Author Index